Novel Diagnostic and Therapeutic Approaches in Temporomandibular Disorders (TMDs) and Myofascial Pain

Novel Diagnostic and Therapeutic Approaches in Temporomandibular Disorders (TMDs) and Myofascial Pain

Editors

Zuzanna Nowak
Aleksandra Nitecka-Buchta

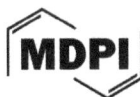

Basel • Beijing • Wuhan • Barcelona • Belgrade • Novi Sad • Cluj • Manchester

Editors

Zuzanna Nowak
Department of
Temporomandibular Disorders
Medical University of Silesia
Katowice
Poland

Aleksandra Nitecka-Buchta
Department of
Temporomandibular Disorders
Medical University of Silesia
Katowice
Poland

Editorial Office
MDPI
St. Alban-Anlage 66
4052 Basel, Switzerland

This is a reprint of articles from the Special Issue published online in the open access journal *Life* (ISSN 2075-1729) (available at: www.mdpi.com/journal/life/special_issues/QFBHSVQI7B).

For citation purposes, cite each article independently as indicated on the article page online and as indicated below:

Lastname, A.A.; Lastname, B.B. Article Title. *Journal Name* **Year**, *Volume Number*, Page Range.

ISBN 978-3-0365-9295-4 (Hbk)
ISBN 978-3-0365-9294-7 (PDF)
doi.org/10.3390/books978-3-0365-9294-7

© 2023 by the authors. Articles in this book are Open Access and distributed under the Creative Commons Attribution (CC BY) license. The book as a whole is distributed by MDPI under the terms and conditions of the Creative Commons Attribution-NonCommercial-NoDerivs (CC BY-NC-ND) license.

Contents

About the Editors vii

Preface ix

Zuzanna Nowak
Editorial for "Novel Diagnostic and Therapeutic Approaches in Temporomandibular Disorders and Myofascial Pain" Special Issue in *Life*
Reprinted from: *Life* **2023**, *13*, 2049, doi:10.3390/life13102049 1

Brendan Moxley, William Stevens, Joel Sneed and Craig Pearl
Novel Diagnostic and Therapeutic Approaches to Temporomandibular Dysfunction: A Narrative Review
Reprinted from: *Life* **2023**, *13*, 1808, doi:10.3390/life13091808 3

Marta Carlota Diaz-Saez, Alfonso Gil-Martínez, Inae Caroline Gadotti, Gonzalo Navarro-Fernández, Javier Gil-Castillo and Hector Beltran-Alacreu
Reliability and Responsiveness of a Novel Device to Evaluate Tongue Force
Reprinted from: *Life* **2023**, *13*, 1192, doi:10.3390/life13051192 15

Bruno Macedo de Sousa, Antonio López-Valverde, Francisco Caramelo, María João Rodrigues and Nansi López-Valverde
Medium-Term Effect of Treatment with Intra-Articular Injection of Sodium Hyaluronate, Betamethasone and Platelet-Rich Plasma in Patients with Temporomandibular Arthralgia: A Retrospective Cohort Study
Reprinted from: *Life* **2022**, *12*, 1739, doi:10.3390/life12111739 28

José A. Blanco-Rueda, Antonio López-Valverde, Antonio Márquez-Vera, Roberto Méndez-Sánchez, Eva López-García and Nansi López-Valverde
Preliminary Findings of the Efficacy of Botulinum Toxin in Temporomandibular Disorders: Uncontrolled Pilot Study
Reprinted from: *Life* **2023**, *13*, 345, doi:10.3390/life13020345 38

Leonardo Sette Vieira, Priscylla Ruany Mendes Pestana, Júlio Pascoal Miranda, Luana Aparecida Soares, Fabiana Silva and Marcus Alessandro Alcantara et al.
The Efficacy of Manual Therapy Approaches on Pain, Maximum Mouth Opening and Disability in Temporomandibular Disorders: A Systematic Review of Randomised Controlled Trials
Reprinted from: *Life* **2023**, *13*, 292, doi:10.3390/life13020292 48

Frauke Müggenborg, Ester Moreira de Castro Carletti, Liz Dennett, Ana Izabela Sobral de Oliveira-Souza, Norazlin Mohamad and Gunnar Licht et al.
Effectiveness of Manual Trigger Point Therapy in Patients with Myofascial Trigger Points in the Orofacial Region—A Systematic Review
Reprinted from: *Life* **2023**, *13*, 336, doi:10.3390/life13020336 67

Caroline M. Speksnijder, Nadiya E. A. Mutsaers and Sajjad Walji
Functioning of the Masticatory System in Patients with an Alloplastic Total Temporomandibular Joint Prostheses Compared with Healthy Individuals: A Pilot Study
Reprinted from: *Life* **2022**, *12*, 2073, doi:10.3390/life12122073 95

Ricardo Luiz de Barreto Aranha, Renata de Castro Martins, Ligia Cristelli Paixão and Mauro Henrique Nogueira Guimarães de Abreu
Professional Factors Associated with Case Resolution without Referrals of Orofacial Pain Cases to Secondary Dental Care by Telehealth in Brazil: A Cross-Sectional Study in 2019 and 2020
Reprinted from: *Life* **2022**, *13*, 29, doi:10.3390/life13010029 . . . . **106**

Łukasz Lassmann, Zuzanna Nowak, Jean-Daniel Orthlieb and Agata Żółtowska
Complicated Relationships between Anterior and Condylar Guidance and Their Clinical Implications—Comparison by Cone Beam Computed Tomography and Electronic Axiography—An Observational Cohort Cross-Sectional Study
Reprinted from: *Life* **2023**, *13*, 335, doi:10.3390/life13020335 . . . . **116**

Amjad Obaid Aljohani, Mohammed Ghazi Sghaireen, Muhammad Abbas, Bader Kureyem Alzarea, Kumar Chandan Srivastava and Deepti Shrivastava et al.
Comparative Evaluation of Condylar Guidance Angles Measured Using Arcon and Non-Arcon Articulators and Panoramic Radiographs—A Systematic Review and Meta-Analysis
Reprinted from: *Life* **2023**, *13*, 1352, doi:10.3390/life13061352 . . . . **133**

Jae Sung Park and Kwan Park
Operative Findings of over 5000 Microvascular Decompression Surgeries for Hemifacial Spasm: Our Perspective and Current Updates
Reprinted from: *Life* **2023**, *13*, 1904, doi:10.3390/life13091904 . . . . **148**

Kyung Rae Cho, Sang Ku Park and Kwan Park
Lateral Spread Response: Unveiling the Smoking Gun for Cured Hemifacial Spasm
Reprinted from: *Life* **2023**, *13*, 1825, doi:10.3390/life13091825 . . . . **159**

Hyun-Seok Lee and Kwan Park
Penetrating Offenders in Hemifacial Spasm: Surgical Tactics and Prognosis
Reprinted from: *Life* **2023**, *13*, 2021, doi:10.3390/life13102021 . . . . **171**

About the Editors

Zuzanna Nowak

Zuzanna Nowak a didactic and research assistant at Medical University of Silesia. Her main focus is on a modern diagnostic and therapeutic approach, natural and minimally invasive treatments, needling therapies, as well as the influence of lifestyle on painful TMD and regeneration abilities.

Aleksandra Nitecka-Buchta

Aleksandra Nitecka-Buchta is the President of the Polish Association of Temporomandibular Disorders, currently working in Medical University of Silesia. Her main focus is to promote modern diagnostic and therapeutic procedures in TMD, researching novel tools to aid the process.

Preface

This Special Issue aimed to cover a diverse scope of topics, from diagnostics to the management of temporomandibular disorders and myofascial pain, with a special focus on innovations in those areas. Intense research progress in the subject as well as technological development, access to knowledge, and novel digital tools allow developing more precise, reproducible, and dedicated diagnostic and therapeutic protocols. We are thrilled to hear about new tools and equipment assisting the diagnostic and treatment process, innovative therapeutic methods, new substances and medications used, as well as novel modifications of already widely used methods.

Zuzanna Nowak and Aleksandra Nitecka-Buchta
Editors

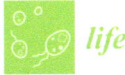

Editorial

Editorial for "Novel Diagnostic and Therapeutic Approaches in Temporomandibular Disorders and Myofascial Pain" Special Issue in *Life*

Zuzanna Nowak

Department of Temporomandibular Disorders, Medical University of Silesia in Katowice, Traugutta sq. 2, 41-800 Zabrze, Poland; zuzannaewanowak33@gmail.com

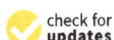

Citation: Nowak, Z. Editorial for "Novel Diagnostic and Therapeutic Approaches in Temporomandibular Disorders and Myofascial Pain" Special Issue in *Life*. *Life* **2023**, *13*, 2049. https://doi.org/10.3390/life13102049

Received: 26 September 2023
Revised: 9 October 2023
Accepted: 11 October 2023
Published: 13 October 2023

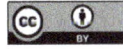

Copyright: © 2023 by the author. Licensee MDPI, Basel, Switzerland. This article is an open access article distributed under the terms and conditions of the Creative Commons Attribution (CC BY) license (https://creativecommons.org/licenses/by/4.0/).

In the dynamic and complex field of temporomandibular disorders (TMDs), keeping our knowledge up to date is of great importance. The following Special Issue focuses on novel as well as established therapies [1–6], with an additional glimpse at diagnostic improving tools and novel approaches [4,7,8], as well as epidemiological data [9].

Diagnosing and screening for TMDs is enduringly a relevant problem for general practitioners. Many patients must visit several specialists, often from various fields, before finding help. Moxley et al., based on the recent literature, pointed to the possibility of introducing an artificial neural network-based program to aid the diagnostic process [4]. Kreiner et al., who created the program, showed its significant advantage over the diagnostic abilities of inexperienced general dental practitioners, as it has a sensitivity and specificity close to 100% [10]. Another method described the assessment of personal salivary endocannabinoid profiles for patients, which could be useful for screening purposes. Another approach was suggested by Diaz-Saez et al., who attempted to assess the intra- and inter-rater reliability of a novel device to evaluate tongue force [7]. In contrast to the methods described above, it is a highly specialistic tool to aid in the search for possible additional TMD risk factors, such as tongue dysfunction.

The understanding of TMDs gradually evolves toward a more biopsychosocial approach where patients' pain and disabilities are no longer attributed to strictly mechanical disruptions but may originate, in fact, from more complex causes, and their treatment should be adequate [11,12]. It turns out that conventional treatments like occlusal splint therapy, intramuscular and intracapsular injections, manual therapy, and pharmacotherapy can be greatly improved by supplementing them with elements attributed to lifestyle medicine that increase general well-being. Regulating sleep patterns, breathing, dietary habits, and exercising, as well as learning stress management, benefits patients. Such actions allow proper tissue regeneration and an increased pain tolerance threshold, which creates a proper environment for patients' recovery at the root of the problem. Following general health improvement, a closer look at the orofacial area and local interventions are still necessary.

Physiotherapy remains a successful local treatment for muscular TMDs. Vieira et al. showed, in a quality systematic review, the evidence for the effectiveness of manual therapy in managing TMDs [1]. Although this approach is nothing novel, there is ongoing research to develop better protocols, as described by Moxley et al. [4]. Similarly, needling therapies constantly reappear in the literature. In this Special Issue, de Sousa et al. and Blanco-Rueda et al. presented their clinical findings as researchers and clinicians still lack standardized protocols for effective therapies [3,5]. With a growing amount of research, the goal should be to determine indications and contraindications for certain substances, the number of sessions for which they should be administered, and their long term effects. A noticeable trend within the studies points towards the use of more natural compounds like collagen, platelet derived plasma (PRP), and hyaluronic acid, which show great effectiveness and safety in needling therapies. In some cases, a last resort treatment has to be applied when patients are qualified for total joint replacement. The indications for such surgery are very limited; however, its benefits for patients in need are enormous, as shown by Speksnijder et al. in their clinical pilot study [6].

The following Special Issue presents a brief cross section through selected topics related to TMDs, bringing some novel insights as well as contributing to topical domains. It is an interesting read that should inspire further investigation within the complex subject of TMDs and point to directions for further clinical research.

Funding: There is no specific funding to declair.

Conflicts of Interest: The author declares no conflict of interest.

References

1. Vieira, L.S.; Pestana, P.R.M.; Miranda, J.P.; Soares, L.A.; Silva, F.; Alcantara, M.A.; Oliveira, V.C. The Efficacy of Manual Therapy Approaches on Pain, Maximum Mouth Opening and Disability in Temporomandibular Disorders: A Systematic Review of Randomised Controlled Trials. *Life* **2023**, *13*, 292. [CrossRef] [PubMed]
2. Müggenborg, F.; Carletti, E.M.d.C.; Dennett, L.; de Oliveira-Souza, A.I.S.; Mohamad, N.; Licht, G.; von Piekartz, H.; Armijo-Olivo, S. Effectiveness of Manual Trigger Point Therapy in Patients with Myofascial Trigger Points in the Orofacial Region— A Systematic Review. *Life* **2023**, *13*, 336. [PubMed]
3. Blanco-Rueda, J.A.; López-Valverde, A.; Márquez-Vera, A.; Méndez-Sánchez, R.; López-García, E.; López-Valverde, N. Preliminary Findings of the Efficacy of Botulinum Toxin in Temporomandibular Disorders: Uncontrolled Pilot Study. *Life* **2023**, *13*, 345. [CrossRef] [PubMed]
4. Moxley, B.; Stevens, W.; Sneed, J.; Pearl, C. Novel Diagnostic and Therapeutic Approaches to Temporomandibular Dysfunction: A Narrative Review. *Life* **2023**, *13*, 1808. [CrossRef] [PubMed]
5. de Sousa, B.M.; López-Valverde, A.; Caramelo, F.; Rodrigues, M.J.; López-Valverde, N. Medium-Term Effect of Treatment with Intra-Articular Injection of Sodium Hyaluronate, Betamethasone and Platelet-Rich Plasma in Patients with Temporomandibular Arthralgia: A Retrospective Cohort Study. *Life* **2022**, *12*, 1739. [CrossRef] [PubMed]
6. Speksnijder, C.M.; Mutsaers, N.E.A.; Walji, S. Functioning of the Masticatory System in Patients with an Alloplastic Total Temporomandibular Joint Prostheses Compared with Healthy Individuals: A Pilot Study. *Life* **2022**, *12*, 2073. [CrossRef] [PubMed]
7. Diaz-Saez, M.C.; Gil-Martínez, A.; Gadotti, I.C.; Navarro-Fernández, G.; Gil-Castillo, J.; Beltran-Alacreu, H. Reliability and Responsiveness of a Novel Device to Evaluate Tongue Force. *Life* **2023**, *13*, 1192. [CrossRef] [PubMed]
8. Lassmann, Ł.; Nowak, Z.; Orthlieb, J.-D.; Żółtowska, A. Complicated Relationships between Anterior and Condylar Guidance and Their Clinical Implications—Comparison by Cone Beam Computed Tomography and Electronic Axiography—An Observational Cohort Cross-Sectional Study. *Life* **2023**, *13*, 335. [PubMed]
9. Aranha, R.L.d.B.; Martins, R.d.C.; Paixão, L.C.; de Abreu, M.H.N.G. Professional Factors Associated with Case Resolution without Referrals of Orofacial Pain Cases to Secondary Dental Care by Telehealth in Brazil: A Cross-Sectional Study in 2019 and 2020. *Life* **2023**, *13*, 29. [CrossRef] [PubMed]
10. Kreiner, M.; Viloria, J. A novel artificial neural network for the diagnosis of orofacial pain and temporomandibular disorders. *J. Oral Rehabil.* **2022**, *49*, 884–889. [CrossRef] [PubMed]
11. Greene, C.; Manfredini, D. Treating Temporomandibular Disorders in the 21st Century: Can We Finally Eliminate the "Third Pathway"? *J. Oral Facial Pain Headache* **2020**, *34*, 206–216. [CrossRef] [PubMed]
12. Manfredini, D.; Saracutu, O.I.; Cagidiaco, E.F.; Ferrari, M. EPA Consensus Project Paper: The Relationship Between Prosthodontic Rehabilitations and Temporomandibular Disorders. *Eur. J. Prosthodont. Restor. Dent.* **2023**. [CrossRef]

Disclaimer/Publisher's Note: The statements, opinions and data contained in all publications are solely those of the individual author(s) and contributor(s) and not of MDPI and/or the editor(s). MDPI and/or the editor(s) disclaim responsibility for any injury to people or property resulting from any ideas, methods, instructions or products referred to in the content.

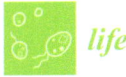

Review

Novel Diagnostic and Therapeutic Approaches to Temporomandibular Dysfunction: A Narrative Review

Brendan Moxley [1,*], William Stevens [1], Joel Sneed [1] and Craig Pearl [2]

[1] School of Dentistry, The University of Texas Health Science Center at Houston, Houston, TX 77054, USA; william.t.stevens@uth.tmc.edu (W.S.); joel.p.sneed@uth.tmc.edu (J.S.)

[2] Department of Oral and Maxillofacial Surgery, The University of Texas Health Science Center at Houston, Houston, TX 77054, USA; craig.b.pearl@uth.tmc.edu

* Correspondence: brendan.moxley@uth.tmc.edu

Abstract: Temporomandibular dysfunction (TMD) is a burgeoning area of study within the dental field. TMD is caused by abnormalities in the temporomandibular joint or muscles of mastication and can lead to pain, loss of function, and other complications. As this area of patient care receives increased focus, the ability to accurately diagnose TMD becomes paramount. The aim of this review is to summarize novel diagnostic and therapeutic techniques that have been proposed within the last approximately 3 years in order to inform readers of the cutting-edge advances in the field of TMD diagnosis and management, while also analyzing the clinical relevance of each study. A PubMed search was completed on 1 March 2023, using MeSH terms related to TMD diagnosis and treatment. The search yielded seven articles that pertained to the aim of this review article. The main findings from each study are summarized in this review article. These novel methods of diagnosing and treating TMD may improve our ability to assess and treat patients suffering from TMD.

Keywords: novel diagnosis; temporomandibular dysfunction; therapeutic

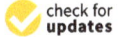

Citation: Moxley, B.; Stevens, W.; Sneed, J.; Pearl, C. Novel Diagnostic and Therapeutic Approaches to Temporomandibular Dysfunction: A Narrative Review. *Life* **2023**, *13*, 1808. https://doi.org/10.3390/life13091808

Academic Editor: Yingchu Lin

Received: 20 July 2023
Revised: 19 August 2023
Accepted: 23 August 2023
Published: 25 August 2023

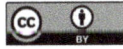

Copyright: © 2023 by the authors. Licensee MDPI, Basel, Switzerland. This article is an open access article distributed under the terms and conditions of the Creative Commons Attribution (CC BY) license (https://creativecommons.org/licenses/by/4.0/).

1. Introduction

Temporomandibular dysfunction (TMD) is the second most common musculoskeletal disorder that causes pain and disability, affecting nearly 5% of Americans (~16 million people) [1–4]. TMD is a condition that can be symptom-free, but more often causes patients pain, discomfort, and dysfunction that can be profoundly debilitating. The treatment costs and quality of life burden can be significant on these patients [5].

In fact, the proportion of TMD patients who experience at least one psychological comorbidity is as high as 75% [6]. TMD is caused by dysfunction of the muscles of mastication and/or the temporomandibular joint (TMJ) itself, and can lead to symptoms such as pain, joint noises, impaired jaw function, and locking. This condition can be hard to diagnose, and even harder to treat, as the manifestations of TMD are varied. TMD patients may present overlapping symptoms with other chronic pain conditions, including headache, fibromyalgia, and neurological conditions. The mechanism of this is not certain, but is likely through the phenomenon of central sensitization, such as allodynia and hyperalgesia [7–10]. There are numerous established methods of diagnosing TMD, although none have a 100% success rate. There are also numerous established therapeutic methods for treating TMD, with more being proposed every year, as this review article will demonstrate; however, no therapeutic method demonstrates a satisfactorily high rate of success.

Currently, the "gold standard" for TMD diagnosis is a Magnetic Resonance Imagine (MRI) scan; however, many patients will suffer from TMD despite no obvious pathological or mechanical disruptions [11]. Thus, TMD can be divided into three groups. Group I includes TMD caused by muscle disorders, including myofascial pain with and without limitations in mouth opening. Group II includes TMD caused by disc displacement with or without reductions and limitations in mouth opening. Group 3 includes arthralgia, arthritis, and arthrosis [12].

As for TMD management, treatment depends on etiology, whether pathological, mechanical, musculoskeletal, or idiopathic. However, in the absence of malignant pathology, conservative management protocols are usually recommended before surgical intervention, which is considered a last-resort treatment. Popular conservative management includes the prescription of muscle relaxants, the use of an occlusal splint, diet modification, and home physiotherapy with patient education [1].

Due in part to the relatively low success rate of existing diagnostic and therapeutic approaches in TMD, novel techniques are constantly being proposed. In this paper, an updated review of the latest techniques is described.

2. Materials and Methods

An article by Wu et al. assessed the established and novel therapeutic remedies available to TMD patients up to July of 2020. The aim of this article is to highlight novel diagnostic and therapeutic approaches that have been published since then. In doing so, the PICO question to be addressed is, "for patients suffering from TMD, do the novel diagnostic and therapeutic approaches proposed in the scientific literature since July of 2020 suggest efficacy in accurately diagnosing and managing their TMD compared with established techniques?" We conducted an electronic search of the PubMed database between 1 July 2020 and 1 March 2023 using the MeSH terms "diagnosis and TMD, therapeutic treatment and TMD, new treatment and TMD, new diagnostics and TMD". In addition to excluding by date, exclusion criteria were papers that were not published in English or those that were not pertinent to TMD diagnosis or treatment (see Table 1).

Table 1. Inclusion and exclusion criteria for the narrative review.

Inclusion Criteria	Exclusion Criteria
MeSH terms "diagnosis and TMD, therapeutic treatment and TMD, new treatment and TMD, new diagnostics and TMD"	Papers not pertinent to TMD Diagnosis or treatment
Published between 1 July 2020 and 1 March 2023	Papers not published in English

3. Results

In total, 40 results were returned upon conducting the PubMed search, as described above (see Figure 1). Five papers on novel TMD diagnosis were analyzed as fitting the criteria for this paper. Additionally, four papers on novel TMD therapeutics were analyzed as fitting the criteria for this study. The topics of each of the papers on TMD diagnosis were AI neural networks, salivary endocannabinoid profiles, electronic signal analysis, a novel MRI scoring system for TMD, and novel functional indices of masticatory activity. The topics of the papers relating to TMD therapeutics include aromatherapy massage, masticatory muscle relaxation techniques, radial extracorporeal shock wave therapy, and light and LASER therapies (see Figure 1).

3.1. Novel Diagnostic Approaches to Temporomandibular Dysfunction

3.1.1. Novel Artificial Neural Network for TMD Diagnosis

At this time, artificial intelligence (AI) is primarily used within the medical field to aid in the diagnosis and treatment of life-threatening conditions such as cardiovascular disease and cancer. Although TMD has a similar prevalence to these conditions in the general population, the use of artificial intelligence for the diagnosis and treatment of TMD is still in its infancy. While TMD is not itself a life-threatening condition, TMD can present with similar symptoms to life-threatening conditions. In fact, 4% of acute myocardial infarctions present with pain in the craniofacial structures as the only symptom [13]. The complexity of diagnosing TMD, in conjunction with the fact that many orofacial pain symptoms arise from other parts of the body, make proper TMD diagnosis a significant challenge for the general practitioner.

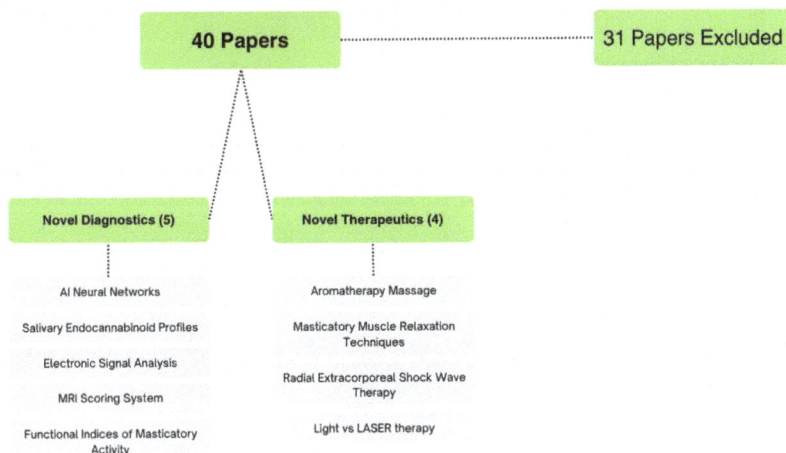

Figure 1. A graphical representation of the literature review conducted.

Given the successful use of AI for the diagnosis and treatment of other areas of medicine, Kreiner et al. attempted to develop an algorithm to diagnose orofacial pain and TMD with equal or higher accuracy than a general dentist [13]. Kreiner et al. created an artificial neural network (ANN) which is a subset of AI. This program allows the input of multiple pieces of information (patient symptoms, diagnostic imaging, etc.) and creates an output (diagnosis). The Kreiner ANN was given the same patient scenarios as 12 general dentists and asked to determine whether the patient's pain was of orofacial origin, and if so, to properly diagnose the condition. The neural network outperformed the dentists on average. The neural network was clearly superior at diagnosing pain from outside the orofacial region (e.g., referred cardiac pain, neuropathic pain). For example, only 25% of clinicians could diagnose the cases of referred orofacial pain from myocardial infarctions. The clinicians frequently chose diagnoses of "occlusal trauma", "bruxism", "periodontal disease", and "I do not know" instead. Only two clinicians could accurately diagnose the patient suffering from migraine symptoms. Only half of the clinicians correctly diagnosed TMD, while the ANN was able to correctly identify all cases. For pain of odontogenic origin (e.g., pulpitis), there was no significant difference between the ANN and the general dentists.

This study found that the novel ANN showed high diagnostic accuracy for the diagnosis of TMD. The results showed that the ANN had a sensitivity of 96.9% and a specificity of 95.5% for the diagnosis of TMD. These results indicate that the ANN was highly accurate in identifying patients with TMD and distinguishing them from patients without TMD. This level of accuracy was found to be comparable to or better than other diagnostic tools currently used for TMD diagnosis, such as clinical examination and imaging.

The results suggest that the ANN could be a useful tool for the diagnosis of orofacial pain and TMD. The ANN has several advantages over traditional diagnostic tools, including the ability to quickly and accurately analyze large amounts of data and identify patterns and relationships that might be missed by human observers. Further research could focus on improving the ANN's diagnostic algorithms and exploring other potential applications for ANN technology in dentistry and medicine.

Overall, this study demonstrates the promise of novel diagnostic tools using artificial intelligence. A simple neural network with only five layers of coding was able to outperform a dozen clinicians on diagnoses ranging from TMD to migraines to referred cardiac pain. More testing is needed before drawing conclusions about the widespread applicability of this ANN, and more AI algorithms like it. However, this is an area that contains vast potential for simplifying and streamlining the otherwise complicated task of accurately diagnosing patients with TMD.

3.1.2. Salivary Endocannabinoid Profiles

Each individual possesses a unique endocannabinoid (eCB) profile within their saliva. It has been suggested that this eCB profile may indicate the presence of underlying conditions that cause pain, such as temporomandibular disorder. The eCB profile of patients diagnosed with certain orofacial pain disorders has not been thoroughly studied. A study by Heiliczer et al. attempted to classify certain eCB profiles according to patients with current diagnoses of post-traumatic neuropathy, trigeminal neuralgia, temporomandibular disorders, migraine, tension-type headaches, and burning mouth syndrome [14]. Correlation analyses between eCB levels, a current and specific diagnosis, and pain characteristics were conducted.

The study enrolled 126 participants, including 83 patients with chronic orofacial pain or headache disorders and 43 healthy controls (see Figure 2). Saliva samples were collected from all participants, and salivary levels of endocannabinoids and related compounds were analyzed using liquid chromatography–tandem mass spectrometry. The results showed significant differences in salivary endocannabinoid profiles between the patient group and the control group. Specifically, the patient group exhibited significantly lower levels of anandamide and 2-arachidonoylglycerol (AG), two endocannabinoids with known analgesic and anti-inflammatory properties. The group of patients who currently suffer from migraines had significantly lower levels of an eCB called PEA in their saliva. There was a significantly increased level of AEA in the saliva of patients who suffer from burning mouth syndrome. There were not significantly increased or decreased levels of any specific eCBs in the temporomandibular disorder or post-traumatic neuropathy groups of this study.

Heiliczer et al. suggest that these findings could have several clinical implications. For example, salivary endocannabinoid profiles could be used as a diagnostic tool for chronic orofacial pain and headache disorders. Additionally, the findings suggest that endocannabinoid-based therapies, such as cannabinoid receptor agonists or inhibitors of endocannabinoid degradation, could be effective in treating these conditions. Heiliczer et al. also noted several limitations of the study, including the relatively small sample size and the lack of longitudinal data. Future studies could address these limitations by enrolling larger cohorts and following patients over time to assess the long-term effectiveness of endocannabinoid-based therapies.

Overall, the study suggests that salivary endocannabinoid profiles could be a useful tool for the diagnosis and management of chronic orofacial pain and headache disorders. The findings also support the potential therapeutic value of endocannabinoid-based therapies in these conditions. Further research is needed to confirm these findings and to explore the underlying mechanisms of endocannabinoid signaling in chronic pain and headache disorders. The fact that salivary samples of patients with certain orofacial pain disorders demonstrated signature eCB patterns suggests that more research should be conducted in this field. The potential to elucidate a certain eCB marker that correlates with temporomandibular disorder exists and would aid in the diagnosis of TMD patients going forward.

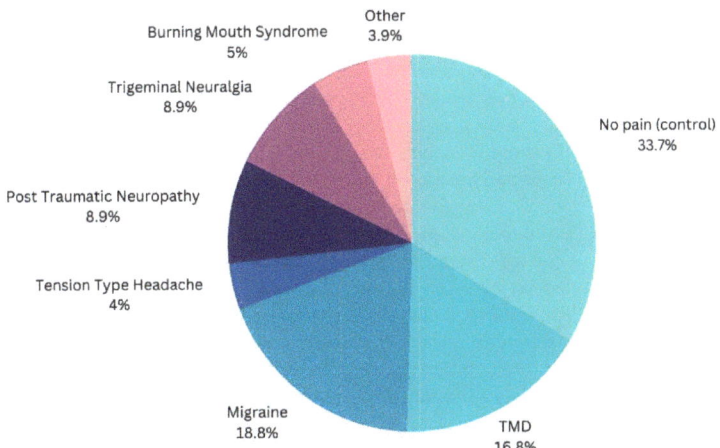

Figure 2. The percentages of each of subcategories of the 126 participants are displayed.

3.1.3. Signal Analysis to Diagnose TMJ Hypermobility

Frequently, certain noises emanating from the temporomandibular joint (TMJ) lead patients and clinicians to assume that temporomandibular dysfunction (TMD) must be present. These noises often including clicking, popping, and crepitus, among others. These noises can occur during speaking, eating, yawning, and other daily activities. However, these noises do not always coincide with disorders, and can lead to misdiagnoses. In fact, the noises caused by TMJ hypermobility are often errantly assumed to be caused by TMD [15]. Grochala et al. conducted a study of noises emanating from the TMJ using a novel technique called signal analysis [16]. This is a non-invasive technique that uses an electronic stethoscope to record noises associated with the TMJ during the process of opening and closing.

The researchers enrolled 47 patients who experienced noises emanating from their temporomandibular joints. The participants completed the official and commonly used research diagnostic criteria for temporomandibular disorder (RDC/TMD) questionnaire to determine whether they likely had TMD or TMJ hypermobility. Next, a Littmann 3200 electronic stethoscope was used simultaneously on both sides of the head to record TMJ sounds in function. These recordings were transferred to a computer for analysis of the signals produced during opening and closing. The research revealed time–frequency features in acoustic signals that are characteristic to TMJ hypermobility.

In this study, signal analysis was used to identify characteristic features of TMJ hypermobility, such as abnormal movement patterns and increased joint laxity. Grochala et al. developed a set of signal processing algorithms that were able to accurately distinguish between patients with TMJ hypermobility and control subjects based on these features. The signals were analyzed using several signal processing techniques, including Fourier transform, Hilbert transform, and wavelet transform. These techniques enable the decomposition of complex signals into their component frequencies and amplitudes, which can then be analyzed to identify patterns and anomalies.

The results showed that the new diagnostic method was able to accurately distinguish between patients with TMJ hypermobility and control subjects. Specifically, the method had a sensitivity of 98.8% and a specificity of 100%, indicating that it was highly accurate in identifying patients with TMJ hypermobility and excluding individuals without the condition. The authors suggest that this novel diagnostic method could have several clinical implications. For example, it could be used to identify patients with TMJ hypermobility who might be at risk of developing more severe TMJ disorders or who might benefit from early intervention to prevent further damage. Additionally, the method could be used to monitor the effectiveness of TMJ treatments over time. The authors note several limitations of the study, including the relatively small sample size and the lack of validation in other patient populations. Further research is needed to confirm the diagnostic accuracy of this new method and to assess its potential clinical utility.

Signal analysis is a powerful tool for diagnosing and monitoring TMJ disorders because it enables the objective measurement of joint movement and function. This can be especially useful in cases where clinical examination alone may be insufficient to diagnose or monitor the progression of the condition. Additionally, signal analysis can provide valuable insights into the underlying biomechanical mechanisms of TMJ disorders, which can inform the development of new treatments and interventions. By creating a database of certain signals unique to patients with TMD versus those with TMJ hypermobility, practitioners may be able to compare the sounds of undiagnosed patients with the signals unique to certain diagnoses, and more accurately diagnose new patients. This is an area of research that still needs extensive study and data collection before it can be definitively used as a diagnostic aid; however, the potential benefit exists.

3.1.4. A Novel MRI Scoring System for TMD Diagnosis

Of the many diagnostic tools used by clinicians to diagnose TMD, magnetic resonance imaging (MRI) is widely considered the gold standard [17]. Not only does this imaging modality confer a high level of resolution of hard and soft tissue structures in the TMJ, but it can also produce imaging of the joint in motion. However, MRI is only useful for diagnosis if there is a reliable system for assessing the imaging and relating it to a diagnosis. In 2018, Wurm et al. proposed a novel MRI-based scoring system to diagnose TMD. This system offers a standardized evaluation using three main variables that assess key relevant structural changes within the TMJ [18]. This system includes an assessment of the articular disc, the direction of disc luxation, and osseous joint alterations. Although this novel system has potential to be a useful diagnostic tool, the inter-rater reliability of the system has not been assessed.

In 2022, Willenbrock et al. conducted a study to assess the inter- and intra-rater reliability of the Wurm et al. MRI scoring system [19]. Willenbrock et al. enrolled 60 patients with suspected uni- and bilateral TMD for assessment by two experienced radiologists. Using MRI of these patients' TMJs, the radiologists scored each patient on the Wurm et al. scoring system. Inter-rater and intra-rater reliability were assessed using two different methods: intraclass correlation coefficient (ICC) and weighted kappa coefficient. The results showed high reliability for both methods, with ICC values ranging from 0.85 to 0.99 and kappa values ranging from 0.76 to 1.00. No significant differences were found between both observers for the articular disc and direction of disc luxation scores. Although significant differences were found for the assessment of subtle osseous changes, these differences were minor.

The correlation between the MRI-based scores and clinical assessments of TMD severity was also evaluated. The clinical assessments included pain intensity, jaw opening, and joint sounds. The results showed a significant correlation between the MRI-based scores and all three clinical assessments, indicating that the scoring system was able to accurately reflect the severity of TMD. Willenbrock et al. noted that the new scoring system has several advantages over existing systems. For example, it is based on MRI, which enables the non-invasive assessment of TMJ abnormalities. Additionally, the system includes multiple categories of abnormalities, which provides a more comprehensive assessment of TMJ health. However, Willenbrock et al. also noted some limitations of the system. For example, the system requires specialized training to use, which may limit its accessibility to some clinicians. Additionally, the system may not be able to detect some types of TMJ abnormalities that are not visible on MRI scans.

In conclusion, Willenbrock et al.'s study concluded that the novel Wurm et al. scoring system is reliable enough to use as a tool in the process of diagnosing patients with suspected TMD. The high reliability and validity of the system suggest that it could be a useful tool for clinicians in diagnosing and managing TMDs. Further research is needed to validate the system in larger patient populations and to explore its potential clinical applications.

3.1.5. Novel Functional Indices of Masticatory Muscle Activity

It is well known that for muscle activity to occur, specific electrical signal pathways within the musculature must occur. This includes the muscles surrounding the TMJ during functional movements and at rest. The practice of measuring electromyography has been applied to diagnosing bruxism [20], tension-type headaches [21], Down syndrome [22], different occlusal features [23], motor neuron disease [24], and in TMD patients [25]. Ginszt et al. hypothesized that analyzing masticatory muscle activity in patients with signs of TMD using novel functional indices could aid in more accurate diagnoses [26]. This team conducted a study in which 78 women were divided equally into two groups based on an existing diagnosis of TMD or a healthy adult. In order to record the bioelectrical activity of facial musculature, surface electromyography was used. The bioelectric activity of the temporalis anterior, the superficial masseter, and anterior bellies of the digastric muscles was recorded during functional clenching, functional opening, opening, and at rest. The data collected were analyzed using a wavelet transformer to extract the time–frequency characteristics of the surface electromyography signals. Ginszt et al. developed three functional indices: the muscle activation index, muscle activity rhythm index, and muscle contraction force index.

Statistical analysis of the results demonstrated significant differences between the control group and TMD group in various categories. The results showed that the muscle activation index was highest during clenching and lowest during chewing soft food. The muscle activity rhythm index was highest during chewing hard food and lowest during clenching. The muscle contraction force index was highest during chewing hard food and lowest during chewing soft food. It was found that the control group had higher values in all functional clenching indices. The most significant difference occurred on the left side during clenching activity. It was found that there was considerable difference within the range of motion during maximum active mouth opening. There were also significant differences in some measurements in the resting position.

Although this study yielded statistically significant results between TMD and non-TMD patients, the applicability of these results is still unreliable. Measuring electromyographic activity is a complex process, and the results cannot be predictably applied to patient diagnoses and treatment recommendations at this time. There is potential for further research in this area that could elucidate specific diagnosable trigger points and muscle activity particular to TMD patients. Ginszt et al. posits that in order to verify and confirm the validity and effectiveness of the use of the functional indices, replication studies must be performed.

3.2. Novel Therapeutic Approaches to Temporomandibular Dysfunction

A PubMed search using the inclusion and exclusion criteria described in the Introduction yielded very few results for novel therapeutic tools published since July 2020. In total, four papers will be reviewed, but the first two articles described below are of limited applicability, relevance, and/or reliability. They have been included in this review article for the purpose of completeness.

Novel TMD Treatment Using Aromatherapy Massage with Lavender Oil

A study was published in the Journal of Craniofacial and Sleep Practice that investigated the effects of massage therapy on alleviating TMD pain symptoms. This therapy theoretically reduces pain via activation of the pain–gate pathway, stimulates the parasympathetic center, and re-establishes muscular length and flexibility, improves local blood circulation, and increases the production of endogenous opioids [27]. This area of study has not received extensive study, and there is not a large body of evidence supporting its efficacy.

Benli et al. conducted a randomized controlled trial to investigate the effects of aromatherapy massage with lavender oil on pain reduction and maximal mouth opening in patients with myogenous TMD compared with a control group. For this study, 90 patients were selected based on stringent eligibility criteria: 30 patients were placed in the test group, which received aromatherapy massage with lavender oil; 30 patients were placed in the placebo group, and received massage therapy with sweet almond oil; 30 patients were placed in the control group, and received no massage therapy. All patients abstained from taking analgesic medication during the trial. Efforts were made to adequately control for other variables; however, a detailed description of those measures is outside the scope of this review.

The findings indicated that the aromatherapy massage group showed significant differences compared with control and placebo groups in terms of maximal mouth opening and the evaluated pain parameters (as measured by visual analog scale). At the beginning of the trial, there was no difference in the two measurements between all groups. Immediately after the treatment, both groups that received aromatherapy massage demonstrated statistically significant improvements in pain reduction and maximal opening compared with the control group. The group that received lavender oil treatment demonstrated significant improvements compared with the placebo group that received almond oil. At two months post-procedure, both massage groups again demonstrated significant improvements compared with the control group. Similarly, the group that received lavender oil demonstrated more pain reduction and greater maximal opening than the almond oil group. However, the difference in results compared with the control group declined compared with measurements taken immediately after treatment. The limited results seemed to suggest that the beneficial effects of treatment waned after a short period of time. These results suggest that there may be merit to further investigation into the use of both massage therapy and use of lavender oil as adjunctive, conservative treatment for pain reduction and increased maximal opening in TMD patients.

3.3. Novel Manual Techniques in Masticatory Muscle Relaxation in TMD Treatment

A study was published in the International Journal of Environmental Research and Public Health that investigates the degree of relaxation of muscles of mastication achieved by manual release techniques. This study by Urbański et al. enrolled patients who are currently undergoing prosthetic treatment to relieve TMD with a dominant muscular component [28]. Sixty patients were randomly assigned to a group that received post-isometric relaxation treatment or a group that received myofascial release treatment. Both groups received ten treatment sessions and were assessed using surface electromyography measurements of the anterior temporal and masseter muscles as well as the intensity of spontaneous masticatory muscle pain assessed via the visual analog scale.

The results from the study demonstrated that both groups exhibited decreased electrical activity in the temporalis and masseter muscles after treatment. Both treatment groups also exhibited a significant drop in the intensity of spontaneous pain in the masticatory muscle group. There was no significant difference in results between the two treatment groups. Urbański et al. suggest that both post-isometric relaxation treatment and myofascial release treatment are appropriate adjunctive treatments for TMD patients receiving prosthetic treatment. The authors also discussed the mechanisms by which manual techniques may exert their therapeutic effects. They suggested that manual techniques may help to release tension and adhesions in the masticatory muscles, increase blood flow and oxygen supply to the muscles, and stimulate the release of endorphins and other pain-relieving substances.

Overall, Urbański et al. concluded that manual techniques can be a valuable adjunctive therapy in the treatment of TMDs. They suggested that manual techniques should be considered as part of a comprehensive treatment plan that includes patient education, stress management, and other therapies, such as physical therapy and pharmacological interventions. While this area of treatment demonstrates potential for certain patients, more research is recommended before definitively adopting this treatment modality for TMD patients.

3.3.1. Radial Extracorporeal Shock Wave Therapy for TMD

Radial Extracorporeal Shock Wave Therapy (rESWT) is an established treatment modality for treating a variety of musculoskeletal conditions. It involves using a machine with a tip that appears similar to an ultrasound. It administers shock waves to the painful, tense area for approximately 3 min every week, and has been shown to effectively reduce pain in the area over time. In this study, this technique was tested in patients with temporomandibular disorders to determine its efficacy in treating the pain exhibited by these patients.

The study design included two groups: the first with eight patients who underwent a series of physical exercises combined with rESWT, and the second group of seven patients who served as a control as they underwent the same series of exercises but with sham rESWT. The treatment regiment included 20 min of bilateral manual physical therapy followed by 3 min of rESWT, one session a week for four weeks. Efficacy was measured using two data points: the patient's self-reported pain intensity according to the visual analogue scale (VAS), as well as a surface electromyography evaluation (sEMG) of the anterior temporalis and masseter muscles to assess muscle function. The sEMG test was performed using four surface electrodes to detect the electrical activity of the masticatory muscles. As these patients presented with trigger points, reduced electrical activity was desired in the post-test for these patients as compared with the pre-test [29].

The results of the study were that the rESWT group exhibited statistically significant pain reduction compared with the group receiving sham rESWT. Additionally, while some providers question the efficacy of the sEMG test in clinical use, there were several statistically significant data points between the two groups for this test as well. The authors state that, to the best of their knowledge, this is the first study on rESWT in this application, so further studies are warranted to confirm the efficacy of these findings, especially since this technique demonstrates conflicting evidence in other areas of the body [30].

3.3.2. Light Therapy vs. LASER in Pain Reduction in TMD

Both red light therapy and LASER are techniques for treating TMD that have been shown to be effective when compared with a control group in previous studies; however, this study compared the two techniques to each other due to their similar mechanism of action [31].

In terms of the mechanism of action, red light therapy works by providing heat to the tender area, which causes vasodilatation of the adjacent blood vessels and increased blood supply. The increased blood supply washes away the inflammatory mediators, which improves patient symptoms. The mechanism of action of LASER therapy is similar, although it is theorized that LASER therapy also increases cell metabolism and protein synthesis. The biggest difference between the mechanism of the two techniques, however, is the specific wavelength of the energy delivered, with LASER being higher energy that is administered for a shorter duration.

Patients were randomly assigned to one of three groups: group A served as the control because the LED light device was applied to the trigger points without turning them on; group B received the LED light device that was turned on for 5 min; and group C received low-level LASER therapy for 30 s. The VAS pain score and presence of trismus and trigger points was assessed in four visits over 4 weeks.

The results of the study are that patients receiving either light therapy or LASER showed statistically significant improvements in pain when compared with a control (consistent with previously published literature); however, there were no differences between LASER or light therapy groups when comparing the two treatments with each other. Regarding tenderness, both techniques were effective in reducing the number of trigger points, but the LASER technique was statistically significant, while the red light therapy was insignificant. However, LASER devices are more expensive and more invasive, so the lower cost and higher biosafety of the LED device may make it more clinically viable as a technique [32,33].

4. Discussion

The field of TMD diagnosis and treatment is rapidly developing as our understanding of the different etiologies of TMD progresses. Although numerous diagnostic and treatment modalities have been established, room exists for improvement and innovation in this area. Since July 2020, five novel diagnostic modalities and two novel therapeutic methods have been proposed. The novel diagnostic modalities of an artificial neural network for TMD diagnosis demonstrated the ability to diagnosis TMD and other myofascial pain syndromes with equal or superior accuracy compared with clinicians. The use of salivary endocannabinoid profiles demonstrated potential as a method to non-invasively screen patients for TMD and other conditions that elicit distinct endocannabinoid profiles. The use of signal analysis to diagnose TMJ hypermobility could potentially reduce the number of patients who are erroneously diagnosed with TMD when, in fact, they have hypermobile temporomandibular joints. The repeated testing of a novel MRI scoring system demonstrated efficacy of the system and lends support to the continued use of it as part of the TMD diagnosis algorithm. Finally, the use of novel functional indices of masticatory muscle activity demonstrates potential as an adjunctive tool for accurate TMD diagnosis.

Furthermore, since July 2020, four novel therapeutic methods have been proposed. The use of aromatherapy massage with lavender oil as a treatment modality for TMD demonstrated positive results. The use of manual techniques in masticatory muscle relaxation to treat TMD also demonstrated potential as an adjunctive treatment modality. However, these studies were limited by small sample sizes and reduced follow-up, so further research is indicated before these therapeutic modalities are adopted as standard treatments. Radial extracorporeal shock wave therapy, red light therapy, and LASER therapy are not new treatment modalities for musculoskeletal problems generally, but studies published within the last 3 years suggest efficacy for managing TMD.

Gender and age were not defined as exclusion criteria for this narrative review; however, TMD has been shown to present in higher frequency and severity in females than males, with peak severity between ages of 20 and 40, which is consistent with the demographic data of the patients enrolled in each study reviewed [34–37].

Although some studies confer more evidence than others, these studies represent the expanding boundaries of this area of patient care. There were limitations to the scope of this review. In some cases, the same novel approach had multiple publications within the last three years, especially in the topic of artificial intelligence (AI) for TMD diagnosis [35–37]. Additionally, although best efforts were undertaken to analyze all novel diagnostic and therapeutic approaches to temporomandibular dysfunction, there are likely some research articles that were not included.

In terms of clinical utility, further studies are warranted for all described novel diagnostic and therapeutic approaches before clinical adoption is recommended. The only therapeutic approaches that are potentially clinically relevant at the current stage are radial extracorporeal shock wave therapy and red light or LASER therapy due to the abundant literature on these techniques in other parts of the body confirming their safety and efficacy, combined with preliminary evidence suggesting that this safety and efficacy extends to the temporomandibular region as well. However, all approaches are potentially suitable in the academic setting if tested as the subject of further investigation.

5. Conclusions

Temporomandibular dysfunction is a condition that affects a significant proportion of the population. TMD carries societal cost burdens as well as a substantially reduced quality of life for many patients. The articles included in this review represent the boundaries that are being expanded in an effort to better care for this patient population. Although this field has achieved considerable progress in recent years, further research is recommended to advance the care of patients suffering from TMD.

Author Contributions: Conceptualization, C.P.; methodology, C.P.; investigation, W.S.; resources, C.P.; writing—original draft preparation, W.S., B.M. and J.S.; writing—review and editing, C.P.; visualization, B.M.; supervision, C.P.; project administration, C.P. All authors have read and agreed to the published version of the manuscript.

Funding: This research received no external funding.

Institutional Review Board Statement: Ethical review and approval were waived for this study due to this paper being a review of previously published research with appropriate IRB approval.

Informed Consent Statement: Not applicable.

Data Availability Statement: Not applicable.

Conflicts of Interest: The authors declare no conflict of interest.

References

1. Wu, M.; Cai, J.; Yu, Y.; Hu, S.; Wang, Y.; Wu, M. Therapeutic agents for the treatment of temporomandibular joint disorders: Progress and perspective. *Front. Pharmacol.* **2021**, *11*, 596099. [CrossRef] [PubMed]
2. de Sire, A.; Marotta, N.; Ferrillo, M.; Agostini, F.; Sconza, C.; Lippi, L.; Respizzi, S.; Giudice, A.; Invernizzi, M.; Ammendolia, A. Oxygen-ozone therapy for reducing pro-inflammatory cytokines serum levels in musculoskeletal and temporomandibular disorders: A comprehensive review. *Int. J. Mol. Sci.* **2022**, *5*, 2528. [CrossRef] [PubMed]
3. Valesan, L.F.; Da-Cas, C.D.; Réus, J.C.; Denardin, A.C.S.; Garanhani, R.R.; Bonotto, D.; Januzzi, E.; de Souza, B.D.M. Prevalence of temporomandibular joint disorders: A systematic review and meta-analysis. *Clin. Oral Investig.* **2021**, *2*, 441–453. [CrossRef]
4. Mishra, R. Global Burden of Temporomandibular Disorder (TMD): A Systematic Review of TMD Prevalence and Incidence (1990–January 2019). Ph.D. Thesis, National Academies of Sciences, Engineering, and Medicine, Washington, DC, USA, 2020.
5. Seo, H.; Jung, B.; Yeo, J.; Kim, K.W.; Cho, J.H.; Lee, Y.J.; Ha, I.H. Healthcare utilisation and costs for temporomandibular disorders: A descriptive, cross-sectional study. *BMJ Open* **2020**, *10*, e036768. [CrossRef]
6. Ferrillo, M.; Migliario, M.; Marotta, N.; Fortunato, F.; Bindi, M.; Pezzotti, F.; Ammendolia, A.; Giudice, A.; Foglio Bonda, P.L.; de Sire, A. Temporomandibular disorders and neck pain in primary headache patients: A retrospective machine learning study. *Acta Odontol. Scand.* **2023**, *3*, 151–157. [CrossRef]
7. Minervini, G.; Mariani, P.; Fiorillo, L.; Cervino, G.; Cicciù, M.; Laino, L. Prevalence of temporomandibular disorders in people with multiple sclerosis: A systematic review and meta-analysis. *Cranio* **2022**, *10*, 1–9. [CrossRef] [PubMed]
8. Ferrillo, M.; Giudice, A.; Marotta, N.; Fortunato, F.; Di Venere, D.; Ammendolia, A.; Fiore, P.; de Sire, A. Pain management and rehabilitation for central sensitization in temporomandibular disorders: A comprehensive review. *Int. J. Mol. Sci.* **2022**, *23*, 12164. [CrossRef] [PubMed]
9. Li, J.H.; Yang, J.L.; Wei, S.Q.; Li, Z.L.; Collins, A.A.; Zou, M.; Wei, F.; Cao, D.Y. Contribution of central sensitization to stress-induced spreading hyperalgesia in rats with orofacial inflammation. *Mol. Brain* **2020**, *13*, 106. [CrossRef]
10. La Touche, R.; Paris-Alemany, A.; Hidalgo-Pérez, A.; López-de-Uralde-Villanueva, I.; Angulo-Diaz-Parreño, S.; Muñoz-García, D. Evidence for central sensitization in patients with temporomandibular disorders: A systematic review and meta-analysis of observational studies. *Pain Pract.* **2018**, *3*, 388–409. [CrossRef]
11. Xiong, X.; Ye, Z.; Tang, H.; Wei, Y.; Nie, L.; Wei, X.; Liu, Y.; Song, B. MRI of temporomandibular joint disorders: Recent advances and future directions. *J. Magn. Reson. Imaging* **2021**, *54*, 1039–1052. [CrossRef] [PubMed]
12. Schiffman, E.; Ohrbach, R.; Truelove, E.; Look, J.; Anderson, G.; Goulet, J.P.; List, T.; Svensson, P.; Gonzalez, Y.; Lobbezoo, F.; et al. Diagnostic Criteria for Temporomandibular Disorders (DC/TMD) for Clinical and Research Applications: Recommendations of the International RDC/TMD Consortium Network* and Orofacial Pain Special Interest Group. *J. Oral Facial Pain Headache* **2014**, *28*, 6–27. [CrossRef] [PubMed]
13. Kreiner, M.; Viloria, J. A novel artificial neural network for the diagnosis of orofacial pain and temporomandibular disorders. *J. Oral Rehabil.* **2022**, *49*, 884–889. [CrossRef] [PubMed]
14. Heiliczer, S.; Wilensky, A.; Gaver, M.; Georgiev, O.; Hamad, S.; Nemirovski, A.; Hadar, R.; Sharav, Y.; Aframian, D.J.; Tam, J.; et al. Salivary Endocannabinoid Profiles in Chronic Orofacial Pain and Headache Disorders: An Observational Study Using a Novel Tool for Diagnosis and Management. *Int. J. Mol. Sci.* **2022**, *23*, 13017. [CrossRef]
15. Taşkesen, F.; Cezairli, B. Efficacy of prolotherapy and arthrocentesis in management of temporomandibular joint hypermobility. *Cranio* **2023**, *41*, 423–431. [CrossRef]
16. Grochala, J.; Grochala, D.; Kajor, M.; Iwaniec, J.; Loster, J.E.; Iwaniec, M. A Novel Method of Temporomandibular Joint Hypermobility Diagnosis Based on Signal Analysis. *J. Clin. Med.* **2021**, *10*, 5145. [CrossRef]

17. Abdalla-Aslan, R.; Shilo, D.; Nadler, C.; Eran, A.; Rachmiel, A. Diagnostic correlation between clinical protocols and magnetic resonance findings in temporomandibular disorders: A systematic review and meta-analysis. *J. Oral Rehabil.* **2021**, *48*, 955–967. [CrossRef] [PubMed]
18. Wurm, M.C.; Behrends, T.K.; Wüst, W.; Wiesmüller, M.; Wilkerling, A.; Neukam, F.W.; Schlittenbauer, T. Correlation between pain and MRI findings in TMD patients. *J. Cranio-Maxillofac. Surg.* **2018**, *46*, 1167–1171. [CrossRef]
19. Willenbrock, D.; Lutz, R.; Wuest, W.; Heiss, R.; Uder, M.; Behrends, T.; Wurm, M.; Kesting, M.; Wiesmueller, M. Imaging temporomandibular disorders: Reliability of a novel MRI-based scoring system. *J. Cranio-Maxillofac. Surg.* **2022**, *50*, 230–236. [CrossRef]
20. Yamaguchi, T.; Mikami, S.; Maeda, M.; Saito, T.; Nakajima, T.; Yachida, W.; Gotouda, A. Portable and wearable electromyographic devices for the assessment of sleep bruxism and awake bruxism: A literature review. *Cranio* **2023**, *41*, 69–77. [CrossRef]
21. Rastogi, R.; Chaturvedi, D.K.; Satya, S.; Arora, N.; Gupta, M.; Yadav, V.; Chauhan, S.; Sharma, P. Chronic TTH analysis by EMG and GSR biofeedback on various modes and various medical symptoms using IoT. In *Big Data Analytics for Intelligent Healthcare Management*; Academic Press: Cambridge, MA, USA, 2019; pp. 87–150.
22. Giannasi, L.C.; Politti, F.; Dutra, M.T.S.; Tenguan, V.L.S.; Silva, G.R.C.; Mancilha, G.P.; da Silva, D.B.; Oliveira, L.V.F.; Oliveira, C.S.; Amorim, J.B.O.; et al. Intra-Day and Inter-Day Reliability of Measurements of the Electromyographic Signal on Masseter and Temporal Muscles in Patients with Down Syndrome. *Sci. Rep.* **2020**, *10*, 7477. [CrossRef]
23. Vozzi, F.; Favero, L.; Peretta, R.; Guarda-Nardini, L.; Cocilovo, F.; Manfredini, D. Indexes of Jaw Muscle Function in Asymptomatic Individuals with Different Occlusal Features. *Clin. Exp. Dent. Res.* **2018**, *4*, 263–267. [CrossRef] [PubMed]
24. Chen, M.; Zhang, X.; Zhou, P. A novel validation approach for high-density surface EMG decomposition in motor neuron disease. *IEEE Trans. Neural Syst. Rehabil. Eng.* **2018**, *6*, 1161–1168. [CrossRef] [PubMed]
25. Szyszka-Sommerfeld, L.; Sycińska-Dziarnowska, M.; Spagnuolo, G.; Woźniak, K. Surface electromyography in the assessment of masticatory muscle activity in patients with pain-related temporomandibular disorders: A systematic review. *Front. Neurol.* **2023**, *14*, 1184036. [CrossRef] [PubMed]
26. Ginszt, M.; Zieliński, G. Novel Functional Indices of Masticatory Muscle Activity. *J. Clin. Med.* **2021**, *10*, 1440. [CrossRef]
27. Benli, M.; Olson, J.; Huck, O.; Oezcan, M. A novel treatment modality for myogenous temporomandibular disorders using aromatherapy massage with lavender oil: A randomized controlled clinical trial. *Cranio* **2023**, *41*, 48–58. [CrossRef]
28. Urbański, P.; Trybulec, B.; Pihut, M. The Application of Manual Techniques in Masticatory Muscles Relaxation as Adjunctive Therapy in the Treatment of Temporomandibular Joint Disorders. *Int. J. Environ. Res. Public Health* **2021**, *18*, 12970. [CrossRef]
29. Marotta, N.; Ferrillo, M.; Demeco, A.; Drago Ferrante, V.; Inzitari, M.T.; Pellegrino, R.; Pino, I.; Russo, I.; de Sire, A.; Ammendolia, A. Effects of Radial Extracorporeal Shock Wave Therapy in Reducing Pain in Patients with Temporomandibular Disorders: A Pilot Randomized Controlled Trial. *Appl. Sci.* **2022**, *12*, 3821. [CrossRef]
30. Lange, T.; Deventer, N.; Gosheger, G.; Lampe, L.P.; Bockholt, S.; Schulze Boevingloh, A.; Schulte, T.L. Effectiveness of Radial Extracorporeal Shockwave Therapy in Patients with Acute Low Back Pain—Randomized Controlled Trial. *J. Clin. Med.* **2021**, *10*, 5569. [CrossRef]
31. Al-Quisi, A.F.; Jamil, F.A.; Abdulhadi, B.N.; Muhsen, S.J. The reliability of using light therapy compared with LASER in pain reduction of temporomandibular disorders: A randomized controlled trial. *BMC Oral Health* **2023**, *2*, 91. [CrossRef]
32. Daggett, C.; Daggett, A.; McBurney, E.; Murina, A. Laser safety: The need for protocols. *Cutis* **2020**, *2*, 87–92. [CrossRef]
33. Liu, H.; Daly, L.; Rudd, G.; Khan, A.P.; Mallidi, S.; Liu, Y.; Cuckov, F.; Hasan, T.; Celli, J.P. Development and evaluation of a low-cost, portable, LED-based device for PDT treatment of early-stage oral cancer in resource-limited settings. *Lasers Surg. Med.* **2019**, *4*, 345–351. [CrossRef]
34. Alrizqi, A.H.; Aleissa, B.M. Prevalence of Temporomandibular Disorders Between 2015–2021: A Literature Review. *Cureus* **2023**, *4*, e37028. [CrossRef] [PubMed]
35. Jha, N.; Lee, K.S.; Kim, Y.J. Diagnosis of temporomandibular disorders using artificial intelligence technologies: A systematic review and meta-analysis. *PLoS ONE* **2022**, *8*, e0272715. [CrossRef] [PubMed]
36. Reda, B.; Contardo, L.; Prenassi, M.; Guerra, E.; Derchi, G.; Marceglia, S. Artificial intelligence to support early diagnosis of temporomandibular disorders: A preliminary case study. *J. Oral Rehabil.* **2023**, *1*, 31–38. [CrossRef] [PubMed]
37. Diniz de Lima, E.; Souza Paulino, J.A.; Lira de Farias Freitas, A.P.; Viana Ferreira, J.E.; Barbosa, J.D.S.; Bezerra Silva, D.F.; Bento, P.M.; Araújo Maia Amorim, A.M.; Melo, D.P. Artificial intelligence and infrared thermography as auxiliary tools in the diagnosis of temporomandibular disorder. *Dentomaxillofac. Radiol.* **2022**, *2*, 20210318. [CrossRef]

Disclaimer/Publisher's Note: The statements, opinions and data contained in all publications are solely those of the individual author(s) and contributor(s) and not of MDPI and/or the editor(s). MDPI and/or the editor(s) disclaim responsibility for any injury to people or property resulting from any ideas, methods, instructions or products referred to in the content.

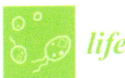

Article

Reliability and Responsiveness of a Novel Device to Evaluate Tongue Force

Marta Carlota Diaz-Saez [1,2,3], Alfonso Gil-Martínez [1,2,4,*], Inae Caroline Gadotti [5], Gonzalo Navarro-Fernández [2], Javier Gil-Castillo [6] and Hector Beltran-Alacreu [7]

1. Physiotherapy Department, Centro Superior de Estudios Universitarios La Salle, Universidad Autónoma de Madrid, C/La Salle, 28023 Madrid, Spain
2. CranioSPain Research Group, Centro Superior de Estudios Universitarios La Salle, Universidad Autónoma de Madrid, C/La Salle, 28023 Madrid, Spain
3. Programa de Doctorado en Medicina y Cirugía, Universidad Autónoma de Madrid, C/Francisco Tomás y Valiente 5, 28049 Madrid, Spain
4. Hospital Universitario La Paz-Carlos III. Institute for Health Research (IdiPaz), Paseo la Castellana, 261, 28046 Madrid, Spain
5. Department of Physical Therapy, Nicole Wertheim College of Nursing and Health Sciences, Florida International University, 11865 SW 26th St Suite H3, Miami, FL 33199, USA
6. Neural Rehabilitation Group, Cajal Institute, Spanish National Research Council (CSIC), Av. Doctor Arce, 37, 28002 Madrid, Spain
7. Toledo Physiotherapy Research Group (GIFTO), Faculty of Physical Therapy and Nursing, Universidad de Castilla-La Mancha, Avenida de Carlos III s/n, 45071 Toledo, Spain
* Correspondence: alfonso.gil@lasallecampus.es; Tel.: +34-666137908

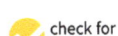

Citation: Diaz-Saez, M.C.; Gil-Martínez, A.; Gadotti, I.C.; Navarro-Fernández, G.; Gil-Castillo, J.; Beltran-Alacreu, H. Reliability and Responsiveness of a Novel Device to Evaluate Tongue Force. *Life* 2023, 13, 1192. https://doi.org/10.3390/life13051192

Academic Editors: Zuzanna Nowak and Aleksandra Nitecka-Buchta

Received: 13 March 2023
Revised: 21 April 2023
Accepted: 11 May 2023
Published: 16 May 2023

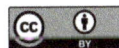

Copyright: © 2023 by the authors. Licensee MDPI, Basel, Switzerland. This article is an open access article distributed under the terms and conditions of the Creative Commons Attribution (CC BY) license (https://creativecommons.org/licenses/by/4.0/).

Abstract: Background: Measurements of tongue force are important in clinical practice during both the diagnostic process and rehabilitation progress. It has been shown that patients with chronic temporomandibular disorders have less tongue strength than asymptomatic subjects. Currently, there are few devices to measure tongue force on the market, with different limitations. That is why a new device has been developed to overcome them. The objectives of the study were to determine the intra- and inter-rater reliability and the responsiveness of a new low-cost device to evaluate tongue force in an asymptomatic population. Materials and Methods: Two examiners assessed the maximal tongue force in 26 asymptomatic subjects using a developed prototype of an Arduino device. Each examiner performed a total of eight measurements of tongue force in each subject. Each tongue direction was measured twice (elevation, depression, right lateralization, and left lateralization) in order to test the intrarater reliability. Results: The intrarater reliability using the new device was excellent for the measurements of the tongue force for up (ICC > 0.94), down (ICC > 0.93) and right (ICC > 0.92) movements, and good for the left movement (ICC > 0.82). The SEM and MDC values were below 0.98 and 2.30, respectively, for the intrarater reliability analysis. Regarding the inter-rater reliability, the ICC was excellent for measuring the tongue up movements (ICC = 0.94), and good for all the others (down ICC = 0.83; right ICC = 0.87; and left ICC = 0.81). The SEM and MDC values were below 1.29 and 3.01, respectively, for the inter-rater reliability. Conclusions: This study showed a good-to-excellent intra- and inter-reliability and good responsiveness in the new device to measure different directions of tongue force in an asymptomatic population. This could be a new, more accessible tool to consider and add to the assessment and treatment of different clinical conditions in which a deficit in tongue force could be found.

Keywords: feedback; muscle strength; neurofeedback; rehabilitation; reproducibility of results tongue

1. Introduction

The tongue is a muscle that is part of the stomatognathic system and plays an important role in phonation, breathing, and eating [1,2]. The tongue has been classified as a muscular hydrostat structure due to its ability of movement and deformation without a bone holder preserving its volume [2]. The tongue performs five main movements: elevation, depression, protrusion, right lateralization, and left lateralization, and their multiple combinations. These movements are important during eating function for the intraoral manipulation of food and swallowing [3]. During chewing, the tongue muscles must coordinate with the masticatory muscles and the temporomandibular joints (TMJ). During breathing, tongue extrinsic muscles move the hyoid bone in the craniocaudal direction, allowing the pharynx to open. In addition, tongue muscles are coordinated with suprahyoid and infrahyoid muscles during swallowing and phonation. Therefore, muscle balance, understood as a phenomenon in which agonist and antagonist muscles work in coordination during voluntary movements or unexpected body perturbations, is important for tongue function. This phenomenon allows maintaining neural control of movements on a specific functional level and avoid excessive muscle control work. Likewise, it seems that coactivation could increase stiffness and movement speed, increasing the stability in kinematic chain cases. Thereby, any disturbance in muscle balance or dysfunction related to the tongue can lead to dysphagia, dysarthria or breathing difficulties [4].

Different studies have shown that the function of the tongue can be compromised in different clinical conditions such as oropharyngeal cancers [5], post-stroke sequalae [6], sequalae associated with Parkinson Disease [7], scleroderma [4], and chronic temporomandibular disorders (TMDs) [8]. For example, tongue weakness was shown to be associated with TMD patients with orofacial restricted mobility [9]. In addition, the aging process may also contribute to tongue disturbances. In this way, it has been reported that older adults have less tongue force than younger adults [10] and it is well known that deficient tongue force can compromise the behavior and efficiency of mastication and swallowing [11].

Due to the above-described factors, measurements of tongue force are important in clinical practice during both the diagnostic process and rehabilitation process [7,12,13]. Currently, there are few devices to measure tongue force on the market. The four most used and studied devices are the Kay Swallowing Workstation (KSW) [14], the Madison Oral Strengthening Therapeutic (MOST) [15], the Iowa Oral Performance Instrument (IOPI) [16], and the OroPress device [17]. The KSW (KayPENTAX Corporation, Lincoln Park, NJ, USA) device is a computerized system with three sensors which allow performing multiple simultaneous measurements in different tongue positions on the palate including pressure measurements during swallowing [18]. However, it is not portable due to its large size and it is very expensive. White et al. reported an excellent intrarater reliability in the KSW device in a healthy population (ICC = 0.92) [19]. The MOST device is a portable device with four or five sensors inside one intraoral piece with a small amount of pliable Reprosil Dental Putty (DENTSPLY International, York, PA, USA), which allows measurements of tongue isometric pressure against the hard palate in five different positions (anterior, middle, posterior, right, and left). The intraoral piece provides stability to the sensors, and it is easy to use by patients. The MOST device has not demonstrated its reliability and validity yet [20]. However, due to its price, it is less accessible for professionals and patients. Likewise, the IOPI (IOPI Northwest Company, LLC, Carnation, WA, USA) is the most used device in research because it is easy to use, it is portable, and has a silicon air-filled bulb, which allows measuring isometric tongue pressure against the hard palate. However, it has poor sensor stability which may cause measurement errors [21], and to date, there are no studies on validity and inter-rater reliability with the use of this device. Although a good inter-rater reliability to measure the maximum isometric tongue force with the IOPI was found (ICC > 0.75) [22], it has been shown to be less reliable than the other devices due to artifacts on the measurements [21]. Finally, the OroPress device is composed of a biomedical interface pressure transducer (BIPT-MS58 series, Measurement Specialities Ltd., Bevaix, Switzerland), an earpiece, and a wireless transmission module which transmits data to a remote laptop or notebook computer for real-time viewing and recording. This system measures the isometric and swallowing pressure applied by the tongue directly at the sensor tongue interface compared to those which apply the pressure indirectly through a column of air or fluid. It is characterized as being portable, having low-cost sensors, and being able to capture pressure while swallowing food or fluids. Oropress demonstrated good-to-excellent ICC values (ICC = 0.86) for its reliability [17]. Nevertheless, this device only has a pilot study trying to demonstrate its validity [17]. A bigger sample is needed to develop a good study of validity, and an intra- and inter-rater reliability study must also be carried out. This is very important to corroborate the safety, the psychometric properties, and the clinical utility of all these devices.

In order to overcome the limitations of the devices and improve the features, a validated, portable, handy, and lower-cost prototype device to measure tongue force was developed. The prototype has an intuitive interface, and it has been developed to assess and train tongue force in different movements, allowing its use not only for professionals, but also for patients for clinical and home rehabilitation. The software includes videogames with biofeedback for training at home which could increase the patient's adherence to the treatment [23]. The new device promotes patient independence in the rehabilitation process and reduces social and health care costs [24]. This new instrument, unlike the others developed up to now, proposes accurate assessments and future treatments based on gamification (Table 1). Moreover, compared to current tongue force instruments, this new device has already demonstrated good validity values and a high intrarater reliability, ensuring its safe use in the clinic [25]. Nevertheless, as a first step in the validation process, good inter-rater reliability for this device is also needed. Reliability is defined as the probability that a system, instrument, or device could perform a specific function in certain circumstances. It refers not only to the agreement but also the consistency between measurements. Moreover, random and systematic errors are needed to obtain reliability data and ensure accurate results. For this reason, devices must demonstrate a good stability and reliability before their use or commercialization. This makes the device safer during its use in a variety of clinical and research settings as well as by any type of person (professionals, patients, or patients' relatives) and ensures the security to be used with patients and different environmental conditions. According to this, it is established that this type of study should be developed in healthy subjects at first for trying to protect vulnerable individuals and could ensure that the device is safe for its condition. After that, reliability studies must be performed in patients for demonstrating the clinical usefulness [26].

Table 1. Feature comparison between the new device, the IOPI, the KSW, and the MOST instruments.

	Easy Portability	Individualized Exercises	Visual Feedback and Videogames	Home Training	Patient Follow-Up	Price of the Device
NEW DEVICE	X	X	X	X	X	EUR 42,544
IOPI	X			X		EUR 800–2000
KSW						Not available
MOST	X					Not available
OROPRESS	X		X (feedback only)			Not available

The main objectives of this study were to determine the intra- and inter-rater reliability and the minimum detectable change (responsiveness) in the maximum tongue force measurements using a newly developed device. The authors of the study wanted to demonstrate that this device could measure with the same reliability independently of the professional or patient who is using it. Since current commercial systems do not have enough evidence of their validity or inter-rater reliability and due to the high costs of technologies such as fluoroscopy, currently applied screening techniques are very subjective and depend on the training and experience of the therapist. This makes the devices less reliable. For this reason, demonstrating the reliability and sensitivity of our system would help in developing more objective assessments, regardless of the therapist performing the measurements.

2. Materials and Methods

An intra- and inter-rater reliability single-blind study with repetitive measurements was conducted based on the guidelines for reporting reliability and agreement studies (GRRAS) [27]. This study was approved by the Ethics Committee from the Centro Superior de Estudios Universitarios La Salle (CSEULS) of the Universidad Autónoma de Madrid (project code: CSEULS-PI-036/2019). Subjects were recruited from the CSEULS of the Universidad Autónoma de Madrid. Participants were recruited through nonprobability sampling.

2.1. Subjects

A total of 26 asymptomatic subjects older than 18 participated in this study. The sample size was calculated based on the intraclass correlation coefficient (ICC) values obtained in previous studies [28–31]. An ICC of 0.90 was estimated based on the hypothesis. A sample of 26 subjects with 2 measurements per subject was needed to achieve 80% power (β = 0.2) to detect an ICC of 0.90, with a significance level of 0.05.

Subjects were excluded if they presented TMD, cancer, or an active infection of the neck/head/mouth, had a history of orofacial or cervical surgery, had temporomandibular/orofacial/cervical acute pain before or during the test, were undergoing physical therapy for the neck or craniofacial region, had more than 6 points out of 10 on the subjective perception of fatigue scale, or had neurological disorders and rheumatic systemic disorders.

2.2. Instrumentation

The new low-cost prototype device, introduced in a previous article [23], was specifically designed and developed to measure tongue force objectively and accurately. The device consists of a physical part and associated software. The physical part consists of a hardware system that measures the pressure exerted on a piezoelectric sensor (FSR 402, Interlink Electronics Inc., Irvine, CA, USA) [32] and transmits the information with an Arduino UNO via a wired connection to a personal computer, where the software is located (Figure 1). This type of sensor is a very thin and flexible piezoelectric that does not cause any discomfort to the patient. The software is responsible for processing and displaying the information in real time. In addition, the software facilitates the recording of the demographic information of the subjects and the information recorded by the sensor is stored in a database for the subsequent extraction of reports (Figure 2).

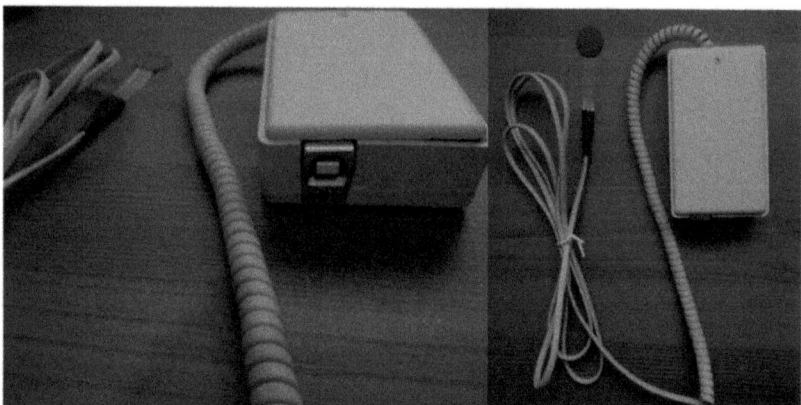

Figure 1. Prototype tongue force device (inferior and upper views). Small casing protecting the backplane, extralong cable, and piezoelectric sensor.

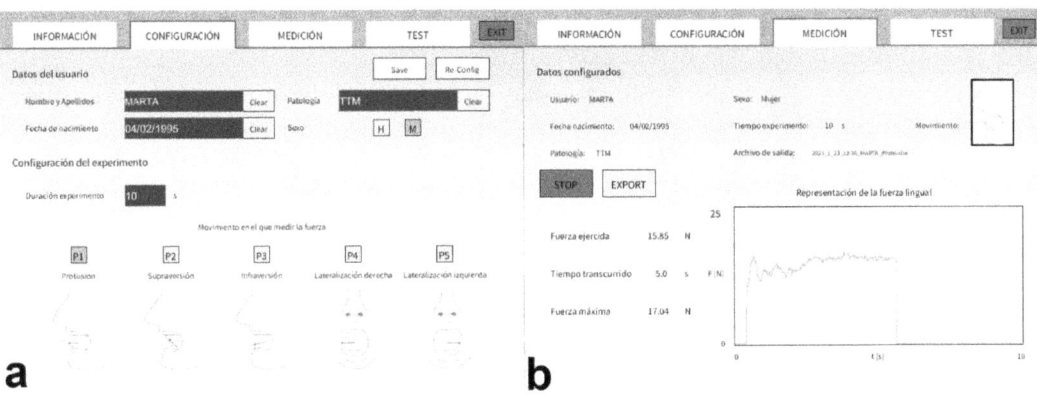

Figure 2. Spanish prototype device interface view. (**a**): Configuration screen view for the main characteristics and personal data of the patient, and the duration of the experiment; (**b**): Measurement screen view for the specific movement that is being measured with the time, maximum force, force exerted during each second, and a feedback representation of the force exerted.

The interface has a user-centered design for ease of use in the clinical environment. The device can measure the pressure exerted on the sensor by placing it in different positions. Depending on the positioning of the sensor, it is possible to measure the force exerted in the following movements: lip to lip, tongue elevation (tongue against the anterior part of the hard palate), tongue depression (tongue against the jaw), right tongue lateralization (tongue against the right cheek), left tongue lateralization (tongue against the left cheek), and their combinations.

2.3. Procedure

Two experienced physical therapists with more than 3 years' experience working in the cervico-craniofacial area were trained on how to perform the maximum tongue force test and the whole intervention. The biomedical engineer that developed the device specifically helped and trained both physical therapists on how to use the new device. The tongue force test was performed on each participant in a sitting position for the tongue movements mentioned above in Section 2.2. Two measurements of each tongue movement were performed by each rater. The GraphPad Quickcals website was used to randomize which assessor had to go first on the measurements. The measurements were performed on the same day for both raters. Each rater was blind to the other rater's measurements. The subjects and raters were not able to see the results between the 2 measurements performed for each movement.

A single-use hypoallergenic protective measure made of nitrile was used to cover the sensor during the measurements for each subject (Figure 3). The single-use protection was not changed during the whole test, only between different participants. The subjects were asked to sit with their back against the chair, feet on the ground, and head in its natural position. The tongue sensors were placed by the subjects following the instructions given by the rater according to the movement tested. During the maximum tongue force test, the subjects were then asked to exert the maximum tongue force against the sensor for 10 s. A 5 min resting period was used between each measurement. Firstly, for the lip-to-lip movement, the sensor was placed between the lips, not including the teeth. Secondly, the sensor was placed behind the superior incisors in the anterior part of the hard palate for the tongue elevation movement. Thirdly, the subjects placed the sensor behind the inferior incisors in the jaw for the tongue depression movement. Finally, right and left tongue lateralization movements were developed by placing the sensor in the anterior part of the right and left cheeks, respectively. The whole procedure is described in Figure 4.

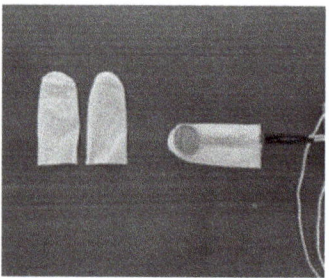

Figure 3. Single-use hypoallergenic protection covering the whole sensor to protect it.

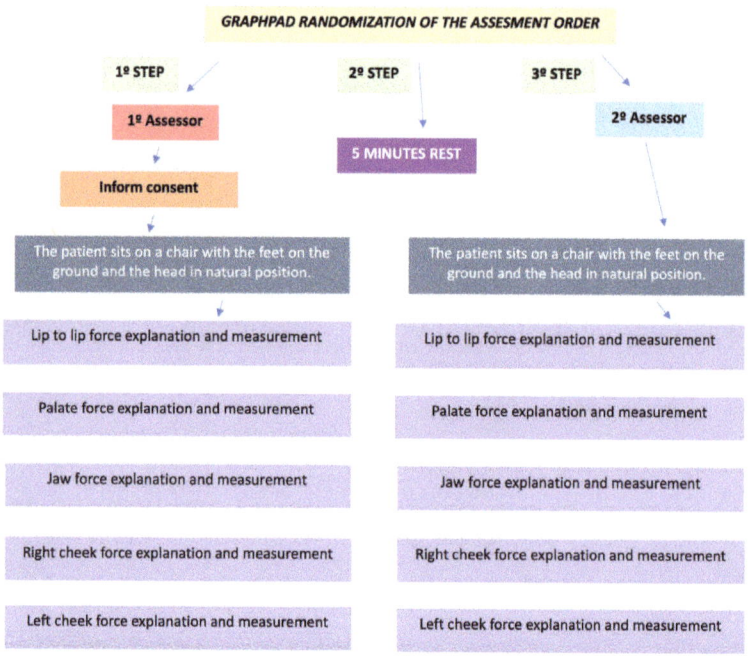

Figure 4. Descriptive graphic of the procedure.

2.4. Analysis and Sample Size

The sample size was calculated based on the intraclass correlation coefficient (ICC) values obtained in previous studies [28–31]. An ICC of 0.90 was estimated based on the hypothesis. A sample of 26 subjects with 2 measurements per subject was needed to achieve 80% power ($\beta = 0.2$) to detect an ICC of 0.90, with a significance level of 0.05.

The interclass correlation coefficient and standard error of measurement (SEM) were used to calculate the reliability. The $ICC_{3,1}$ was designated as the two-way analysis of variance mixed model for the absolute agreement of single measures. The $ICC_{3,2}$ was designated the same way as the $ICC_{3,1}$ but using the average of the two measures of each rater to determine the inter-rater reliability [33]. Intraclass correlation coefficient values greater than 0.75 indicate good reliability, those between 0.50 and 0.75 indicate moderate agreement, and those below 0.50 indicate poor agreement [33]. A 95% confidence interval (CI) was also calculated, and $p < 0.05$ was used as the level of statistical significance.

Bland–Altman plots were constructed using mean differences between measurements [34]. Limits of agreement (LOA) were calculated as mean differences ± (standard deviation multiplied by 1.96) [35]. Calculation of the occurrence of systematic or random changes in the data means that it was performed through a calculation of 95% confidence intervals (CI) of the mean differences between the values of the measurements.

The responsiveness was determined with minimal detectable change at 90%, which was calculated as SEM $\times$ 1.65 $\times$ $\sqrt{2}$ [36,37]. The MDC_{90} expresses the minimal change required to be 90% confident that the change observed between two measurements reflects a real change (sensitive measure) and not a measurement error.

3. Results

A total of 26 subjects were included in the reliability analysis (57.7% men and 42.3% women). The average age of the sample was 25.69 years old with a standard deviation of 7.46 years old. In relation to body mass index, it was 26.1 (25.7–26.5; 95%CI) in men and 24.1 (23.7–24.7; 95%CI) in women. In addition, the percentage of participants with or in the process of completing tertiary education was 63%. According to the Shapiro–Wilk test, the data were normally distributed ($p > 0.05$).

3.1. Intrarater Reliability Results

The descriptive data for intrarater reliability, $ICC_{3,1}$, SEM, MDC_{90}, and Bland–Altman analysis with the 95%CI and LOA are summarized in Table 2. Good-to-excellent intrarater reliability for all tongue movements was found for both raters ($ICC_{3,1} \geq 0.80$). The SEM was <0.70 for rater A and <0.98 for rater B. The MDC was between 1.10 and 1.64 for rater A and between 0.96 and 2.30 for rater B.

Table 2. Intrarater reliability ($n = 26$).

Outcome Measurements (Newtons)	Mean ± SD	Mean ± SD			
	1st Measure	2nd Measure	ICC (95%CI)	SEM	MDC 90%
Rater A					
Elevation	6.92 ± 4.26	6.87 ± 3.94	0.97 (0.93–0.99)	0.70	1.64
Depression	6.02 ± 3.39	6.09 ± 3.43	0.96 (0.91–0.98)	0.68	1.58
Right	2.58 ± 1.77	2.45 ± 1.84	0.93 (0.85–0.97)	0.47	1.10
Left	2.11 ± 1.21	2.25 ± 1.40	0.84 (0.68–0.92)	0.52	1.21
Rater B					
Elevation	6.19 ± 4.78	6.46 ± 4.07	0.95 (0.89–0.98)	0.98	2.30
Depression	5.17 ± 2.91	5.00 ± 2.87	0.94 (0.88–0.98)	0.70	1.64
Right	2.12 ± 1.69	2.37 ± 1.69	0.94 (0.87–0.97)	0.41	0.96
Left	1.83 ± 1.09	2.10 ± 1.22	0.82 (0.65–0.92)	0.49	1.14
	Bland–Altman				
	Mean difference ± SD	95%CI	LOA (Inf-Sup)		
Rater A					
Elevation	0.06 ± 1.05	(−0.34 to 0.46)	(−2.00 to 2.12)		
Depression	−0.07 ± 0.98	(−0.45 to 0.31)	(−2.00 to 1.85)		
Right	0.13 ± 0.68	(−0.13 to 0.39)	(−1.20 to 1.46)		
Left	−0.14 ± 0.73	(−0.42 to 0.14)	(−1.57 to 1.29)		
Rater B					
Elevation	−0.27 ± 1.42	(−0.82 to 0.28)	(−3.05 to 2.51)		
Depression	0.16 ± 0.97	(−0.21 to 0.53)	(−1.74 to 2.06)		
Right	−0.24 ± 0.60	(−0.47 to −0.01)	(−1.42 to 0.94)		
Left	−0.27 ± 0.69	(−0.54 to −0.005)	(−1.62 to 1.08)		

Abbreviations: ICC: intraclass correlation coefficient; CI: confidence interval; SEM: standard error of measurement; MDC: minimum detectable change; SD: standard deviation; LOA: limits of agreement.

3.2. Inter-Rater Reliability Results

The descriptive data for inter-rater reliability, $ICC_{3,2}$, SEM, MDC, and Bland–Altman analysis with the 95%CI and LOA are summarized in Table 3. Good-to-excellent intrarater reliability for all tongue movements was found for both raters ($ICC_{3,2} \geq 0.80$). The SEM was <1.29. The MDC was between 1.20 and 3.01. Graphical representations of the Bland–Altman plot are shown in Figure 5.

Table 3. Inter-rater reliability ($n = 26$).

Outcome Measurements (in Newtons)	Mean ± SD	Mean ± SD			
	Rater A	Rater B	ICC (95%CI)	SEM	MDC 90%
Elevation	6.89 ± 4.07	6.32 ± 4.38	0.94 (0.86–0.97)	1.03	2.40
Depression	6.05 ± 3.37	5.08 ± 2.85	0.83 (0.57–0.93)	1.29	3.01
Right	2.52 ± 1.77	2.24 ± 1.66	0.87 (0.73–0.94)	0.61	1.43
Left	2.18 ± 1.26	1.97 ± 1.10	0.81 (0.63–0.91)	0.51	1.20
		Bland–Altman			
	Mean difference ± SD	95%CI	LOA (Inf-Sup)		
Elevation	0.57 ± 1.43	(0.02 to 1.12)	(−2.23 to 3.37)		
Depression	0.97 ± 1.65	(0.33 to 1.60)	(−2.26 to 4.20)		
Right	0.27 ± 0.86	(−0.06 to 0.60)	(−1.42 to 1.96)		
Left	0.21 ± 0.71	(−0.06 to 0.48)	(−1.18 to 1.60)		

Abbreviations: ICC: intraclass correlation coefficient; CI: confidence interval; SEM: standard error of measurement; MDC: minimum detectable change; SD: standard deviation; LOA: limits of agreement.

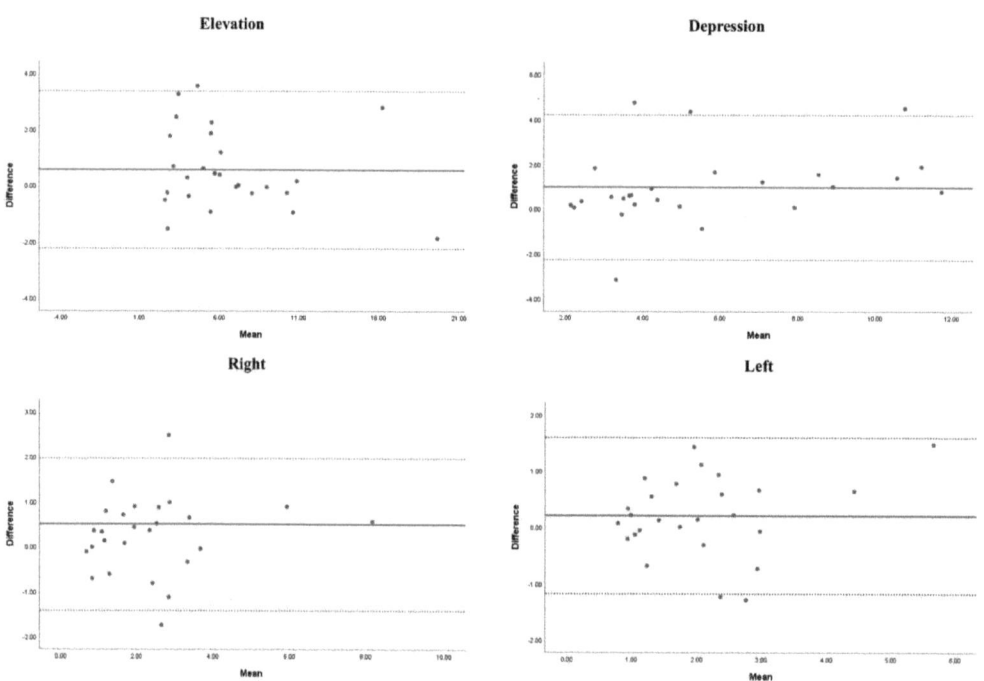

Figure 5. Graphical representations of the Bland–Altman plot. The red line is the mean difference. The green lines represent the Limits of Agreement (LOA).

4. Discussion

As far as the authors know, this is the first study evaluating the maximum tongue force in four different directions of tongue movement. According to the results, a good-to-excellent intra- and inter-rater reliability was found for all movements. The measurements were also responsive to detect real changes.

This was also the first study testing the reliability of a device with a force-sensitive resistor (FSR) sensor to measure the maximum tongue force. Although the MOST device is composed of the same type of sensor, its reliability has not been tested [20]. There is currently no gold standard for maximum tongue force outcome measurements. That is why the results from this study are compared with the devices that are often used in clinical practice and research.

The present study has demonstrated an excellent intrarater reliability for maximum tongue force measurements of the superior, inferior, and right tongue movements ($ICC_{3,1} > 0.93$) and a good intrarater reliability for measurements of the left tongue movement ($ICC_{3,1} > 0.82$). The measurements of the superior tongue movement obtained the highest $ICC_{3,1}$ values (>0.95). These values were slightly greater than those found for the reliability measurements of tongue force in superior movements using the IOPI device, which ranged from 0.77 to 0.90 [38]. Likewise, better ICC values were obtained when compared to the study by White et al., who reported an excellent intrarater reliability for the KSW device in a healthy population (ICC = 0.92) [19]. In reference to the Oropress reliability results, similar ICC values were found (ICC = 0.86) when compared to the present study [17].

An excellent inter-rater reliability for measurements of the tongue force in elevation ($ICC_{3,2} = 0.94$) and a good inter-rater reliability for measurements of the tongue force in depression and right and left lateralization ($ICC_{s3,1} = 0.83$, 0.87 and 0.81, respectively) were found in the current study. Youmans and Stierwalt (2006) obtained a 94% inter-rater agreement (r = 0.94) during the maximum isometric force measurement using the IOPI device [39]. The IOPI device is commonly used; however, it is only used to measure tongue force in one direction (tongue elevation). Additionally, the IOPI analysis protocols are different from the ones utilized in the present study. While the common IOPI protocol for analysis uses the highest value obtained during the three tests or the mean of the two best tests, the current study used the mean of the two measurements. Nevertheless, researchers cannot define the analysis with any of the devices since there is no defined protocol. Similarly to the IOPI device, the KSW instrument only measures superior tongue force movement and commonly collects the higher measure of the three tests performed.

The inter-rater reliability of tongue force measurements using the IOPI device in subjects with different conditions was reported to be good to excellent (ICC > 0.75) [22], with the exception of a study evaluating dysarthria patients in which a moderate reliability was found (ICC = 0.535) [22,38]. However, there are no recent studies available on the evaluation of the inter-rater reliability for the IOPI in healthy subjects, and the authors of this paper believe that this should be the first step prior to measurement and use in patients. Likewise, there is no inter-rater reliability research for measuring tongue force with the KSW device. The KSW device uses the same type of sensor as the IOPI, a silicon air-filled bulb. The main difference is that the KSW bulb is fixed to the palate, providing more stability and reliability. Probably due to its multiple functions, the KSW device is used more for research evaluating tongue force during swallowing. According to Fei et al., the KSW device is more reliable than the IOPI when evaluating tongue force during the function of swallowing [40].

Regarding responsiveness, the SEM values were low for elevation, depression, and right and left tongue movements (1.03, 1.09, 0.60, and 0.51, respectively). The MDC values were also low for elevation, depression, and right and left tongue movements: 2.40, 3.01, 1.43, and 1.20, respectively. Therefore, the new device was able to capture real change in tongue measures in all directions. Although we can assure good reliability and responsiveness for the device presented in this study in an asymptomatic population, we cannot guarantee the same findings in symptomatic subjects yet. Only one previous study determined the SEM and the MDC of the IOPI device in asymptomatic subjects [38]. This study estimated these values using standard deviation (SD), while the present study based the calculation on the root mean square (RMS) [40]. The SD was used to estimate the SEM, avoiding possible uncertainties due to the selected ICC type [35]. Therefore, the evaluation of the SEM varies between studies. Additionally, a Bland–Altman method was used to evaluate agreement, including the LOA. A good LOA was found, and the SEM, MDC, and LOA revealed a good level of concordance. These values are very important for the use of the device in clinical practice as they ensure that any improvement in tongue force is due to the treatment rather than measurement errors.

This study demonstrated that the newly developed tongue force device is reliable for measuring the maximum tongue force in different directions within and in between professionals. The new device overcomes some limitations from the tongue devices commonly used in the literature. This validated, safe, portable, and easy-to-use device can allow patients to perform tongue exercises at home, and the ability of the device to display the tongue activity in real time may increase their motivation to progress with their rehabilitation program. All these features add to the fact that it is a low-cost instrument. We recommend that future studies are needed to test the tongue force device including both healthy subjects and patients. Additionally, future studies must include in silico/computational simulation to ensure that the force data used from the device is accommodated correctly [41].

4.1. Limitations

This study presents some limitations. Nonprobability sampling is always a limitation of a study. Ideally, a sufficiently large population would have been accessible for probability sampling. The reliability of the developed tongue force device was tested on healthy young subjects mainly (at an average of 25.7 years of age) and, therefore, these results should be taken with caution when transferring them to other populations. Further studies should test the device in different age groups in order to generalize the results. Likewise, future studies should include subjects with different health conditions. The results showed a significant statistical difference in some values of the Bland–Altman plot. These differences are close to 0 and all mean difference values are below the MCD in all cases. This led us to assume those results are statistically significant but not clinically relevant. The minimal clinically important difference (MCID) should be evaluated in future studies. Likewise, the values of other populations must be established and validated in future studies as with any measurement device or questionnaire.

4.2. Clinical Implications

From a neurophysiological point of view, it is known that the cerebral cortex has areas where information (input and output) from the V (trigeminal nerve), VII (facial nerve), and XII (hypoglossal nerve) cranial nerves is integrated [42]. In this way, these cranial nerves control the muscles of mastication, facial gestures, and the tongue, respectively, in order to achieve the optimal functionality of the entire system during speech and mastication, among other functions. Additionally, we have already published an observational study which showed significant differences in the maximum tongue force between asymptomatic women and those with chronic temporomandibular disorder, corroborating the necessity for the assessment of the tongue force in this pathology [43]. In this article, a decrease in tongue strength of about 30% on average across all directions was found in the group of patients with chronic TMD. In line with this, clinical experience shows that many patients with TMD (especially the chronic type) have lingual alternations both in terms of flexibility (length) and strength in various directions.

This new device to measure tongue force allows obtaining objective measurements of tongue force in clinical practice in order to help clinicians with the diagnosis process and treatment progression. This will give clinicians and patients real data to observe the changes during the treatment. Moreover, the new tongue force device has a diagnostic interface and treatment interface with different games to train the force at home and in the clinic. This training with games will motivate the patients and increase the adherence to the treatment. This offers an accessible device for patients and clinicians due to the fact that the few that are available in the market have this limitation and are much more expensive. Moreover, its validity has been proved in a previous study that has been recently published [25]. This could be a new tool to consider and add for the assessment and treatment of these patients. Likewise, as a new tool in the treatment of TMD, it could decrease the sociosanitary costs that this pathology implies for the sanitary system due to its chronicity.

5. Conclusions

This study showed a good-to-excellent intra- and inter-reliability for the newly developed device to measure the maximum tongue force in four different directions in an asymptomatic population. The measurements with the new device were also able to detect real changes, suggesting a more sensitive measure (good responsiveness in the device). These results confirmed that the device is suitable for objective and precise tongue measurements independently of the subject that is using this tool. The new prototype device seems to be an improved tongue force measurement tool that is safe, validated, and more accessible than others on the market.

Author Contributions: Conceptualization, A.G.-M.; methodology, A.G.-M. and J.G.-C.; software, J.G.-C.; formal analysis, G.N.-F.; investigation, M.C.D.-S.; data curation, G.N.-F. and J.G.-C.; writing—original draft preparation, M.C.D.-S.; writing—review and editing, H.B.-A., A.G.-M. and I.C.G.; visualization, H.B.-A. and A.G.-M.; supervision, H.B.-A. and A.G.-M.; project administration, H.B.-A. and A.G.-M. All authors have read and agreed to the published version of the manuscript.

Funding: This research received no external funding.

Institutional Review Board Statement: The study was conducted in accordance with the guidelines for reporting reliability and agreement studies (GRRAS) [27]. This study was approved by the Ethics Committee from the Centro Superior de Estudios Universitarios La Salle (CSEULS) of the Universidad Autónoma de Madrid (project code: CSEULS-PI-036/2019). Subjects were recruited from the Centro Superior de Estudios Universitarios La Salle (CSEULS) of the Universidad Autónoma de Madrid.

Informed Consent Statement: Informed consent was obtained from all subjects involved in the study. Written informed consent has been obtained from the patient(s) to publish this paper.

Data Availability Statement: Not applicable.

Acknowledgments: The authors would like to thank Estela Sánchez and Mª Dolores Pérez (members of Innovation Support Unit in Hospital Universitario La Paz) who assisted us in drafting and submitting the application for protection for this new device. Moreover, we want to thank Daniel Mañoso for his help with the English translation.

Conflicts of Interest: The authors declare no conflict of interest.

References

1. Inoue, T.; Nakayama, K.; Ihara, Y.; Tachikawa, S.; Nakamura, S.; Mochizuki, A.; Takahashi, K.; Iijima, T. Coordinated control of the tongue during suckling-like activity and respiration. *J. Oral Sci.* **2017**, *59*, 183–188. [CrossRef]
2. Sanders, I.; Mu, L. A Three-dimensional atlas of human tongue muscles. *Anat. Rec.* **2013**, *296*, 1102–1114. [CrossRef]
3. Dotiwala, A.K.; Samra, N.S. *Anatomy, Head and Neck, Tongue*; StatPearls Publishing: Tampa, FL, USA, 2018.
4. Bordoni, B.; Morabito, B.; Mitrano, R.; Simonelli, M.; Toccafondi, A. The Anatomical Relationships of the Tongue with the Body System. *Cureus* **2018**, *10*, e3695. [CrossRef] [PubMed]
5. Van den Steen, L.; Van Gestel, D.; Vanderveken, O.; Vanderwegen, J.; Lazarus, C.; Daisne, J.F.; Van Laer, C.; Specenier, P.; Van Rompaey, D.; Mariën, S.; et al. Evolution of self-perceived swallowing function, tongue strength and swallow-related quality of life during radiotherapy in head and neck cancer patients. *Head Neck.* **2019**, *41*, 2197–2207. [CrossRef]
6. Crincoli, V.; Fatone, L.; Fanelli, M.; Rotolo, R.P.; Chialà, A.; Favia, G.; Lapadula, G. Orofacial Manifestations and Temporomandibular Disorders of Systemic Scleroderma: An Observational Study. *Int. J. Mol. Sci.* **2016**, *17*, 1189. [CrossRef]
7. Pitts, L.L.; Morales, S.; Stierwalt, J.A.G. Lingual pressure as a clinical indicator of swallowing function in Parkinson's disease. *J. Speech Lang. Heart Res.* **2018**, *61*, 257–265. [CrossRef] [PubMed]

8. Melchior, M.d.O.; Magri, L.V.; Mazzetto, M.O. Orofacial myofunctional disorder, a possible complicating factor in the management of painful temporomandibular disorder. *Braz. J. Pain* **2018**, *1*, 80–86.
9. Pizolato, A.R.; Fernandes, F.S.D.F.; Gavião, M.B.D. Deglutition and temporomandibular disorders in children. *Minerva Dent. Oral Sci.* **2009**, *58*, 567–576.
10. Yamaguchi, K.; Hara, K.; Nakagawa, K.; Yoshimi, K.; Ariya, C.; Nakane, A.; Furuya, J.; Tohara, H. Ultrasonography Shows Age-related Changes and Related Factors in the Tongue and Suprahyoid Muscles. *J. Am. Med. Dir. Assoc.* **2020**, *22*, 766–772. [CrossRef] [PubMed]
11. Nakazawa, Y.; Kikutani, T.; Igarashi, K.; Yajima, Y.; Tamura, F. Associations between tongue strength and skeletal muscle mass under dysphagia rehabilitation for geriatric out patients. *J. Prosthodont. Res.* **2019**, *64*, 188–192. [CrossRef]
12. Printza, A.; Goutsikas, C.; Triaridis, S.; Kyrgidis, A.; Haidopoulou, K.; Constantinidis, J.; Pavlou, E. Dysphagia diagnosis with questionnaire, tongue strength measurement, and FEES in patients with childhood-onset muscular dystrophy. *Int. J. Pediatr. Otorhinolaryngol.* **2019**, *117*, 198–203. [CrossRef] [PubMed]
13. Van den Steen, L.; Vanderwegen, J.; Guns, C.; Elen, R.; De Bodt, M.; Van Nuffelen, G. Tongue-Strengthening Exercises in Healthy Older Adults: Does Exercise Load Matter? A Randomized Controlled Trial. *Dysphagia* **2018**, *34*, 315–324. [CrossRef] [PubMed]
14. Anil, M.A.; Balasubramaniam, R.K.; Babu, S.; Varghese, A.L.; Hussain, Z.R.; Dsouza, D.F. Does Tongue-Hold Maneuver Affect Respiratory–Swallowing Coordination? Evidence from Healthy Adults. *J. Nat. Sci. Biol. Med.* **2019**, *10*, 68–71. [CrossRef]
15. Ulrich Sommer, J.; Birk, R.; Hörmann, K.; Stuck, B.A. Evaluation of the maximum isometric tongue force of healthy volunteers. *Eur. Arch. Oto-Rhino-Laryngol.* **2014**, *271*, 3077–3084. [CrossRef]
16. Park, J.-S.; Kim, H.-J.; Oh, D.-H. Effect of tongue strength training using the Iowa Oral Performance Instrument in stroke patients with dysphagia. *J. Phys. Ther. Sci.* **2015**, *27*, 3631–3634. [CrossRef]
17. McCormack, J.; Casey, V.; Conway, R.; Saunders, J.; Perry, A. OroPress a new wireless tool for measuring oro-lingual pressures: A pilot study in healthy adults. *J. Neuroeng. Rehabil.* **2015**, *12*, 32. [CrossRef]
18. Ball, S.; Idel, O.; Cotton, S.; Perry, A. Comparison of Two Methods for Measuring Tongue Pressure During Swallowing in People with Head and Neck Cancer. *Dysphagia* **2006**, *21*, 28–37. [CrossRef] [PubMed]
19. White, R.; Cotton, S.M.; Hind, J.; Robbins, J.; Perry, A. A Comparison of the Reliability and Stability of Oro-lingual Swallowing Pressures in Patients with Head and Neck Cancer and Healthy Adults. *Dysphagia* **2008**, *24*, 137–144. [CrossRef]
20. Hewitt, A.; Hind, J.; Kays, S.; Nicosia, M.; Doyle, J.; Tompkins, W.; Gangnon, R.; Robbins, J. Standardized Instrument for Lingual Pressure Measurement. *Dysphagia* **2007**, *23*, 16–25. [CrossRef]
21. Adams, V.; Mathisen, B.; Baines, S.; Lazarus, C.; Callister, R. A Systematic Review and Meta-analysis of Measurements of Tongue and Hand Strength and Endurance Using the Iowa Oral Performance Instrument (IOPI). *Dysphagia* **2013**, *28*, 350–369. [CrossRef]
22. Berggren, K.N.; Hung, M.; Dixon, M.M.; Bounsanga, J.; Crockett, B.; Foye, M.D.; Gu, Y.; Campbell, C.; Butterfield, R.J.; Johnson, N.E. Orofacial strength, dysarthria, and dysphagia in congenital myotonic dystrophy. *Muscle Nerve* **2018**, *58*, 413–417. [CrossRef]
23. Constantinescu, G.; Rieger, J.; Mummery, K.; Hodgetts, W. Flow and Grit by Design: Exploring Gamification in Facilitating Adherence to Swallowing Therapy. *Am. J. Speech-Lang. Pathol.* **2017**, *26*, 1296–1303. [CrossRef] [PubMed]
24. Frändin, K.; Grönstedt, H.; Helbostad, J.L.; Bergland, A.; Andresen, M.; Puggaard, L.; Harms-Ringdahl, K.; Granbo, R.; Hellström, K. Long-Term Effects of Individually Tailored Physical Training and Activity on Physical Function, Well-Being and Cognition in Scandinavian Nursing Home Residents: A Randomized Controlled Trial. *Gerontology* **2016**, *62*, 571–580. [CrossRef] [PubMed]
25. Diaz-Saez, M.C.; Beltran-Alacreu, H.; Gil-Castillo, J.; Navarro-Fernández, G.; Cebrián Carretero, J.L.; Gil-Martínez, A. Validity and Intra Rater Reliability of a New Device for Tongue Force Measurement. *Int. J. Interact. Multimed. Artif. Intell.* **2022**. [CrossRef]
26. Portney, L.G.W.M. *Foundations of Clinical Research: Applications to Practice*; Prentice-Hall: Englewood Cliffs, NJ, USA, 2000.
27. Kottner, J.; Audigé, L.; Brorson, S.; Donner, A.; Gajewski, B.J.; Hróbjartsson, A.; Roberts, C.; Shoukri, M.; Streiner, D.L. Guidelines for Reporting Reliability and Agreement Studies (GRRAS) were proposed. *J. Clin. Epidemiol.* **2011**, *64*, 96–106. [CrossRef]
28. Walter, S.D.; Eliasziw, M.; Donner, A. Sample size and optimal designs for reliability studies. *Stat. Med.* **1998**, *17*, 101–110. [CrossRef]
29. Donner, A.; Eliasziw, M. Sample size requirements for reliability studies. *Stat. Med.* **1987**, *6*, 441–448. [CrossRef]
30. Shoukri, M.M.; Asyali, M.H.; Donner, A. Sample size requirements for the design of reliability study: Review and new results. *Stat. Methods Med. Res.* **2004**, *13*, 251–271. [CrossRef]
31. Adam Bujang, M.; Baharum, N. A simplified guide to determination of sample size requirements for estimating the value of intraclass correlation coefficient: A review. *Arch. Orofac. Sci.* **2017**, *12*, 1–11.
32. *State-of-the-Art Pointing Solutions for the OEM. Force Sensing Resistor Integration Guide and Evaluation Parts Catalog*; Interlinks Electronics: Camarillo, CA, USA, 2002.
33. Weir, J.P. Quantifying Test-Retest Reliability Using the Intraclass Correlation Coefficient and the SEM. *J. Strength Cond. Res.* **2005**, *19*, 231.
34. Bunce, C. Correlation, Agreement, and Bland–Altman Analysis: Statistical Analysis of Method Comparison Studies. *Am. J. Ophthalmol.* **2009**, *148*, 4–6. [CrossRef] [PubMed]
35. Bland, J.; Altman, D. Comparing methods of measurement: Why plotting difference against standard method is misleading. *Lancet* **1995**, *346*, 1085–1087. [CrossRef] [PubMed]
36. Haley, S.M.; Fragala-Pinkham, M.A. Interpreting Change Scores of Tests and Measures Used in Physical Therapy. *Phys. Ther.* **2006**, *86*, 735–743. [CrossRef]

37. Wyrwich, K.W. Minimal Important Difference Thresholds and the Standard Error of Measurement: Is There a Connection? *J. Biopharm. Stat.* **2004**, *14*, 97–110. [CrossRef] [PubMed]
38. Adams, V.; Mathisen, B.; Baines, S.; Lazarus, C.; Callister, R. Reliability of Measurements of Tongue and Hand Strength and Endurance Using the Iowa Oral Performance Instrument with Healthy Adults. *Dysphagia* **2013**, *29*, 83–95. [CrossRef]
39. Youmans, S.R.; Stierwalt, J.A.G. Measures of Tongue Function Related to Normal Swallowing. *Dysphagia* **2006**, *21*, 102–111. [CrossRef]
40. Fei, T.; Cliffe, R.; Sarah, P.; Sonja, E.H.; Clemence MP pigeon Catriona, T. Age-related Differences in Tongue-Palate Pressures for Strength and Swallowing Tasks. *Dysphagia* **2013**, *28*, 575–581. [CrossRef]
41. Jamari, J.; Ammarullah, M.I.; Santoso, G.; Sugiharto, S.; Supriyono, T.; Permana, M.S.; Winarni, T.I.; van der Heide, E. Adopted walking condition for computational simulation approach on bearing of hip joint prosthesis: Review over the past 30 years. *Heliyon* **2022**, *8*, e12050. [CrossRef]
42. Yamada, Y.; Yamamura, K.; Inoue, M. Coordination of cranial motoneurons during mastication. *Respir. Physiol. Neurobiol.* **2005**, *147*, 177–189. [CrossRef]
43. Diaz-Saez, M.C.; Beltran-Alacreu, H.; Gil-Castillo, J.; Gil-Martínez, A. Differences between Maximum Tongue Force in Women Suffering from Chronic and Asymptomatic Temporomandibular Disorders—An Observational Study. *Life* **2023**, *13*, 229. [CrossRef]

Disclaimer/Publisher's Note: The statements, opinions and data contained in all publications are solely those of the individual author(s) and contributor(s) and not of MDPI and/or the editor(s). MDPI and/or the editor(s) disclaim responsibility for any injury to people or property resulting from any ideas, methods, instructions or products referred to in the content.

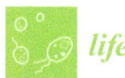

Article

Medium-Term Effect of Treatment with Intra-Articular Injection of Sodium Hyaluronate, Betamethasone and Platelet-Rich Plasma in Patients with Temporomandibular Arthralgia: A Retrospective Cohort Study

Bruno Macedo de Sousa [1,*], Antonio López-Valverde [2], Francisco Caramelo [3], María João Rodrigues [1] and Nansi López-Valverde [4,5]

1. Institute for Occlusion and Orofacial Pain, Faculty of Medicine, University of Coimbra, Polo I-Edifício Central Rua Larga, 3004-504 Coimbra, Portugal
2. Department of Surgery, University of Salamanca, Instituto de Investigación Biomédica de Salamanca (IBSAL), P.º de San Vicente, 58-182, 37007 Salamanca, Spain
3. Laboratory of Biostatistics and Medical Informatics, Institute for Clinical and Biomedical Research (iCBR), School of Medicine, University of Coimbra, Polo 3, Azinhaga de Santa Comba, 3000-548 Coimbra, Portugal
4. Department of Medicine and Medical Specialties, Faculty of Health Sciences, Universidad Alcalá de Henares, 28871 Madrid, Spain
5. Instituto de Investigación Biomédica de Salamanca (IBSAL), Avda. Alfonso X El Sabio S/N., 37007 Salamanca, Spain
* Correspondence: bsousa@fmed.uc.pt

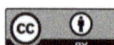

Simple Summary: Temporomandibular disorders are a major public health problem affecting approximately 10% of the population, currently the second most common musculoskeletal condition after chronic low back pain, and causing disability and pain in patients who suffer from them, limiting the individual's daily activities and quality of life. Intra-articular injections have been proposed as a specific treatment for joint inflammation and degeneration and have been shown to increase mouth opening and decrease pain associated with these disorders, although long-term follow-up is scarce in the literature. Our study compared the efficacy on TMJ pain of intra-articular injections of betamethasone, sodium hyaluronate and platelet-rich plasma in a sample of 114 patients, with a three-year follow-up, and found that both platelet-rich plasma and sodium hyaluronate led to significant pain-free time after treatment; betamethasone was less effective.

Abstract: Temporomandibular joint disorders are associated with pain and reduced jaw mobility. The aim of this study was to compare the long-term effect on pain of intra-articular TMJ injections of betamethasone, sodium hyaluronate and platelet-rich plasma. The sample was made up of 114 patients, who were randomly distributed into three groups at least three years ago and who achieved a total remission of pain after treatment. We found that the median number of months without pain was, according to each group, as follows: platelet-rich plasma: 33; sodium hyaluronate: 28; betamethasone: 19. Both platelet-rich plasma and sodium hyaluronate lead to significant pain-free time after treatment; when we compare bethametasone with the two other substances, it proved to be very ineffective.

Keywords: temporomandibular disorders; arthralgia; sodium hyaluronate; betamethasone; platelet-rich plasma

1. Introduction

Temporomandibular joint disorder (TMD) is a significant public health disorder affecting between 5% and 12% of the population on average. After persistent low back pain, TMD is the second most prevalent musculoskeletal disorder causing discomfort and impairment. [1] The Diagnostic Criteria (DC) for TMD is intended for use in any clinical setting and supports the full range of diagnostic activities from screening to definitive evaluation and diagnosis. Using this, TMD could be divided into muscle disorders (including myofascial pain with or without referral and with or without mouth opening limitation) and intra-articular disorders (including disc displacement with or without reduction and mouth opening limitation, arthralgia, arthritis and degenerative joint disorders) [2].

The most common clinical manifestations are pain, mouth opening limitation, muscle or joint tenderness on palpation, changes of mandibular movements, joint sounds and otologic complaints like tinnitus or vertigo [3].

Temporomandibular joint disorders (TMJDs) is a collective term that refers to a range of pathologies affecting the jaw joints and associated structures, resulting in internal joint space dysregulation, bony changes and degenerative pathologies. TMJDs are characterized by pain, joint noise, limited range of motion, impaired jaw function, deviation when opening and closing the mouth and open locking. They are a very common pathological agent affecting about 10% of the population, and are twice as frequent in women than in men [4–6].

In clinical practice, different treatments have been proposed to alleviate joint pain and disc displacement, including conservative therapies such as non-steroidal anti-inflammatory drugs (NSAIDs), mandibular rest, splints and physiotherapy, as well as surgical procedures such as arthrocentesis, disc repositioning or discectomy in patients who do not respond to conservative treatments. A conservative approach should always be taken primarily [7,8].

In 1953, Horton et al. were the first to propose intra-articular administration of corticosteroids (CS) for the treatment of temporomandibular joint osteoarthritis (TMJO) [9]. Since then, several investigators have confirmed that intra-articular injections of hydrocortisone, prednisolone and betamethasone reduce joint pain. It is commonly accepted that therapy with intra-articular corticosteroid injections is a procedure used mainly in patients who have not achieved satisfactory results with other less invasive approaches [10,11].

Sodium hyaluronate (SH), a hyaluronic acid (HA) derivative, is a material of high molecular density and high viscosity, essential for joint lubrication and cartilage protection, which would reduce granulation tissue formation and intra-articular adhesions, having been proposed as an additional therapy with similar therapeutic effects [12,13]. There is speculation as to whether SH not only acts as a viscosupplement in reducing mechanical friction, but also plays a role in inflammatory mediators in the osteoarthritic phase, controlling the proteolytic activation of plasminogen activator and preventing the release of proinflammatory mediators such as IL-1b or the indirect activation of metalloproteinases [14].

Platelet-rich plasma (PRP) is an autologous blood product obtained by peripheral venipuncture and subsequent centrifugation. The concentrated plasma product contains a high concentration of platelets, which play important roles in tissue homeostasis and control of inflammation, as well as in inhibition of chondrocyte apoptosis, bone and vascular remodeling and collagen synthesis. Certain studies have compared the clinical results of intra-articular injection of PRP with other conservative treatment methods such as corticosteroid injection [15–17].

Platelets are enucleated cells derived from megakaryocytes [18]. When platelets are activated, the growth factors contained in the α-granules react in a localized and specific manner. These growth factors, in addition to coagulation factors, cytokines, chemokines and other proteins contained in platelets, have been shown to induce proliferation of chondrocytes and chondrogenic mesenchymal stem cells (MSCs), which promote the secretion of cartilaginous matrix from chondrocytes and reduce the catabolic effects of proinflammatory cytokines [19–23].

The aim of this study was to analyze how long a patient could remain pain free after being treated with one of three intra-articular infiltrations—betamethasone, SH or PRP—as a continuation of a previous study [23] that assessed the short-term effect of these three infiltrations. From that research we selected the patients who achieved complete pain remission after treatment and followed them for three years. No patient dropped out.

2. Materials and Methods

2.1. Patients

A sample of 114 patients who were diagnosed with TMJ arthralgia was selected, according to the original version of the diagnostic criteria for TPMJDs, such as local pain modified with movement and pain on palpation, and who were treated with intra-articular injection of PRP, SH or betamethasone, achieving no pain after treatment and who were followed up for at least 3 years, in order to study the duration of the treatment effect. The patients were recruited and treated, after the conservative approach showed no effect, in consultations within the framework of the Occlusal Rehabilitation Course of the University of Coimbra, organized by the Faculty of Medicine. All patients agreed to participate in the research and signed the consent forms. This study was conducted in accordance with the Declaration of Helsinki and was approved by the ethics committee of the Faculty of Medicine of the University of Coimbra (Coimbra, Portugal). This study was approved on 25 June 2017 by the institutional review board (IRB 06-2017-096). No patient has dropped out from the study.

2.2. Inclusion and Exclusion Criteria

Inclusion: All patients with a clinical history of more than 6 months of TMJP that is modified by mandibular movement in function or parafunction; pain present on clinical examination on opening, lateral movements or palpation; and without previous effective treatment. All patients included in this study have achieved, after treatment, a grade 0 according to the Visual Analogic Scale (VAS).

Exclusion: patients who had received effective previous treatment for TMJ dysfunction; patients suffering from any rheumatic pathology such as rheumatoid arthritis or psoriatic arthritis (including juvenile arthritis); patients undergoing hypnosis; pregnant or breastfeeding women; patients under 18 years of age; and patients who had partial or no relief of the pain condition and had to receive another treatment.

Prior to treatment, patients were randomly assigned to three groups: patients receiving an intra-articular injection of PRP, betamethasone or SH.

2.3. Treatments

The following protocol was followed: after disinfection of the preauricular area, patients were injected with 1 mL of articaine (40 mg/mL) and adrenaline (10 µg/mL). A 23-gauge needle was used to inject 1 mL of betamethasone (Diprofos Depot®, Schering-Plough Labo, Heist-Op-Den-Berg Belgium 14 mg/2 mL) or 1 mL of SH (Hyalart®, Grunenthal GmbH, Achen, Germany, 20 mg/2 mL). The exact puncture point was determined by tracing the canthus-tragus line and measuring 10 mm from the tragus and 2 mm below the line. The zygomatic arch was palpated, and patients were asked to open their mouth to move the condyle forward. The position of the needle was from outside to inside, top to bottom, and back to front. Patients were informed that they might experience discomfort in the region. No analgesic or anti-inflammatory drugs were prescribed. During the whole process, all patients were always followed by the same professional. Alternatively, after signing the informed consent, patients were randomly assigned to the corresponding treatment group. Each patient's treatment was assigned by means of a randomization list automatically generated before the start of the study in which the treatment approach was determined.

In the PRP group, injections were preceded by drawing the patient's peripheral blood from the cubital vein into a glass tube with sodium citrate as anticoagulant. After mixing the blood with the citrate, with rotating movements, the tubes were centrifuged at 3200 rpm for 12 min. After careful aspiration of the platelet-rich plasma into a syringe, 2 mL of PRP was injected into the TMJ following the procedure described above for betamethasone and sodium hyaluronate injections.

2.4. Statistics

The statistical analysis focused on the description of the data using absolute and relative frequencies for qualitative and mean variables, minimum and maximum standard deviation for quantitative variables. Sex was evaluated between the different groups by Fisher's exact test and age by the Kruskal-Wallis test. Pain-free time was compared between the groups by means of the ANCOVA test in which age was used as a covariate and sex as an additional factor. Weibull analysis was also performed to determine the median time without pain. The assumption of normality was evaluated by the Shapiro-Wilk test.

In the statistical analysis, a significance level of 0.05 was considered, having been performed on the IBM® SPSS® v26 platform and on MATLAB (R2019b).

3. Results

The sample of this study was composed of 114 individuals, 27 men and 87 women randomly distributed in 3 groups.

In the betamethasone group there were 8 men and 26 women, the mean age was 41.2 years, the youngest being 18 years and the oldest 66 years.

In the SH group the gender distribution was 9 men and 30 women. With respect to age, the minimum was also 18 years, while the maximum was 65 years.

Finally, in the PRP group, composed of 10 men and 31 women, the age range was 18 to 66 years, with a mean of 37.6.

The maximum number of months of follow-up of the patients was 36 months (3 years). It is important to mention that 33 of the 41 patients treated with PRP were permanently pain-free. The same result was obtained by 19 of 39 patients treated with SH. The worst result was observed in the betamethasone group, in which only 9 of the 34 patients were able to remain pain-free for the entire 36-month period.

The following table shows the statistics of age and sex in the three groups defined by the substance injected (Table 1).

Table 1. Age and sex statistics in the three groups.

	PRP (41)	SH (39)	Betamethasone (34)A	p
sex (M/F)	10/31 (24.4%/75.6%)	9/30 (23.1%/76.9%)	8/26 (23.5%/76.5%)	1.000 [§]
age $\bar{x} \pm sd$ (min/max)	37.6 ± 15.0 (18/66)	39.1 ± 13.1 (18/65)	41.2 ± 15.3 (18/66)	0.570 [£]

[§] Fisher; [£] Kruskal-Wallis exact test.

Statistics on pain-free time are presented in Table 2. Figure 1 shows the distribution of pain-free times for the three groups. The results emphasize the contrast between betamethasone and the two other substances.

Table 2. Pain-free time for PRP, SH and betamethasone.

	PRP (41)	SH (39)	Betamethasone (34)A	p
time $\bar{x} \pm sd$ (min/max)	32.0 ± 9.0 (3/36)	26.8 ± 11.4 (1/36)	20.4 ± 11.2 (2/36)	0.005 [#]

[#] ANCOVA (age: $p = 0.827$; gender: $p = 0.403$).

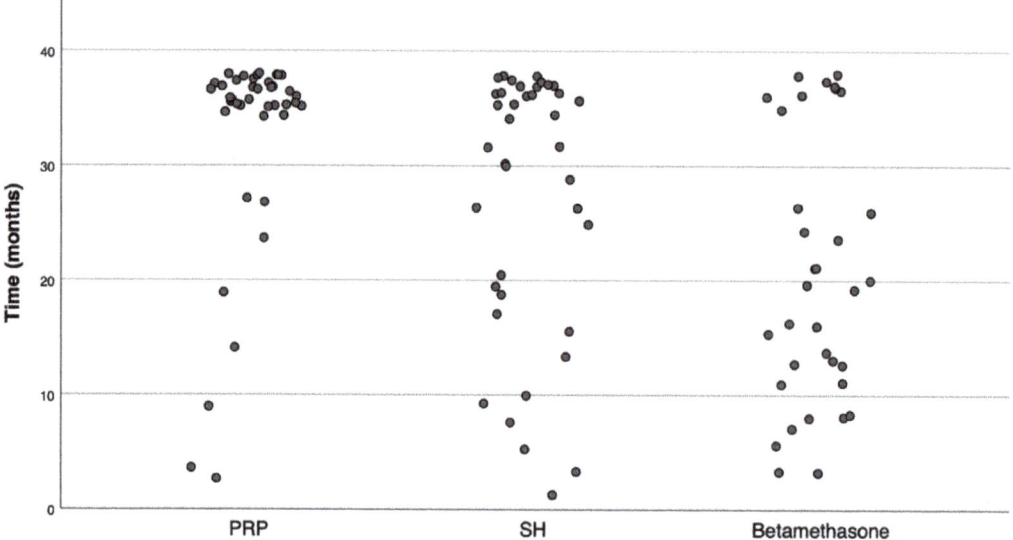

Figure 1. Distribution of pain-free times.

Statistically significant differences are observed ($p = 0.005$) between the groups in terms of administered substances, but neither age ($p = 0.827$) nor sex ($p = 0.403$) have an impact on pain-free time. To compare the groups among themselves, the Dunn-Sidak post-hoc test was chosen, whose results were:

- PRP vs. SH: $p = 0.048$
- PRP vs. Betamethasone: $p < 0.001$
- SH vs. Betamethasone: $p = 0.069$

The following figures show the probability curve of pain-free time obtained by Weibull analysis (Figures 2–4).

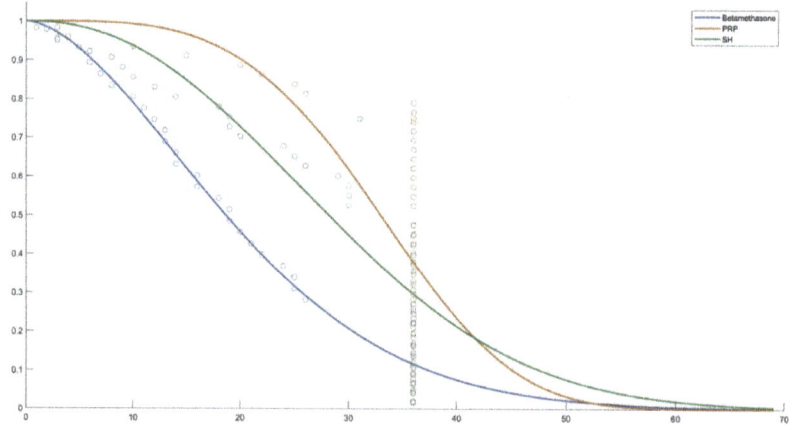

Figure 2. Probability curve for the three substances used.

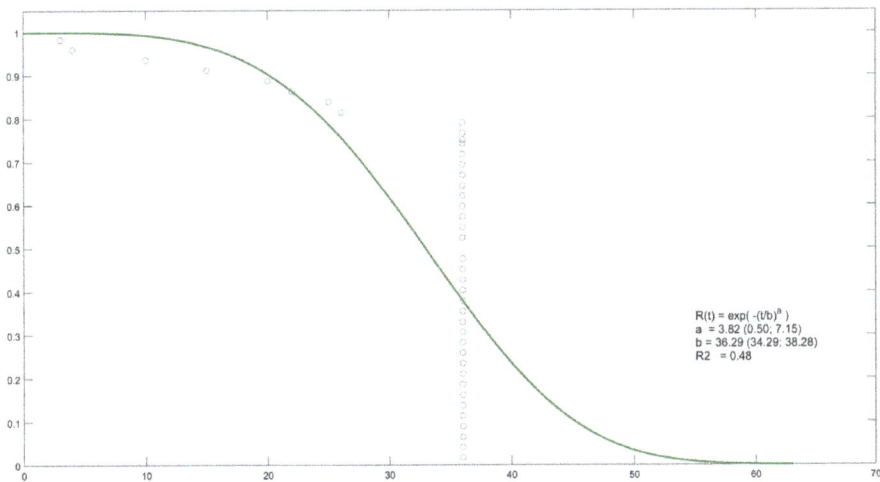

Figure 3. Probability curve for PRP.

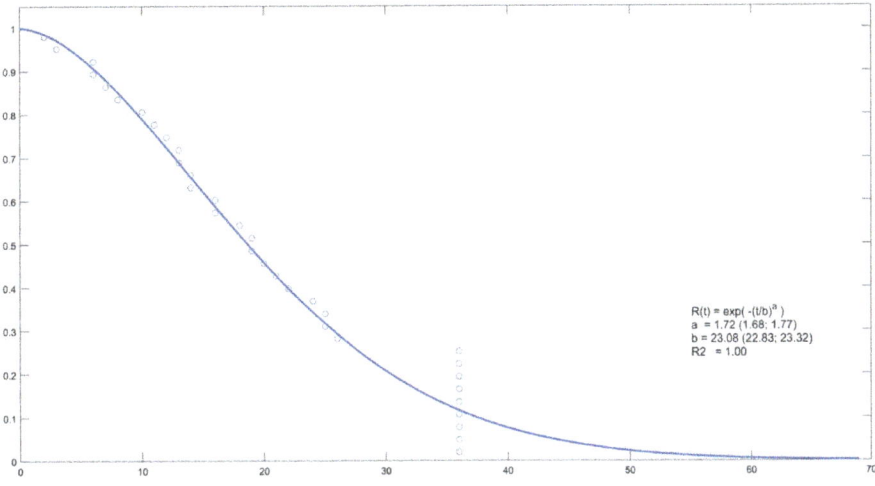

Figure 4. Probability curve for SH.

4. Discussion

The TMJ is the only double joint in which two separate joints must move in a coordinated manner. if an imbalance is caused it can result in pathological states of one or both sides of the joint. In modern society, increasingly stressful eating habits and lifestyles make an increasing percentage of the population susceptible to TMD [24]. Intra-articular injection therapy is used particularly in patients who do not obtain favorable results with other conservative methods. The aim of this study was to analyze the effects of three intra-articular infiltrations (betamethasone, SH and PRP) on TMJ joint pain following the same protocol of a previous randomized clinical trial that evaluated the short-term effect of these three substances [23].

Several previous studies have demonstrated the efficacy of intra-articular infiltrations of betamethasone, HA and PRP [4,6,13,25–32], despite the fact that most research relates infiltrations to more invasive procedures, such as arthrocentesis, which is especially useful in TMJDs and can be performed as an outpatient treatment under local anesthesia.

Currently, arthrocentesis generally uses two needles, one for serum inflow and one for outflow, although techniques using a single needle have been described [33], but there is no evidence of superiority of the latter [34].

Moreover, it should be noted that this type of treatment does not require the use of complex or expensive equipment [35].

Most studies point to the short-term benefits of this type of treatment, with a paucity of long-term studies [36]. Intra-articular betamethasone injections have been the most widely followed [37,38].

Gokçe et al. [11], in a study of 60 patients, compared clinically and radiologically the effects of PRP, HA and corticosteroid injections in osteoarthritis of the TMJ, finding no significant (short-term) differences in the assessment of crepitus or pain. Jüni et al. [39], in a Cochrane review of 27 trials with 1767 participants, drew attention to the use of intra-articular corticosteroids, their benefits and safety, highlighting the uncertainty of their clinical benefits, together with the low methodological quality of the included RCTs. They further highlighted the lack of benefit after 6 months of follow-up, coinciding with our study, in which both PRP and SH led to significant time without pain after treatment, while betamethasone was less effective.

Comparative randomized studies of intra-articular injections of HA (SH) or corticosteroids (betamethasone) into the TMJ have not demonstrated substantial differences between the two therapies. Follow-ups of one or two years reported sustained and substantial reductions in TMJ symptoms and increased joint mobility [28,38]; Tanaka et al. [40] used HA injections to increase synovial fluid viscosity and decrease inflammatory markers, but despite short-term clinical improvement, their research did not provide evidence to support the hypothesis that HA can modify the arthritic environment and reverse or slow long-term cartilage deterioration. Hegab et al. demonstrate that HA injections have similar effects to PRP injections at mid-term follow-up; however, PRP allows for better results in long-term follow-up, with no recurrence of joint pain and sound at 12 months [41]; Al-Delayme et al. reported the efficacy of PRP injection as a primary treatment for nonreducing disc displacement but limited the period of clinical benefit to 6 months, after which an additional injection may be necessary [42].

PRP has an effect on chondrogenic differentiation and tissue remodeling. It has been studied more in other joints than in the TMJ [43]. Given the anti-inflammatory potential of PRP, several studies and meta-analyses have explored the curative effect of intra-articular PRP injection in the treatment of patients with joint pathology [44–47].

A study by Joshi Jubert et al. concluded that PRP was effective in relieving pain and improving TMJ function, although the effects of PRP were comparable with the effects of corticosteroids in patients with advanced stage osteoarthritis (OA) [48]. Other studies argued that a single injection of PRP relieved pain and symptoms better than corticosteroids, noting that PRP produced beneficial effects in the treatment of OA, up to 12 months after intra-articular injection [49,50]. Some research has indicated that the benefits of intra-articular PRP injections in the reduction and relief of joint pain may be due to its effect on inflammatory mediators, increasing jaw dynamics and masticatory performance [27,51,52].

In general, the results of the different studies on the use of betamethasone, SH and PRP in the treatment of TMJ diseases coincide with the results of our studies. Our first study [23] compared the effectiveness of intra-articular injections with SH, PRP and betamethasone in the short term (1 week, 1 month and 6 months). In that study, betamethasone and SH intra-articular injections showed the greatest decrease in pain in the first week, but at 6 months, PRP showed the best results. This second, long-term investigation confirmed our first results.

5. Conclusions

In our study, both PRP and SH led to significant pain-free time after treatment; betamethasone was less effective. However, more rigorous randomized controlled trials with long-term follow-up are needed.

Author Contributions: Conceptualization, B.M.d.S. and N.L.-V.; methodology, B.M.d.S. and A.L.-V.; validation, B.M.d.S. and N.L.-V.; formal analysis, F.C.; investigation, B.M.d.S.; data curation, N.L.-V.; writing—original draft preparation, B.M.d.S. and A.L.-V.; supervision, A.L.-V. and M.J.R. All authors have read and agreed to the published version of the manuscript.

Funding: This research received no external funding.

Institutional Review Board Statement: The study was conducted in accordance with the Declaration of Helsinki and was approved by the Ethics Committee of the Faculty of Medicine of the University of Coimbra (Coimbra, Portugal). This study was approved on 25 June 2017 by the institutional review board (IRB 06-2017-096).

Informed Consent Statement: Informed consent was obtained from all subjects involved in the study.

Data Availability Statement: Faculty of Medicine, University of Coimbra Database.

Conflicts of Interest: The authors declare no conflict of interest.

Abbreviations

TMJDs	Temporomandibular joint disorders
NSAIDs	Non-steroidal anti-inflammatory drugs
CS	Corticosteroids
TMJO	Temporomandibular joint osteoarthritis
SH	Sodium hyaluronate
HA	Hyaluronic acid
PRP	Platelet-rich plasma
MSCs	Mesenchymal stem cells
VSA	Visual Analogic Scale

References

1. Valesan, L.F.; Da-Cas, C.D.; Réus, J.C.; Denardin, A.C.S.; Garanhani, R.R.; Bonotto, D.; Januzzi, E.; de Souza, B.D.M. Prevalence of temporomandibular joint disorders: A systematic review and meta-analysis. *Clin. Oral. Investig.* **2021**, *25*, 441–453. [CrossRef] [PubMed]
2. Schiffman, E.; Ohrbach, R.; Truelove, E.; Look, J.; Anderson, G.; Goulet, J.; List, T.; Svensson, P.; Gonzalez, Y.; Lobbezoo, F.; et al. Diagnostic Criteria for Temporomandibular Disorders (DC/TMD) for Clinical and Research Applications: Recommendations of the International RDC/TMD Consortium Network* and Orofacial Pain Special Interest Group. *J. Oral. Facial. Pain Headache* **2014**, *28*, 6–27. [CrossRef] [PubMed]
3. Jin, L.J.; Lamster, I.B.; Greenspan, J.S.; Pitts, N.B.; Scully, C.; Warnakulasuriya, S. Global burden of oral diseases: Emerging concepts, management and interplay with systemic health. *Oral Dis.* **2016**, *22*, 609–619. [CrossRef]
4. Gencer, Z.K.; Özkiris, M.; Okur, A.; Korkmaz, M.; Saydam, L. A comparative study on the impact of intra-articular injections of hyaluronic acid, tenoxicam and betametazon on the relief of temporomandibular joint disorder complaints. *J. Craniomaxillofac. Surg.* **2014**, *42*, 1117–1121. [CrossRef] [PubMed]
5. Nicot, R.; Raoul, G.; Ferri, J.; Schlund, M. Temporomandibular disorders in head and neck cancers: Overview of specific mechanisms and management. *J. Stomatol. Oral Maxillofac. Surg.* **2020**, *121*, 563–568. [CrossRef]
6. Chung, P.Y.; Lin, M.T.; Chang, H.P. Effectiveness of platelet-rich plasma injection in patients with temporomandibular joint osteoarthritis: A systematic review and meta-analysis of randomized controlled trials. *Oral Surg. Oral Med. Oral Pathol. Oral Radiol.* **2019**, *127*, 106–116. [CrossRef]
7. Ouanounou, A.; Goldberg, M.; Haas, D.A. Pharmacotherapy in Temporomandibular Disorders: A Review. *J. Can. Dent. Assoc.* **2017**, *83*, h7. [PubMed]
8. Ferrillo, M.; Nucci, L.; Giudice, A.; Calafiore, D.; Marotta, N.; Minervini, G.; d'Apuzzo, F.; Ammendolia, A.; Perillo, L.; de Sire, A. Efficacy of conservative approaches on pain relief in patients with temporomandibular joint disorders: A systematic review with network meta-analysis. *Cranio* **2022**, *23*, 1–17. [CrossRef]
9. Horton, C.P. Treatment of arthritic temporomandibular joints by intra-articular injection of hydrocortisone. *Oral Surg. Oral Med. Oral Pathol.* **1953**, *6*, 826–829. [CrossRef]
10. McCrum, C. Therapeutic Review of Methylprednisolone Acetate Intra-Articular Injection in the Management of Osteoarthritis of the Knee—Part 1: Clinical Effectiveness. *Musculoskelet. Care* **2017**, *15*, 79–88. [CrossRef]
11. Gokçe Kutuk, S.; Gökçem, G.; Arslan, M.; Özkan, Y.; Kütük, M.; Kursat Arikan, O. Clinical and Radiological Comparison of Effects of Platelet-Rich Plasma, Hyaluronic Acid, and Corticosteroid Injections on Temporomandibular Joint Osteoarthritis. *J. Craniofac. Surg.* **2019**, *30*, 1144–1148. [CrossRef] [PubMed]

12. Santagata, M.; De Luca, R.; Lo Giudice, G.; Troiano, A.; Lo Giudice, G.; Corvo, G.; Tartaro, G. Arthrocentesis and Sodium Hyaluronate Infiltration in Temporomandibular Disorders Treatment. *Clinical and MRI Evaluation. J. Funct. Morphol. Kinesiol.* **2020**, *5*, 18. [CrossRef] [PubMed]
13. Giraddi, G.B.; Siddaraju, A.; Kumar, A.; Jain, T. Comparison Between Betamethasone and Sodium Hyaluronate Combination with Betamethasone Alone After Arthrocentesis in the Treatment of Internal Derangement of TMJ-Using Single Puncture Technique: A Preliminary Study. *J. Maxillofac. Oral Surg.* **2015**, *14*, 403–409. [CrossRef] [PubMed]
14. Iturriaga, V.; Bornhardt, T.; Manterola, C.; Brebi, P. Effect of hyaluronic acid on the regulation of inflammatory mediators in osteoarthritis of the temporomandibular joint: A systematic review. *Int. J. Oral Maxillofac. Surg.* **2017**, *46*, 590–595. [CrossRef] [PubMed]
15. Wu, P.I.; Diaz, R.; Borg-Stein, J. Platelet-Rich Plasma. *Phys. Med. Rehabil. Clin. N. Am.* **2016**, *4*, 825–853. [CrossRef]
16. Bennell, K.; Hunter, D.; Paterson, K. Platelet-rich plasma for the management of hip and knee osteoarthritis. *Curr. Rheumatol. Rep.* **2017**, *19*, 24. [CrossRef]
17. Campbell, K.A.; Saltzman, B.M.; Mascarenhas, R.; Khair, M.M.; Verma, N.N.; Bach, B.R., Jr.; Cole, B.J. Does intra-articular platelet-rich plasma injection provide clinically superior outcomes compared with other therapies in the treatment of knee osteoarthritis? A systematic review of overlapping meta-analyses. *Arthroscopy* **2015**, *31*, 2213–2221. [CrossRef]
18. Machlus, K.; Thon, J.; Italiano, J. Interpreting the developmental dance of the megakaryocyte: A review of the cellular and molecular processes mediating platelet formation. *Br. J. Haematol.* **2014**, *165*, 227–236. [CrossRef]
19. Ludwig, H.; Birdwhistell, K.; Brainard, B.; Franklin, S. Use of a cyclooxygenase-2 inhibitor does not inhibit platelet activation or growth factor release from platelet-rich plasma. *Am. J. Sports Med.* **2017**, *45*, 3351–3357. [CrossRef]
20. Cole, B.; Seroyer, S.; Filardo, G.; Bajaj, S.; Fortier, L. Platelet-rich plasma: Where are we now and where are we going? *Sports Health* **2010**, *2*, 203–210. [CrossRef]
21. Watson, S.; Bahou, W.; Fitzgerald, D.; Ouwehand, W.; Rao, A.; Leavitt, A. Mapping the platelet proteome: A report of the ISTH Platelet Physiology Subcommittee. *J. Thromb. Haemost.* **2005**, *3*, 2098–2101. [CrossRef] [PubMed]
22. Xie, X.; Zhang, C.; Tuan, R. Biology of platelet-rich plasma and its clinical application in cartilage repair. *Arthritis Res. Ther.* **2014**, *16*, 204. [CrossRef] [PubMed]
23. Sousa, B.M.; López-Valverde, N.; López-Valverde, A.; Caramelo, F.; Fraile, J.F.; Payo, J.H.; Rodrigues, M.J. Different Treatments in Patients with Temporomandibular Joint Disorders: A Comparative Randomized Study. *Medicina (Kaunas)* **2020**, *56*, 113. [CrossRef] [PubMed]
24. Boughner, J.C. Implications of vertebrate craniodental evo-devo for human oral health. *J. Exp. Zool. B Mol. Dev. Evol.* **2017**, *328*, 321–333. [CrossRef]
25. Moldez, M.; Camones, V.; Ramos, G.; Padilla, M.; Enciso, R. Effectiveness of Intra-Articular Injections of Sodium Hyaluronate or Corticosteroids for Intracapsular Temporomandibular Disorders: A Systematic Review and Meta-Analysis. *J. Oral Facial Pain Headache* **2018**, *32*, 53–66. [CrossRef]
26. Vingender, S.; Restár, L.; Csomó, K.B.; Schmidt, P.; Hermann, P.; Vaszikó, M. Intra-articular steroid and hyaluronic acid treatment of internal derangement of the temporomandibular joint. *Orv. Hetil.* **2018**, *159*, 1475–1482. [CrossRef]
27. Goiato, M.; Da Silva, E.V.F.; De Medeiros, R.; Túrcio, K.; Dos Santos, D. Are intra-articular injections of hyaluronic acid effective for the treatment of temporomandibular disorders? A systematic review. *Int. J. Oral Maxillofac. Surg.* **2016**, *45*, 1531–1537. [CrossRef]
28. Kopp, S.; Carlsson, G.E.; Haraldson, T.; Wenneberg, B. The short-term effect of intra-articular injection of sodium hyaluronate and corticosteroid on temporomandibular joint pain and dysfunction. *J. Oral Maxillofac. Surg.* **1985**, *43*, 429–435. [CrossRef]
29. Bjørnland, T.; Gjærum, A.A.; Møystad, A. Osteoarthritis of the temporomandibular joint: An evaluation of the effects and complications of corticosteroid injection compared with injection with sodium hyaluronate. *J. Oral Rehabil.* **2007**, *34*, 583–589. [CrossRef]
30. Nardini, L.G.; Masiero, S.; Marioni, G. Conservative treatment of temporomandibular joint osteoarthrosis: Intra-articular injection of sodium hyaluronate. *J. Oral Rehabil.* **2005**, *32*, 729–734. [CrossRef]
31. Nardini, L.G.; Tito, R.; Staffieri, A.; Beltrame, A. Treatment of patients with arthrosis of the temporomandibular joint by infiltration of sodium hyaluronate: A preliminary study. *Eur. Arch. Oto-Rhino- Laryngol.* **2002**, *259*, 279–284. [CrossRef] [PubMed]
32. Hepguler, S.; Akkoc, Y.S.; Pehlivan, M.; Ozturk, C.; Celebi, G.; Saracoglu, A.; Ozpinar, B. The efficacy of intra-articular sodium hyaluronate in patients with reducing displaced disc of the temporomandibular joint. *J. Oral Rehabil.* **2002**, *29*, 80–86. [CrossRef] [PubMed]
33. Laskin, D.M. Needle placement for arthro-centesis. *J. Oral Maxillofac. Surg* **1998**, *56*, 907. [CrossRef]
34. Manfredini, D.; Rancitelli, D.; Ferronato, G.; Guarda-Nardini, L. Arthrocentesis with or without additional drugs in temporomandibular joint inflammatory-degenerative disease: Comparison of six treatment protocols*. *J. Oral Rehabil* **2012**, *39*, 245–251. [CrossRef] [PubMed]
35. Batifol, D. Les différents types d'injection pour traiter les dysfonctions de l'articulation temporomandibulaire [Different types of injection in temporomandibular disorders (TMD) treatment]. *Rev. Stomatol. Chir. Maxillofac. Chir. Orale.* **2016**, *117*, 256–258.
36. Shen, L.; Yuan, T.; Chen, S.; Xie, X.; Zhang, C. The temporal effect of platelet-rich plasma on pain and physical function in the treatment of knee osteoarthritis: Systematic review and meta-analysis of randomized controlled trials. *J. Orthop. Surg. Res.* **2017**, *12*, 16. [CrossRef]

37. Hetland, M.L.; Østergaard, M.; Ejbjerg, B.; Jacobsen, S.; Stengaard-Pedersen, K.; Junker, P.; Lottenburger, T.; Hansen, I.; Andersen, L.S.; Tarp, U.; et al. CIMESTRA study group. Short- and long-term efficacy of intra-articular injections with betamethasone as part of a treat-to-target strategy in early rheumatoid arthritis: Impact of joint area, repeated injections, MRI findings, anti-CCP, IgM-RF and CRP. *Ann. Rheum. Dis.* **2012**, *71*, 851–856. [CrossRef]
38. Kopp, S.; Carlsson, G.E.; Haraldson, T.; Wenneberg, B. Long-term effect of intra-articular injections of sodium hyaluronate and corticosteroid on temporomandibular joint arthritis. *J. Oral Maxillofac. Surg.* **1987**, *45*, 929–935. [CrossRef]
39. Jüni, P.; Hari, R.; Rutjes, A.W.; Fischer, R.; Silletta, M.G.; Reichenbach, S.; da Costa, B.R. Intra-articular corticosteroid for knee osteoarthritis. *Cochrane Database Syst. Rev.* **2015**, *10*, CD005328. [CrossRef]
40. Tanaka, E.; Iwabe, T.; Dalla-Bona, D.A.; Kawai, N.; van Eijden, T.; Tanaka, M.; Kitagawa, S.; Takata, T.; Tanne, K. The effect of experimental cartilage damage and impairment and restoration of synovial lubrication on friction in the temporomandibular joint. *J. Orofac. Pain* **2005**, *19*, 331–336.
41. Hegab, A.F.; Ali, H.E.; Elmasry, M.; Khallaf, M.G. Platelet-Rich Plasma Injection as an Effective Treatment for Temporomandibular Joint Osteoarthritis. *J. Oral Maxillofac. Surg.* **2015**, *73*, 1706–1713. [CrossRef] [PubMed]
42. Al-Delayme, R.M.A.; Alnuamy, S.H.; Hamid, F.T.; Azzamily, T.J.; Ismaeel, S.A.; Sammir, R.; Hadeel, M.; Nabeel, J.; Shwan, R.; Alfalahi, S.J.; et al. The Efficacy of Platelets Rich Plasma Injection in the Superior Joint Space of the Tempromandibular Joint Guided by Ultra Sound in Patients with Non-reducing Disk Displacement. *J. Maxillofac. Oral Surg.* **2017**, *16*, 43–47. [CrossRef] [PubMed]
43. Kilic, S.C.; Gungormus, M. A comparison of effects of platelet-rich plasma, hyaluronic acid, and corticosteroid injections following arthrocentesis on pain during joint palpation after treatment of temporomandibular joint osteoarthritis. *J. Dent. Fac. Atatürk Uni.* **2016**, *26*, 407–412.
44. Vannabouathong, C.; Del, F.G.; Sales, B.; Smith, C.; Li, C.S.; Yardley, D.; Bhandari, M.; Petrisor, B.A. Intra-articular injections in the treatment of symptoms from ankle arthritis: A systematic review. *Foot Ankle Int.* **2018**, *39*, 1141–1150. [CrossRef]
45. Le, A.D.K.; Enweze, L.; DeBaun, M.R.; Dragoo, J.L. Current clinical recommendations for use of platelet-rich plasma. *Curr. Rev. Musculoskelet. Med.* **2018**, *11*, 624–634. [CrossRef]
46. Dallari, D.; Stagni, C.; Rani, N.; Sabbioni, G.; Pelotti, P.; Torricelli, P.; Tschon, M.; Giavaresi, G. Ultrasound-guided injection of platelet-rich plasma and hyaluronic acid, separately and in combination, for hip osteoarthritis: A randomized controlled study. *Am. J. Sports Med.* **2016**, *44*, 664–671. [CrossRef]
47. Chen, P.; Huang, L.; Ma, Y.; Zhang, D.; Zhang, X.; Zhou, J.; Ruan, A.; Wang, Q. Intra-articular platelet-rich plasma injection for knee osteoarthritis: A summary of meta-analyses. *J. Orthop. Surg. Res.* **2019**, *14*, 385. [CrossRef]
48. Joshi Jubert, N.; Rodríguez, L.; Reverté-Vinaixa, M.; Navarro, A. Platelet-rich plasma injections for advanced knee osteoarthritis: A prospective, randomized, double-blinded clinical trial. *Orthop. J. Sports Med.* **2017**, *5*, 232596711668938. [CrossRef]
49. Forogh, B.; Mianehsaz, E.; Shoaee, S.; Ahadi, T.; Raissi, G.R.; Sajadi, S. Effect of single injection of platelet-rich plasma in comparison with corticosteroid on knee osteoarthritis: A double-blind randomized clinical trial. *J. Sports Med. Phys. Fitness.* **2016**, *56*, 901–908.
50. Meheux, C.; McCulloch, P.; Lintner, D.; Varner, K.; Harris, J. Efficacy of intra-articular platelet-rich plasma injections in knee osteoar- thritis: A systematic review. *Arthroscopy* **2016**, *32*, 495–505. [CrossRef]
51. Kütük, N.; Baş, B.; Soylu, E.; Gönen, Z.B.; Yilmaz, C.; Balcioğlu, E.; Özdamar, S.; Alkan, A. Effect of platelet-rich plasma on fibrocartilage, cartilage, and bone repair in temporomandibular joint. *J. Oral Maxillofac. Surg.* **2014**, *72*, 277–284. [CrossRef] [PubMed]
52. Pihut, M.; Szuta, M.; Ferendıuk, E.; Zeńczak-Więckiewicz, D. Evaluation of pain regression in patients with temporomandibular dysfunction treated by intra-articular platelet-rich plasma injections: A preliminary report. *Biomed. Res. Int.* **2014**, *2014*, 132369. [CrossRef] [PubMed]

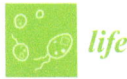

Brief Report

Preliminary Findings of the Efficacy of Botulinum Toxin in Temporomandibular Disorders: Uncontrolled Pilot Study

José A. Blanco-Rueda [1], Antonio López-Valverde [2,*], Antonio Márquez-Vera [1], Roberto Méndez-Sánchez [3], Eva López-García [4] and Nansi López-Valverde [5]

1. Instituto de Investigación Biomédica de Salamanca (IBSAL), University Hospital, 37007 Salamanca, Spain
2. Instituto de Investigación Biomédica de Salamanca (IBSAL), Department of Surgery, University of Salamanca, 37007 Salamanca, Spain
3. Department of Nursing and Physiotherapy, University of Salamanca, 37007 Salamanca, Spain
4. Primary Care, University Hospital "Rio Hortega", 47012 Valladolid, Spain
5. Instituto de Investigación Biomédica de Salamanca (IBSAL), Department of Medicine and Medical Specialties, Universidad Alcalá de Henares, 28801 Madrid, Spain
* Correspondence: alopezvalverde@usal.es

Abstract: Temporomandibular disorders are a common pathology affecting up to 70% of the population, with a maximum incidence in young patients. We used a sample of twenty patients recruited in the Maxillofacial Surgery Service of the University Hospital of Salamanca (Spain), who met the inclusion criteria, with unilateral painful symptomatology of more than three months' duration. All patients were randomly treated by intramuscular and intra-articular injections of botulinum toxin (100 U) in eight predetermined points. Pain symptomatology was assessed by the visual analog scale (VAS) at the different locations, together with joint symptomatology, at baseline and six weeks after treatment. Adverse effects were also evaluated. In 85% of the patients, pain upon oral opening improved and 90% showed improvement in pain upon mastication. A total of 75% of the patients reported improvement in joint clicking/noise. Headaches improved or disappeared in 70% of the patients treated. Despite the limitations of the study and the preliminary results, intramuscular and intra-articular infiltrations with botulinum toxin were effective in the treatment of symptoms associated with temporomandibular disorders (TMDs), with minimal adverse effects.

Keywords: botox; botulin toxin therapy; temporomandibular disorders; masticatory dysfunction syndrome; pilot study

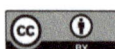

Citation: Blanco-Rueda, J.A.; López-Valverde, A.; Márquez-Vera, A.; Méndez-Sánchez, R.; López-García, E.; López-Valverde, N. Preliminary Findings of the Efficacy of Botulinum Toxin in Temporomandibular Disorders: Uncontrolled Pilot Study. *Life* **2023**, *13*, 345. https://doi.org/10.3390/life13020345

Academic Editors: Zuzanna Nowak and Aleksandra Nitecka-Buchta

Received: 10 January 2023
Revised: 17 January 2023
Accepted: 20 January 2023
Published: 28 January 2023

Copyright: © 2023 by the authors. Licensee MDPI, Basel, Switzerland. This article is an open access article distributed under the terms and conditions of the Creative Commons Attribution (CC BY) license (https://creativecommons.org/licenses/by/4.0/).

1. Introduction

Temporomandibular disorders (TMDs) is a term that refers to a number of pathological conditions and disorders related to the temporomandibular joint (TMJ) and its associated musculoskeletal structures [1]. This set of disorders has previously been referred to as TMJ dysfunction syndrome, functional TMJ alterations, myofascial pain dysfunction syndrome, and temporomandibular pain dysfunction syndrome [2].

It is a common condition, with signs appearing in up to 60–70% of the population, yet only one in four people report the presence of any clinical symptoms, and only 5% of patients seek treatment [3]. Although it can appear at any age, the maximum incidence is observed in young adults, between 20 and 40 years of age, predominantly in women, in a ratio of 4/1 with respect to men [4].

More than 50% of TMDs manifest as myofascial pain, produced by parafunctional habits, such as clenching or bruxism. Its etiology remains poorly understood, but it is likely to be multifactorial and include anatomical, pathophysiological, psychosocial, environmental, biological, and genetic factors, including pre-disposing, triggering, and perpetuating factors [5]. Pain is the most common symptom, along with joint noises and functional limitation [6,7]; however, 40% of patients have an exponential reduction in symptoms and 50–90% have pain relief after conservative and rehabilitative treatment, such as physiotherapy, occlusal splints, orthodontic treatments, electrotherapy, etc. [8,9].

Therefore, multidisciplinary approaches are the ideal treatment option, always with the primary goal of resolving the patient's pain and dysfunction; a recent systematic review suggested that a multidisciplinary approach involving physical medicine and rehabilitation physicians along with dentists is mandatory for the proper diagnosis and treatment of postural disorders in patients with TMDs. [10]

Nonsteroidal anti-inflammatory drugs (NSAIDs), benzodiazepines, antiepileptics, and muscle relaxants are the most commonly used drugs in the treatment of acute pain, with NSAIDs being the most commonly used; however, despite the multiple NSAID options available, only naproxen has been shown to be effective in reducing pain [11]. Muscle relaxants may be prescribed along with NSAIDs if there is evidence of a muscle component, and tricyclic antidepressants are reserved for the treatment of chronic pain [12,13].

Botulinum toxin (BTX) is a neurotoxin produced by the anaerobic bacterium *Clostridium botulinum* with forty different serotypes and is one of the most potent toxins. Despite being considered lethal for many centuries, it was the first toxin used in the history of medicine [14]. Serotype A (the most studied for therapeutic purposes) is the most commonly used, although serotype B is occasionally used [15].

There is a gap in the scientific literature and only a limited number of studies refer to the efficacy of botulinum toxin type A (Botox) and its promising results in the improvement of painful myofascial symptoms [16–20] and although it is not considered a first-choice treatment for the management of TMDs, it could be a therapeutic option in situations where conventional treatments are ineffective.

This uncontrolled pilot study analyzed, after six weeks, the efficacy of intra-articular and facial muscle injections of botulinum toxin type A (Botox) on pain and joint clicking/noise associated with temporomandibular joint dysfunction pathology in a sample of twenty patients. Adverse side effects following botulinum toxin injection were also evaluated.

2. Materials and Methods

2.1. Patients

A sample of 20 patients (n = 20), who met the inclusion criteria for the study, were recruited at the Maxillofacial Surgery Department of the University Hospital of Salamanca. All patients agreed to participate in the research and signed the informed consent form. This study was conducted in accordance with the Helsinki Declaration and was approved by the Salamanca Health Area Drug Research Ethics Committee on 26 April 2021, Reference CEIm:PI 2021 04 734 and was registered in Clinicaltrials.gov (Identifier: NCT05651256).

2.2. Patient Description; Inclusion and Exclusion Criteria

The study included patients diagnosed with TMDs, according to the established diagnostic criteria [1], aged between 18 and 69 years (both included) and with unilateral painful symptomatology of more than three months' duration. Patients previously treated with surgery/arthrocentesis of the TMJ; patients treated in the last six months with surgery in the cervicofacial region; patients who, at the time of inclusion in the study, were being treated in a "Pain Unit"; and patients who had previously received treatment with BTX were excluded. The mean age of the patients was 42.5 years and the distribution by sex was mostly in favor of women, at 17 of the 20 included (85%).

2.3. Treatments

The solution for injection was prepared immediately before the intervention, by dissolving the vials of BTX (Botox® 100 U, Allergan Pharmaceuticals, Westport, Ireland), kept refrigerated at 5 °C, in 1 mL of sterile saline solution at room temperature. Eight injection sites were marked: three located in the masseter muscle, two in the lateral pterygoid muscle, one in the TMJ and two in the temporalis muscle (Figure 1).

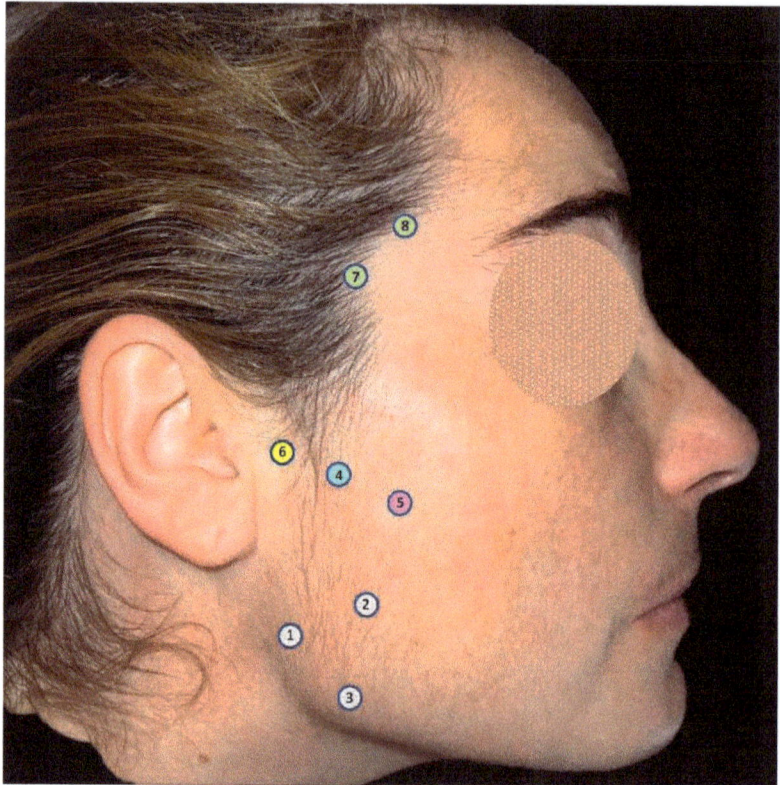

Figure 1. Injection points. 1, 2 and 3, masseter muscle; 4, lateral pterygoid muscle (extra-oral injection); 5, lateral pterygoid muscle (intra-oral injection); 6, TMJ; 7 and 8, anterior temporalis muscle fibers.

All patients included in the study (Figure 2) were randomized to receive a single dose at each injection site of the prepared solution by a single experienced blinded surgeon, 11 patients (55%) on the right side and 9 (45%) on the left side.

A 1 cc marked insulin syringe was used for intramuscular injection of the prepared solution, according to the locations and amounts proposed by Kim et al. and Ho et al. [21,22], with a total dose of 100 U in each patient, distributed at the different injection sites: 40 U in the masseter muscle, (0.1 cc = 10 U), 20 U in the area of greatest hypertrophy (anterior inferior masseter, point 1), 10 U in the direction of the mandibular inferior border (point 2, middle inferior masseter) and 10 U in the area of the posterior inferior masseter (point 3); 20 U in the lateral pterygoid muscle (10 U extraorally between the zygomatic arch and sigmoid notch and 10 U intraorally, behind the maxillary tuberosity) (points 4 and 5); 20 U in the TMJ (point 6), 10mm anterior to the tragus and 2mm below the zygomatic arch; and 20 U in the anterior part of the temporalis muscle (points 7 and 8). The location of the injection point in the lateral pterygoid muscle was performed taking as a reference, in front of the coronoid process, behind the mandibular condyle, above the zygomatic arch and below the mandibular sigmoid notch, penetrating this area with the needle in an anteroposterior and cranial direction, with an angle of 15° with respect to the anterior border of the mandibular condyle; the injection needle in our study reached a depth of 2.5 cm ± 0.5 cm [23–25].

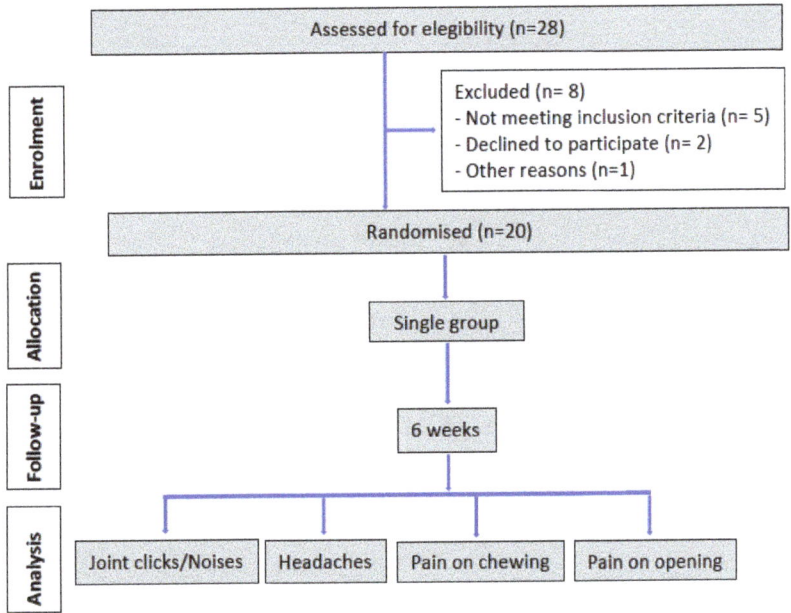

Figure 2. Flow chart of progress through the phases of the study according to the CONSORT statement 2010 [26].

2.4. Pain Measurement

Pain was evaluated in different locations of the craniofacial region (temporalis muscle, masseter muscle, pterygoid muscle, trapezius muscle, externocleidomastoid muscle and temporomandibular joint), before BTX treatment and after six weeks, using the visual analog scale (VAS), in a range from 0 to 10, considering a value of 0 as no pain and 10 as maximum pain.

2.5. Adverse Effect Assessment

Side effects evaluated included warmth, flushing and hematoma at the injection site, swallowing alteration, contralateral muscle contracture or pain and presence of abnormal jaw movements.

3. Results

3.1. Pain Reduction

The average values of pain intensity, in the different locations, before and after treatment, respectively, are presented in Figure 3.

Before treatment, 19 patients (95%) presented with joint clicking/noise, 17 patients (85%) with headaches, 19 patients (95%) with pain upon opening the mouth and 18 (90%) with pain upon chewing.

At six weeks after treatment, 75% of the patients reported an improvement in joint clicks/noises. Regarding headaches, 70% showed an improvement/disappearance, and only 1 patient (5%) showed a very slight improvement. Eighty-five percent of the patients showed improvement in pain on headaches and 90% showed improvement in pain on chewing. Pain intensity decreased in all areas injected with BTX; however, three patients (15%) reported minimal or no decrease in pain intensity in the different locations.

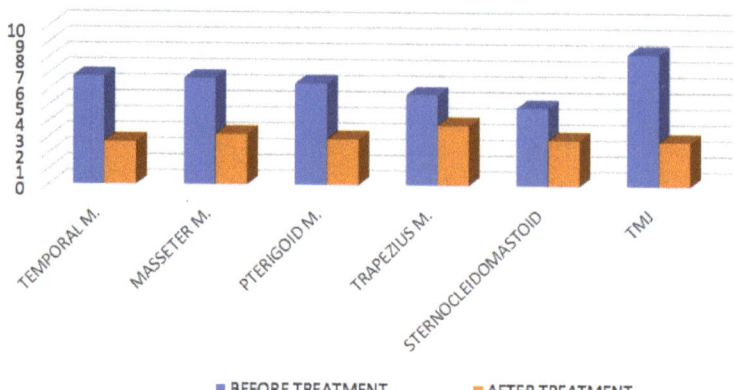

Figure 3. Assessment of pain intensity in the cervicofacial musculature by VAS before and after intramuscular injection of BTX.

3.2. Adverse Events

It is noteworthy that most of the patients did not report having suffered any adverse event after treatment.

The most frequent adverse effect was the appearance of abnormal jaw movements, which was present in four patients (20%); however, two patients (10%) reported that these abnormal movements were only present in the first few days after treatment, while two others reported that they continued to suffer them.

Two of the patients (10%) reported a sensation of flushing/heat in the injection area in the days following treatment, and only one of the patients (5%) reported the appearance of hematoma in the injected area. Three patients (15%) reported the appearance of muscle contracture/pain on the side contralateral to the injection; however, it is noteworthy that swallowing alteration did not appear in any of the patients (Figure 4).

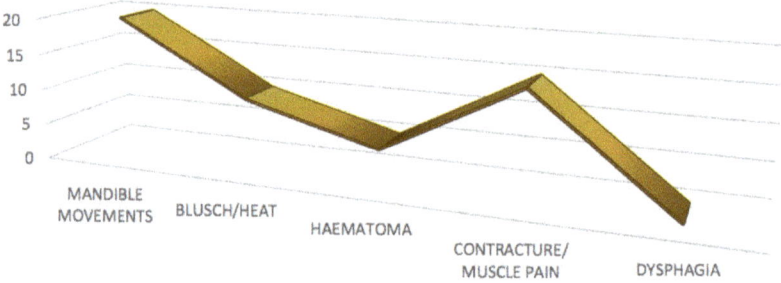

Figure 4. Adverse effects after BTX treatment.

4. Discussion

Botulinum toxin has evolved from being a toxicant to a versatile therapeutic tool for a growing list of pathologies; however, treatment with BTX remains controversial and there are not many studies evaluating its efficacy in the treatment of TMDs, most of them being in favor of its use and its ability to alleviate pain associated with this pathology [27–30].

Freund et al. in 1999 [31] were the first to report preliminary results on the benefits of BTX on pain, function and mouth opening in a sample of 15 patients diagnosed with TMDs. Subsequently, these same investigators, in an expanded sample of 46 patients, demonstrated that intramuscular injections of BTX-A produced significant improvements in pain, function and mouth opening, reducing the severity of symptoms and improving the functional abilities of patients with TMDs, and that these effects would extend beyond its capacity as a muscle relaxant [32]. Recently, several studies and systematic reviews have focused on the benefits of BTX in patients with TMDs [33–37], although there are discrepancies regarding the efficacy of BTX in this pathology, mainly based on methodological errors. Laskin pointed out that many studies do not address the etiology and focus only on symptomatic treatment and that conservative treatments would be equally effective; however, he acknowledges that the etiology of pain and masticatory muscle dysfunction remains unknown [10,38].

Preliminary results of our study found a beneficial effect in 85% of patients with TMDs. These results coincided with those obtained by Sidebottom et al. [27] who, in a prospective study on 62 patients, with a mean age of 42.5 years and (like our study) a preponderance in the sample of the female sex, reported a significant reduction in pain, greater than 90% in 79% of patients treated with a single dose of BTX, concluding that intramuscular injections of BTX, although not guaranteeing complete resolution of myofascial pain, often produce a beneficial effect on symptomatology, and should be considered as an alternative treatment for masticatory myofascial pain in the face of failure of conservative treatments.

The facial areas injected with BTX differ in different studies. Some inject only the masseter muscle [39], others the masseter and temporalis [40,41] and others use injection in the temporalis, masseter, and external pterygoid muscles [42]. Intramuscular injection with BTX in the masseter muscle is often used in the treatment of myofascial syndrome, whose etiological factors lie mainly in fatigue or spasm of the masticatory muscles, with a concomitant arthralgia of the TMJ [27,43]. Schwartz and Freund base the diagnosis of TMDs on two etiologies, one anatomical and the other functional, with two critical areas, the arthrogenic pathology (intracapsular) and the myogenic pathology, originating in the musculature, recommending their simultaneous approach [44]; however, Batifol [45] recommends intra-articular injections exclusively if the pain is chronic. In accordance with these recommendations, our study included patients with a history of pain lasting more than 3 months.

Although BTX was initially only used in the treatment of focal dystonia, it has been shown to provide relief from migraine and tension headaches and neck pain (cervical dystonia), suggesting a possible role in the treatment of TMDs [46–50]; a review by Ihde and Konstantinovic concluded that BTX appears to be relatively safe and effective in the treatment of cervical dystonia and chronic facial pain associated with masticatory hyperactivity [51]. Similarly, Blitzer and Sulica demonstrated its effectiveness in the treatment of torticollis, including as involved muscles the sternocleidomastoid, trapezius, semispinalis capitis, splenius capitis, levator scapulae, and minor paraspinal muscles [52] and that BTX was the most frequently injected substance, intramuscularly, in the treatment of TMDs [53].

Our study, in accordance with these results, found a disappearance of headaches in 70% of the patients treated, although 15% of the patients reported not having found relief from painful symptomatology. In our study, we combined BTX infiltration in the masseter, temporalis, and pterygoid muscles with intra-articular infiltration, obtaining excellent results on pain in the cervicofacial musculature (Figure 3).

On the other hand, intra-articular infiltration of BTX has demonstrated its efficacy in reducing pain [54]. Lora et al. demonstrated in a study in rats the strong antinociceptive effect of intra-articular injection of BTX-A [55]. Intra-articular injection of BTX inhibits inflammatory mediators, reduces neuropeptide release from joint nociceptors and thus reduces neurogenic inflammation and joint pain [56]. Our study found in 85% of treated patients an improvement of pain on mouth opening and 90% showed improvement of pain on chewing. Furthermore, in 75% of the treated patients, an improvement in joint clicking/noise was observed. These results would agree with those obtained by Bakke et al. [57], who, by BTX-A injections into the lateral pterygoid muscle, temporarily reduced the muscle action, but the clicking was permanently eliminated and did not reappear during the 1-year observation period, obtaining a small but clear positional improvement in the disc–condyle relationship. Similarly, other studies [58–60] with BTX-A injections into the lateral pterygoid muscle reported benefits on temporomandibular clicking.

The dose ranges are also discrepant in the different studies. Schwartz and Freund recommend doses like those used by us: 25–50 U in the masseter muscle, 5–25 U in the temporalis muscle and 5–25 in the pterygoid muscle [44]. Batifol recommends for intra-articular injection doses similar to those used in our study [45].

Regarding adverse effects, Ihde and Konstantinovic, in a review identifying randomized clinical trials evaluating patients treated with botulinum toxin, found that the adverse effects were mild and transient [61]; similarly, a systematic review by Machado et al. [62] found no significant difference in adverse effects between BTX-A and a placebo. In our study, only four patients (20%) reported them, reporting their disappearance within a few days.

Despite these results, we are aware of the limitations of the study: on the one hand, the small sample size, although authors such as Sipahi Calis et al. and Patel et al. [42,63] base their studies of the effect of BTX on TMDs on sample sizes similar to ours, at 25 and 20 patients, respectively; on the other hand, the evaluation was performed six weeks after the infiltrations, clearly resulting in a reduced evaluation time. In addition, joint and muscle infiltrations, at the same time, could lead to biases in the results. Nevertheless, we present a pilot study with preliminary results.

5. Conclusions

Despite the limitations of the study and presenting preliminary results, we believe that multiple intramuscular and intra-articular infiltrations with BTX-A, with a total dose of 100 U, are effective (at least temporarily) in relieving TMJ pain and clicking and noises, with minimal adverse effects. Future ongoing controlled studies, with a larger sample of patients and longer-term follow-up, will allow comparison of the results.

Author Contributions: Conceptualization, J.A.B.-R. and N.L-V.; methodology A.L.-V.; validation, N.L.-V. and A.M.-V.; formal analysis, E.L.-G. and R.M.-S.; investigation, J.A.B.-R.; writing—original draft preparation, A.L.-V. and N.L.-V.; writing—review and editing, A.L.-V. and N.L.-V.; supervision, A.L.-V. All authors have read and agreed to the published version of the manuscript.

Funding: This research received no external funding.

Institutional Review Board Statement: This study was conducted in accordance with the Declaration of Helsinki and was approved by the Salamanca Health Area Drug Research Ethics Committee on 26 April 2021, Reference CEIm:PI 2021 04 734.

Informed Consent Statement: Informed consent was obtained from all subjects involved in the study.

Data Availability Statement: https://beta.clinicaltrials.gov/.

Conflicts of Interest: The authors declare no conflict of interest.

References

1. Schiffman, E.; Ohrbach, R.; Truelove, E.; Look, J.; Anderson, G.; Goulet, J.P.; List, T.; Svensson, P.; Gonzalez, Y.; Lobbezoo, F.; et al. Diagnostic Criteria for Temporomandibular Disorders (DC/TMD) for Clinical and Research Applications: Recommendations of the International RDC/TMD Consortium Network* and Orofacial Pain Special Interest Group†. *J. Oral Facial Pain Headache* **2014**, *28*, 6–27. [CrossRef] [PubMed]
2. Okeson, J.P. Current terminology and diagnostic classification schemes. *Oral Surg. Oral Med. Oral Pathol. Oral Radiol. Endodontology* **1997**, *83*, 61–64. [CrossRef] [PubMed]
3. Liu, F.; Steinkeler, A. Epidemiology, diagnosis, and treatment of temporomandibular disorders. *Dent. Clin.* **2013**, *57*, 465–479. [CrossRef] [PubMed]
4. Kobayashi, F.Y.; Gavião, M.B.D.; Montes, A.B.M.; Marquezin, M.C.S.; Castelo, P.M. Evaluation of orofacial function in young subjects with temporomandibular disorders. *J. Oral Rehabil.* **2014**, *41*, 496–506. [CrossRef] [PubMed]
5. Baba, K.; Tsukiyama, Y.; Yamazaki, M.; Clark, G.T. A review of temporomandibular disorder diagnostic techniques. *J. Prosthet. Dent.* **2001**, *86*, 184–194. [CrossRef] [PubMed]
6. Gauer, R.L.; Semidey, M.J. Diagnosis and treatment of temporomandibular disorders. *Am. Fam. Physician.* **2015**, *91*, 378–386.
7. Lomas, J.; Gurgenci, T.; Jackson, C.; Campbell, D. Temporomandibular dysfunction. *Aust. J. Gen. Pract.* **2018**, *47*, 212–215. [CrossRef]

8. Shoohanizad, E.; Garajei, A.; Enamzadeh, A.; Yari, A. Nonsurgical management of temporomandibular joint autoimmune disorders. *AIMS Public Health.* **2019**, *6*, 554–567. [CrossRef] [PubMed]
9. Ferrillo, M.; Marotta, N.; Giudice, A.; Calafiore, D.; Curci, C.; Fortunato, L.; Ammendolia, A.; de Sire, A. Effects of Occlusal Splints on Spinal Posture in Patients with Temporomandibular Disorders: A Systematic Review. *Healthcare* **2022**, *10*, 739. [CrossRef]
10. Ferrillo, M.; Ammendolia, A.; Paduano, S.; Calafiore, D.; Marotta, N.; Migliario, M.; Fortunato, L.; Giudice, A.; Michelotti, A.; de Sire, A. Efficacy of rehabilitation on reducing pain in muscle-related temporomandibular disorders: A systematic review and meta-analysis of randomized controlled trials. *J. Back Musculoskelet. Rehabil.* **2022**, *35*, 921–936. [CrossRef]
11. Ta, L.E.; Dionne, R.A. Treatment of painful temporomandibular joints with a cyclooxygenase-2 inhibitor: A randomized placebo-controlled comparison of celecoxib to naproxen. *Pain* **2004**, *111*, 13–21. [CrossRef] [PubMed]
12. Herman, C.R.; Schiffman, E.L.; Look, J.O.; Rindal, D.B. The effectiveness of adding pharmacologic treatment with clonazepam or cyclobenzaprine to patient education and self-care for the treatment of jaw pain upon awakening: A randomized clinical trial. *J. Orofac. Pain.* **2002**, *16*, 64–70. [PubMed]
13. Hersh, E.V.; Balasubramaniam, R.; Pinto, A. Pharmacologic management of temporomandibular disorders. *Oral Maxillofac Surg. Clin. N. Am.* **2008**, *20*, 197–210. [CrossRef] [PubMed]
14. Park, J.; Park, H.J. Botulinum Toxin for the Treatment of Neuropathic Pain. *Toxins* **2017**, *9*, 260. [CrossRef]
15. Malgorzata, P.; Piotr, C.; Edward, K. The Mechanism of the Beneficial Effect of Botulinum Toxin Type a Used in the Treatment of Temporomandibular Joints Dysfunction. *Mini. Rev. Med. Chem.* **2017**, *17*, 445–450. [CrossRef]
16. Fallah, H.M.; Currimbhoy, S. Use of botulinum toxin A for treatment of myofascial pain and dysfunction. *J. Oral Maxillofac Surg.* **2012**, *70*, 1243–1245. [CrossRef]
17. Patel, J.; Cardoso, J.A.; Mehta, S. A systematic review of botulinum toxin in the management of patients with temporomandibular disorders and bruxism. *Br. Dent. J.* **2019**, *226*, 667–672. [CrossRef]
18. Serrera-Figallo, M.A.; Ruiz-de-León-Hernández, G.; Torres-Lagares, D.; Castro-Araya, A.; Torres-Ferrerosa, O.; Hernández-Pacheco, E.; Gutierrez-Perez, J.L. Use of Botulinum Toxin in Orofacial Clinical Practice. *Toxins* **2020**, *12*, 112. [CrossRef] [PubMed]
19. von Lindern, J.J.; Niederhagen, B.; Bergé, S.; Appel, T. Type A botulinum toxin in the treatment of chronic facial pain associated with masticatory hyperactivity. *J. Oral Maxillofac. Surg.* **2003**, *61*, 774–778. [CrossRef]
20. Muñoz Lora, V.R.M.; Del Bel Cury, A.A.; Jabbari, B.; Lacković, Z. Botulinum Toxin Type A in Dental Medicine. *J. Dent. Res.* **2019**, *98*, 1450–1457. [CrossRef]
21. Kim, N.H.; Park, R.H.; Park, J.B. Botulinum toxin type A for the treatment of hypertrophy of the masseter muscle. *Plast. Reconstr. Surg.* **2010**, *125*, 1693–1705. [CrossRef] [PubMed]
22. Ho, K.Y.; Tan, K.H. Botulinum toxin A for myofascial trigger point injection: A qualitative systematic review. *Eur. J. Pain.* **2007**, *11*, 519–527. [CrossRef] [PubMed]
23. Mesa-Jiménez, J.A.; Sánchez-Gutiérrez, J.; de-la-Hoz-Aizpurua, J.L.; Fernández-de-las-Peñas, C. Cadaveric validation of dry needle placement in the lateral pterygoid muscle. *J. Manip. Physiol. Ther.* **2015**, *38*, 145–150. [CrossRef] [PubMed]
24. Gonzalez-Perez, L.M.; Infante-Cossio, P.; Granados-Nuñez, M.; Urresti-Lopez, F.J. Treatment of temporomandibular myofascial pain with deep dry needling. *Med. Oral Patol. Oral Cir. Bucal.* **2012**, *17*, e781-5. [CrossRef] [PubMed]
25. Kucukguven, A.; Demiryurek, M.D.; Kucukguven, M.B.; Vargel, I. A Novel Injection Technique to the Lateral Pterygoid Muscle for Temporomandibular Disorders: A Cadaveric Study. *Plast. Reconstr. Surg.* **2021**, *148*, 785e–790e. [CrossRef]
26. Moher, D.; Hopewell, S.; Schulz, K.F.; Montori, V.; Gøtzsche, P.C.; Devereaux, P.J.; Elbourne, D.; Egger, M.; Altman, D.G. CONSORT 2010 explanation and elaboration: Updated guidelines for reporting parallel group randomised trials. *Int. J. Surg.* **2012**, *10*, 28–55. [CrossRef]
27. Sidebottom, A.J.; Patel, A.A.; Amin, J. Botulinum injection for the management of myofascial pain in the masticatory muscles. A prospective outcome study. *Br. J. Oral Maxillofac. Surg.* **2013**, *51*, 199–205. [CrossRef]
28. Laskin, D.M. The Use of Botulinum Toxin for the Treatment of Myofascial Pain in the Masticatory Muscles. *Oral Maxillofac. Surg. Clin. N. Am.* **2018**, *30*, 287–289. [CrossRef]
29. Soares, A.; Andriolo, R.B.; Atallah, A.N.; da Silva, E.M. Botulinum toxin for myofascial pain syndromes in adults. *Cochrane Database Syst. Rev.* **2014**, *2014*, CD007533.
30. Zhou, J.Y.; Wang, D. An update on botulinum toxin A injections of trigger points for myofascial pain. *Curr. Pain Headache Rep.* **2014**, *18*, 386. [CrossRef]
31. Freund, B.; Schwartz, M.; Symington, J.M. The use of botulinum toxin for the treatment of temporomandibular disorders: Preliminary findings. *J. Oral Maxillofac. Surg.* **1999**, *57*, 916–920. [CrossRef] [PubMed]
32. Freund, B.; Schwartz, M.; Symington, J.M. Botulinum toxin: New treatment for temporomandibular disorders. *Br. J. Oral Maxillofac. Surg.* **2000**, *38*, 466–471. [CrossRef]
33. Nayyar; Kumar, P.; Nayyar, P.V.; Singh, A. BOTOX: Broadening the Horizon of Dentistry. *J. Clin. Diagn. Res.* **2014**, *8*, ZE25–ZE29. [PubMed]
34. Hoque, A.; McAndrew, M. Use of botulinum toxin in dentistry. *N. Y. State Dent. J.* **2009**, *75*, 52–55. [PubMed]
35. Al-Wayli, H. Treatment of chronic pain associated with nocturnal bruxism with botulinum toxin. A prospective and randomized clinical study. *J. Clin. Exp. Dent.* **2017**, *9*, e112–e117. [CrossRef]
36. Satriyasa, B.K. Botulinum toxin (Botox) A for reducing the appearance of facial wrinkles: A literature review of clinical use and pharmacological aspect. *Clin. Cosmet. Investig. Dermatol.* **2019**, *12*, 223–228. [CrossRef]

37. Srivastava, S.; Kharbanda, S.; Pal, U.S.; Shah, V. Applications of botulinum toxin in dentistry: A comprehensive review. *Natl. J. Maxillofac. Surg.* **2015**, *6*, 152–159.
38. Laskin, D.M. Botulinum toxin A in the treatment of myofascial pain and dysfunction: The case against its use. *J. Oral Maxillofac. Surg.* **2012**, *70*, 1240–1242. [CrossRef]
39. Pihut, M.; Ferendiuk, E.; Szewczyk, M.; Kasprzyk, K.; Wieckiewicz, M. The efficiency of botulinum toxin type A for the treatment of masseter muscle pain in patients with temporomandibular joint dysfunction and tension-type headache. *J. Headache Pain* **2016**, *17*, 29. [CrossRef]
40. Chikhani, L.; Dichamp, J. Bruxisme, syndrome algodysfonctionnel des articulations temporo-mandibulaires et toxine botulique [Bruxism, temporo-mandibular dysfunction and botulinum toxin]. *Ann. Readapt. Med. Phys.* **2003**, *46*, 333–337. [CrossRef]
41. Hosgor, H.; Altindis, S. Efficacy of botulinum toxin in the management of temporomandibular myofascial pain and sleep bruxism. *J. Korean Assoc. Oral Maxillofac. Surg.* **2020**, *46*, 335–340. [CrossRef] [PubMed]
42. Patel, A.A.; Lerner, M.Z.; Blitzer, A. IncobotulinumtoxinA Injection for Temporomandibular Joint Disorder. *Ann. Otol. Rhinol. Laryngol.* **2017**, *126*, 328–333. [CrossRef] [PubMed]
43. Thomas, N.J.; Aronovich, S. Does Adjunctive Botulinum Toxin a Reduce Pain Scores When Combined with Temporomandibular Joint Arthroscopy for the Treatment of Concomitant Temporomandibular Joint Arthralgia and Myofascial Pain? *J. Oral Maxillofac. Surg.* **2017**, *75*, 2521–2528. [CrossRef] [PubMed]
44. Schwartz, M.; Freund, B. Treatment of temporomandibular disorders with botulinum toxin. *Clin. J. Pain* **2002**, *18* (Suppl. S6), S198–S203. [CrossRef]
45. Batifol, D. Les différents types d'injection pour traiter les dysfonctions de l'articulation temporomandibulaire [Different types of injection in temporomandibular disorders (TMD) treatment]. *Rev. Stomatol. Chir. Maxillo-Faciale Chir. Orale* **2016**, *117*, 256–258. [CrossRef]
46. Gadhia, K.; Walmsley, D. The therapeutic use of botulinum toxin in cervical and maxillofacial conditions. *Evid. Based Dent.* **2009**, *10*, 53. [CrossRef]
47. Blumenfeld, A.M.; Stark, R.J.; Freeman, M.C.; Orejudos, A.; Manack Adams, A. Long-term study of the efficacy and safety of OnabotulinumtoxinA for the prevention of chronic migraine: COMPEL study. *J. Headache Pain* **2018**, *19*, 13. [CrossRef]
48. Binder, W.J.; Brin, M.F.; Blitzer, A.; Schoenrock, L.D.; Pogoda, J.M. Botulinum toxin type A (BOTOX) for treatment of migraine headaches: An open-label study. *Otolaryngol. Head Neck Surg.* **2000**, *123*, 669–676. [CrossRef]
49. Freund, B.; Schwartz, M. Treatment of chronic cervical-associated headache with botulinum toxin A: A pilot study. *Headache J. Head Face Pain* **2000**, *40*, 231–236. [CrossRef] [PubMed]
50. Freund, B.; Schwartz, M. Treatment of whiplash associated with neck pain with botulinum toxin-A: A pilot study. *J. Rheumatol.* **2000**, *27*, 481–484.
51. Ihde, S.K.; Konstantinovic, V.S. The therapeutic use of botulinum toxin in cervical and maxillofacial conditions: An evidence-based review. *Oral Surg. Oral Med. Oral Pathol. Oral Radiol. Endodontology* **2007**, *104*, e1–e11. [CrossRef] [PubMed]
52. Blitzer, A.; Sulica, L. Botulinum toxin: Basic science and clinical uses in otolaryngology. *Laryngoscope* **2000**, *111*, 218–226. [CrossRef] [PubMed]
53. Nowak, Z.; Chęeciński, M.; Nitecka-Buchta, A.; Bulanda, S.; Ilczuk-Rypuła, D.; Postek-Stefańska, L.; Baron, S. Intramuscular Injections and Dry Needling within Masticatory Muscles in Management of Myofascial Pain. Systematic Review of Clinical Trials. *Int. J. Environ. Res. Public Health* **2021**, *18*, 9552. [CrossRef] [PubMed]
54. Sari, B.C.; Develi, T. The effect of intraarticular botulinum toxin-A injection on symptoms of temporomandibular joint disorder. *J. Stomatol. Oral Maxillofac. Surg.* **2022**, *123*, e316–e320. [CrossRef] [PubMed]
55. Lora, V.R.; Clemente-Napimoga, J.T.; Abdalla, H.B.; Macedo, C.G.; Canales, G.T.; Barbosa, C.M. Botulinum toxin type A reduces inflammatory hypernociception induced by arthritis in the temporomadibular joint of rats. *Toxicon* **2017**, *129*, 52–57. [CrossRef]
56. Drinovac Vlah, V.; Filipović, B.; Bach-Rojecky, L.; Lacković, Z. Role of central versus peripheral opioid system in antinociceptive and anti-inflammatory effect of botulinum toxin type A in trigeminal region. *Eur. J. Pain* **2018**, *22*, 583–591. [CrossRef] [PubMed]
57. Bakke, M.; Møller, E.; Werdelin, L.M.; Dalager, T.; Kitai, N.; Kreiborg, S. Treatment of severe temporomandibular joint clicking with botulinum toxin in the lateral pterygoid muscle in two cases of anterior disc displacement. *Oral Surg. Oral Med. Oral Pathol. Oral Radiol. Endod.* **2005**, *100*, 693–700. [CrossRef]
58. Emara, A.S.; Faramawey, M.I.; Hassaan, M.A.; Hakam, M.M. Botulinum toxin injection for management of temporomandibular joint clicking. *Int. J. Oral Maxillofac. Surg.* **2013**, *42*, 759–764. [CrossRef]
59. Karacalar, A.; Yilmaz, N.; Bilgici, A.; Baş, B.; Akan, H. Botulinum toxin for the treatment of temporomandibular joint disk disfigurement: Clinical experience. *J. Craniofac. Surg.* **2005**, *16*, 476–481. [CrossRef]
60. Rezazadeh, F.; Esnaashari, N.; Azad, A.; Emad, S. The effects of botulinum toxin A injection on the lateral pterygoid muscle in patients with a painful temporomandibular joint click: A randomized clinical trial study. *BMC Oral Health* **2022**, *22*, 217. [CrossRef]
61. Truong, D.; Brodsky, M.; Lew, M.; Brashear, A.; Jankovic, J.; Molho, E.; Orlova, O.; Timerbaeva, S. Global Dysport Cervical Dystonia Study Group. Long-term efficacy and safety of botulinum toxin type A (Dysport) in cervical dystonia. *Park. Relat. Disord.* **2010**, *16*, 316–323. [CrossRef] [PubMed]

62. Machado, D.; Martimbianco, A.L.C.; Bussadori, S.K.; Pacheco, R.L.; Riera, R.; Santos, E.M. Botulinum Toxin Type A for Painful Temporomandibular Disorders: Systematic Review and Meta-Analysis. *J. Pain* **2020**, *21*, 281–293. [CrossRef] [PubMed]
63. Sipahi Calis, A.; Colakoglu, Z.; Gunbay, S. The use of botulinum toxin-a in the treatment of muscular temporomandibular joint disorders. *J. Stomatol. Oral Maxillofac. Surg.* **2019**, *120*, 322–325. [CrossRef] [PubMed]

Disclaimer/Publisher's Note: The statements, opinions and data contained in all publications are solely those of the individual author(s) and contributor(s) and not of MDPI and/or the editor(s). MDPI and/or the editor(s) disclaim responsibility for any injury to people or property resulting from any ideas, methods, instructions or products referred to in the content.

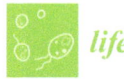

Systematic Review

The Efficacy of Manual Therapy Approaches on Pain, Maximum Mouth Opening and Disability in Temporomandibular Disorders: A Systematic Review of Randomised Controlled Trials

Leonardo Sette Vieira [1], Priscylla Ruany Mendes Pestana [1], Júlio Pascoal Miranda [1], Luana Aparecida Soares [1], Fabiana Silva [2,*], Marcus Alessandro Alcantara [1] and Vinicius Cunha Oliveira [1,3]

[1] Postgraduate Program in Rehabilitation and Functional Performance, Universidade Federal dos Vales do Jequitinhonha e Mucuri (UFVJM), Diamantina 39100-000, Brazil
[2] Cirklo Health Education, Barão de Ubá, Porto Alegre 90450-090, Brazil
[3] Postgraduate Program in Health Sciences, Universidade Federal dos Vales do Jequitinhonha e Mucuri (UFVJM), Diamantina 39100-000, Brazil
* Correspondence: fabisis@gmail.com; Tel.: +55-(51)-99837-9083

Abstract: Temporomandibular disorder (TMD) is a common condition disabling people and bringing up costs. The aim of this study was to investigate the effects of manual therapy on pain intensity, maximum mouth opening (MMO) and disability. Searches were conducted in six databases for randomised controlled trials (RCTs). Selection of trials, data extraction and methodological quality assessment were conducted by two reviewers with discrepancies resolved by a third reviewer. Estimates were presented as mean differences (MDs) or standardized mean differences (SMDs) with 95% confidence intervals (CIs). Quality of the evidence was assessed using the GRADE approach. Twenty trials met the eligibility criteria and were included. For pain intensity, high and moderate quality evidence demonstrated the additional effects of manual therapy at short- (95% CI −2.12 to −0.82 points) and long-term (95% CI −2.17 to −0.40 points) on the 0–10 points scale. For MMO, moderate to high quality evidence was found in favour of manual therapy alone (95% CI 0.01 to 7.30 mm) and its additional effects (95% CI 1.58 to 3.58 mm) at short- and long-term (95% CI 1.22 to 8.40 mm). Moderate quality evidence demonstrated an additional effect of manual therapy for disability (95% CI = −0.87 to −0.14). Evidence supports manual therapy as effective for TMD.

Keywords: temporomandibular joint disorders; temporomandibular joint dysfunction syndrome; musculoskeletal manipulations; manual therapies; systematic review

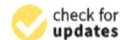

Citation: Vieira, L.S.; Pestana, P.R.M.; Miranda, J.P.; Soares, L.A.; Silva, F.; Alcantara, M.A.; Oliveira, V.C. The Efficacy of Manual Therapy Approaches on Pain, Maximum Mouth Opening and Disability in Temporomandibular Disorders: A Systematic Review of Randomised Controlled Trials. *Life* **2023**, *13*, 292. https://doi.org/10.3390/life13020292

Academic Editors: Zuzanna Nowak and Aleksandra Nitecka-Buchta

Received: 26 December 2022
Revised: 13 January 2023
Accepted: 16 January 2023
Published: 20 January 2023

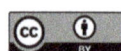

Copyright: © 2023 by the authors. Licensee MDPI, Basel, Switzerland. This article is an open access article distributed under the terms and conditions of the Creative Commons Attribution (CC BY) license (https://creativecommons.org/licenses/by/4.0/).

1. Introduction

Temporomandibular disorders (TMD) can be defined as a group of pathologies of the temporomandibular joint and muscles involved [1]. TMD can be classified as myogenic (i.e., muscle and myofascial origin), arthrogenic, mixed and joint-related disorders (i.e., disc displacements with or without reduction, arthritis or subluxation) according to The Diagnostic Criteria for Temporomandibular Disorders (DC/TMD) [1,2]. It is a common health condition worldwide with an estimated prevalence ranging from 11% to 31%, and is especially high in people with multiple sclerosis [3,4]. After a new episode of TMD, 27% of people persist with significant pain one year later [5–7], and recurrence is common [8]. Its related pain and disability bring direct (e.g., use of medication to alleviate symptoms) and indirect (e.g., productivity loss) costs [9–13]; therefore, effective management of the condition is important.

Management options for TMD include occlusal splints, cognitive behavioural therapy, acupuncture, manual therapy, therapeutic exercises, nonsteroidal anti-inflammatory drugs, surgical treatment and others [14–19]. Counselling and a conservative approach are generally advocated as a first management choice by health professionals for patients with disabling TMD [19]. Previous systematic review suggested that manual therapy may improve pain intensity, function, and oral health-related quality of life in this population [19]; however, their scope and methods adopted might have compromised the effect estimates presented. These consist of the inclusion of trials that did not adequately compare manual therapy to investigate its effectiveness and the inclusion of non-randomised controlled trials (RCTs) [19]. In addition, the evidence needs updating, as new trials have been published since then. Thus, a new systematic review of randomized controlled trials that methodologically isolate manual therapy to assess its isolate or additional effects is needed to inform the current state of the evidence on this topic.

The aim of this systematic review of RCTs was to investigate the efficacy of manual therapy approaches and whether they enhance effects when combined with other active intervention on pain intensity, maximum mouth opening (MMO) and disability in TMD. The quality of evidence was assessed using the Grading of Recommendations Assessment (GRADE) approach [20].

2. Methods

2.1. Study Design

This systematic review of RCTs followed the Cochrane recommendations [21] and the Preferred Reporting Items for Systematic Reviews and Meta-Analyses (PRISMA) checklist [22] (Supplementary File S1: PRISMA checklist). Its protocol was prospectively registered in the International Prospective Registry of Systematic Reviews (PROSPERO) platform (CRD42022372298) and Open Science Framework (DOI: 10.17605/OSF.IO/XSN42).

2.2. Search Strategy and Study Selection

Searches were conducted on MEDLINE, COCHRANE, EMBASE, AMED, PSYCINFO and PEDRO without language or date restrictions up to 3 October 2022. Search terms were related to "randomised controlled trials" and "temporomandibular disorders". A detailed search strategy is in the Supplementary File S2: Search Strategy. In addition, we hand searched identified systematic reviews published in the field for potentially relevant full texts that do not identify in the optimized searches. After searches, the retrieved references were exported to an Endnote® file and duplicates were removed. Then, two independent reviewers (JPM and LAS) screened titles and abstracts and assessed potential full texts. Those trials fulfilling our eligibility criteria were included. The between-reviewer discrepancies were resolved by a third reviewer (VCO).

2.3. Inclusion and Exclusion Criteria

We included RCTs investigating people of both sexes, regardless of age, diagnosed with TMD of any duration or type/classification, i.e., myogenic, arthrogenic, mixed and joint-related disorders. The intervention of interest was any manual therapy approach, i.e., any clinician-applied movement of the joints and other structures such as joint mobilization or manipulation (thrust), massage, myofascial release techniques/soft-tissue mobilization, muscle energy techniques, passive stretching and others, as investigated previously [17], using the hands and/or any assisting device. We compared the intervention of interest with control (i.e., placebo, no intervention, waiting list or sham) to investigate the potential specific effects of manual therapy. To investigate whether manual therapy approaches enhance the estimated effects of other active intervention, we also considered comparisons between manual therapy approaches combined with any other active intervention and the other active intervention standing alone. Our outcomes of interest were pain intensity, maximum mouth opening/MMO (i.e., maximum distance between the edge of the upper incisors and the edge of the lower incisors with or without pain) and oral disability. We considered any valid instrument such as Visual Analog Scale—VAS or Numerical Rating Scales—NRS [23] for pain intensity, ruler and caliper for maximum mouth opening [24], and Jaw Functional Limitation Scale (JFLS) [25] and Mandibular Function Impairment Questionnaire (MFIQ) [26] for disability.

2.4. Data Extraction

Two independent reviewers (JPM and LAS) extracted characteristics and outcome data from included trials. Between-reviewer disagreements were resolved by a third reviewer (VCO). The extracted data include study type; the participants; details about the interventions and comparator; outcomes and time-points for the purpose of this review. For our outcomes of interest, we extracted post-intervention means (first option) or within-group mean changes over time, standard deviations (SDs) and sample sizes for each of our groups of interest to investigate the effects at immediate- short- and long-term. Immediate effects were considered as the point of measure right after a single session of manual therapy. We considered short-term effects follow-ups from one to 12 weeks after randomization and long-term effects as follow-ups over 12 weeks after randomization. If more than one time-point was available within the same follow-up period, the one closer to the end of the intervention was considered. When outcome data were not reported, at first, the authors were contacted. If we received no answer, we imputed when possible following the recommendations [21]. When authors did not respond and imputation was not possible, trials were excluded from the quantitative analysis.

2.5. Risk of Bias Assessment

Two independent reviewers (JPM and LAS) assessed the risk of bias of included trials using the 0–10 PEDRO scale [27]. According to this scale, higher scores represent a higher methodological quality. Discrepancies were resolved by a third reviewer (VCO). When available, we used scores already on the PEDRO database (https://pedro.org.au/, accessed on 10 November 2022).

2.6. Data Analysis

When possible, data were converted to a common scale and meta-analysis was conducted using random-effects models (DerSimonian and Laird method). Mean differences (MDs) and 95% CIs were reported in forest-plots. When it was not possible to convert data to a common scale, estimates were presented as standardized mean differences (SMDs). The clinical importance of the interventions of interest was interpreted by comparing the estimated effect sizes and 95% CI in association with the minimum clinically important difference (MCID) of the outcome of interest, or Minimal Detectable Change (MDC) when MCID was not available. MCID considered for pain intensity was 2 points on the 0–10 points scale [28]; MDC of 5 mm for MMO [29]; MDC of 8 points on the 0–68 on Migraine Functional Impact Questionnaire (MFIQ) or 7 points on the 0–63 on Craniofacial Pain and Disability Inventory (CF-PDI) [29] for disability. We used the Hedges' g effect size measure when estimates were presented as SMD, considering the cut-off points of 0.20, 0.50 and 0.80 for small, medium and large effects, respectively. All analyses were performed in the Comprehensive Meta-analysis software, version 2.2.04 (Biostat, Englewood, NJ, USA). Heterogeneity was assessed using I^2. We planned to perform subgroup and sensitivity analyses to assess the impact of potential sources of heterogeneity and risk of bias on the estimates. All procedures followed the recommended methods [21].

Two independent reviewers (JPM and LAS) assessed the quality of the current evidence using the GRADE system (Classification of Recommendations, Evaluation, Development and Evaluations) [30,31]. Any disagreement was resolved by consensus or a third reviewer (VCO). According to the four-level GRADE system, the evidence may range from high to very low quality, with low levels indicating that future high-quality trials are likely to change estimated effects. In the current review, evidence began from high quality and was downgraded for each of the following issues: serious imprecision when analysed sample less than 400 [32]; serious risk of bias when more than 25% of the analysed participants are from trials with a high risk of bias (i.e., PEDRO scores less than 7 out of 10) [33]; and serious inconsistency when $I^2 > 50\%$, visual inspection of forest plots or when pooling was not possible [21]. We evaluated the publication bias using visual inspection of funnel plots and the Egger's test adopting an $\alpha = 0.1$ when data from at least ten trials were pooled in the same meta-analysis [20,34].

3. Results

A total of 9639 records were retrieved from our searches, 6009 duplicates were removed, and the remaining 3630 titles and abstracts were screened. Then, 63 potential full texts were assessed for eligibility and 20 trials were included [35–54]. The study selection flow diagram is available in Figure 1.

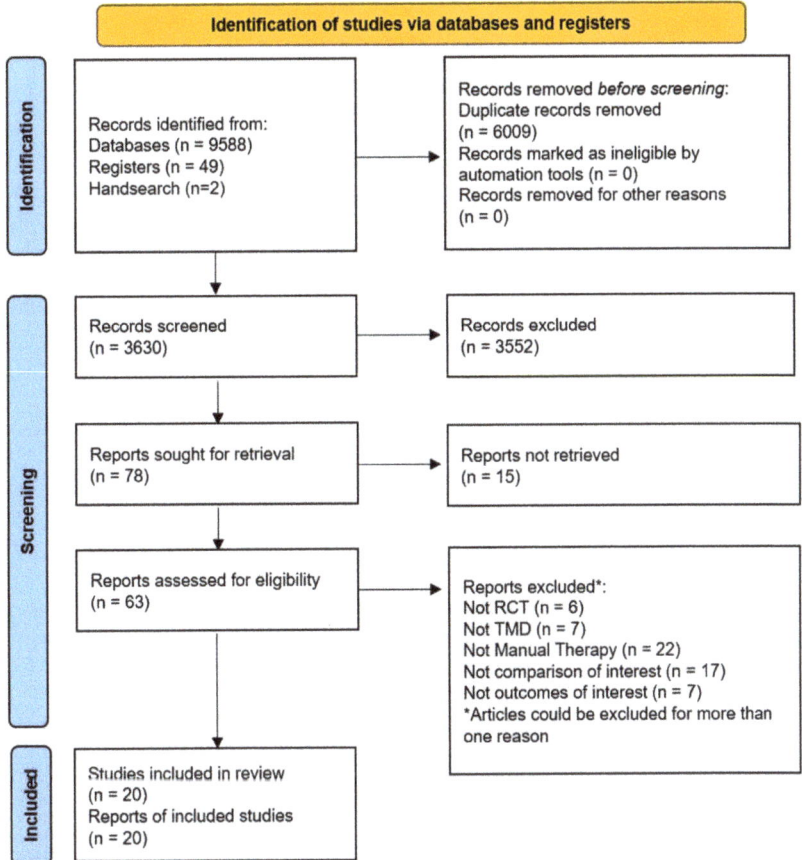

Figure 1. Flow of studies through the literature search and screening. RCT = randomised controlled trial; TMD = Temporomandibular disorders.

3.1. Characteristics of Included Trials and Assessment of Risk of Bias

The included trials were published between 2005 and 2022, conducted in Spain (five trials), Brazil (four trials), Japan (two trials), USA (two trials), Turkey (two trials), Australia (one trial), Iran (one trial), Portugal (one trial), Thailand (one trial) and Croatia (one trial). Most of them (85%) used some version of the Diagnostic Criteria for TMD. Five trials investigated the effects of manual therapy versus control (sham or wait list) and fifteen trials investigated the additional effects of manual therapy on pain intensity (16 trials), MMO (16 trials) and/or disability (7 trials).

The modalities of manual therapy used were manual pressure release techniques (six trials), joint manipulation (four trials), joint mobilization (one trial), soft-tissue mobilization (one trial), stretching (one trial), instrumental-assisted techniques (two trials), massage (one trial), multimodalities (i.e., combination of two or more modalities of manual therapy) (five trials) and not specified (one trial). When outcome data was not adequately provided, we contacted the authors but received no answer, so we reported the findings that were available. Findings from trials with skewed data were reported separately. Further information regards the characteristics of the included trials are presented in Table 1.

Table 1. Characteristics of the included trials (n = 20).

Study	Local	Participants	Intervention	Outcome Time-Points
Alajbeg et al., 2015 [35]	Croatia	12 participants (M = 3; F = 9), mean age of 30.5 ± 14 y/o, with TMJ disc displacement based on DC/TMD and MRI.	EG = Joint mobilization + Massage + Stabilization occlusal splint CG = Stabilization occlusal splint	Pain intensity (0–100 VAS); MMO Short and long-term.
Antunez et al., 2015 [36]	Spain	42 participants (M = 14; F = 28), mean age of 21.2 ± 1.6 y/o; TMD (myofascial pain) based on DC/TMD, for ≥6 months.	EG = Ischemic compression technique on the masseter muscle + stretching of hamstrings CG = PNF stretching of hamstrings	Pain intensity (0–10 VAS); MMO (Caliper); Immediate effects
Blanco et al., 2015 [37]	Spain	60 participants (M = 19; F = 41), mean age 35.2 ± 12 y/o, with TMD (myofascial pain) for ≥6 months based on DC/TMD; restricted cervical mobility.	EG = Suboccipital muscle inhibition + Pressure release massage + stretching. CG = Pressure release massage + stretching	MMO (Caliper); Immediate effects
Brochado et al., 2017 [38]	Brazil	28 participants (M = 1; F = 27), mean age 44.5 ± 17 y/o, with TMD (myogenic and arthrogenic) based on DC/TMD.	EG = Pressure Release Massage + Joint Mobilization + Photobiomodulation. CG = Photobiomodulation	Pain intensity (0–10 VAS) Short and long-term.
Devocht et al., 2013 [39]	USA	39 amateur athletes (M = 8; F = 31), mean age of 33 y/o, with TMD (myofascial pain) based on DC/TMD, for at ≥6 months.	EG = Mechanically assisted manipulation (hand-held spring-loaded instrument)—12 sessions for 2 months. CG = Sham Device	Pain intensity (0–10 NRS) Short and Long-term
Gomes et al., 2014 [40]	Brazil	30 participants (M = 4; F = 26), mean age of 27 ± 1.6 y/o, with severe TMD and bruxism.	EG = Massage + Occlusal splint—3 times week, for 4 weeks. CG = Occlusal splint	Oral Disability (0–100 FPHI) Short-term
Hernanz et al., 2018 [41]	Spain	72 participants (M = 12; F = 60), mean age 42 y/o, with TMD (myofascial pain) based on DC/TMD for ≥6 months.	EG = Pressure Release Technique + Occlusal splint + education CG = Sham + Occlusal splint and education	Pain intensity (0–10 VAS). MMO Short and long-term.
Kalamir et al., 2011 [42]	Australia	60 participants (M = 26; F = 34), age between 18–50 y/o, with TMD based on DC/TMD for ≥3 months.	EG = Intraoral manual pressure—2 times week for 5 weeks CG = Waitlist	Pain intensity (0–10 NRS); MMO (caliper); Short and Long-term

Table 1. Cont.

Study	Local	Participants	Intervention	Outcome Time-Points
Kanhachon et al., 2021 [43]	Thailand	38 academics (M = 4; F = 34), mean age of 25 ± 5 y/o, with pain on the neck, scapular, and jaw for more than 3 months, with a referral pattern.	EG = Active Stretching Release Therapy + hot pack on jaw and scapular areas + education CG = Hot pack on jaw and scapular areas + education	Pain intensity (0–10 VAS); MMO (therabite device)® Immediate, short-term
La Touche et al., 2013 [44]	Spain	32 patients (M = 11; F = 21), mean age 34 y/o, with TMD (myofascial pain)—DC/TMD.	EG = Upper cervical mobilization—3 sessions over 2 weeks. CG = Sham	Pain intensity (0–100 VAS) Immediate, short-term
Leite et al., 2020 [45]	Brazil	48 women, age between 18–45 y/o, with TMD (pain dysfunction) based on DC/TMD, for ≥6 months.	EG = Diacutaneous Fibrolysis—2 sessions week for 4 weeks CG = Sham	Pain intensity (0–100 VAS); MMO (Calliper); Disability (0–68 MFIQ) Short-term
Lucas et al., 2017 [46]	Portugal	20 participants with pain on masticatory muscles and/or TMJ according to DC/TMD.	EG = Manual Therapy + Therapeutic Exercises—2 sessions week for 6 weeks CG = Therapeutic Exercises	Pain intensity (0–10 NRS); MMO Immediate effects
Nagata et al., 2019 [47]	Japan	61 participants (M = 11; F = 50), mean age of 49.6 ± 25 y/o, with TMD based on DC/TMD and MRI.	EG = Joint manipulation + self-exercise + CBT + education. CG = Self-exercise + CBT + education.	Pain intensity (0–10 NRS). MMO (caliper). Immediate, short and long-term
Packer et al., 2015 [48]	Brazil	32 women, mean age 24 ± 5 y/o, with TMD based on DC/TMD	EG = Upper thoracic manipulation CG = Sham	MMO (caliper). Immediate, short-term
Reynolds et al., 2020 [49]	USA	50 participants (M = 7; F = 43), mean age of 24.78 ± 5.4 y/o, with TMD according to DC/TMD.	EG = Cervical HVLAT + suboccipital release + education + home exercises CG = Sham HVLAT + suboccipital release + education + home exercises	Pain intensity (0–10 NRS); MMO (ROM scale). Disability (0–20 JFLS) Immediate, short-term
Rezaie et al., 2022 [50]	Iran	30 participants (M = 13; F = 17), mean age of 28 y/o, with TMD according to DC/TMD, for ≥3 months.	EG = Joint and soft-tissue mobilization on TMJ and cervical spine + Massage + UST + TENS CG: Massage + UST + TENS	Pain intensity (0–10 NRS); MMO (Calliper); Short and long-term
Sahin et al., 2020 [51]	Turkey	42 participants (M = 10; F = 32), mean age of 26.2 y/o, with TMD according to DC/TMD and trigger-point in the masseter muscle.	EG = Ischemic compression technique + Postural and Rocabado's 6 × 6 exercises. CG =Postural and Rocabado's 6 × 6 exercises	Pain intensity (0–10 VAS). MMO (Ruler). Disability (JFLS-8) Short-term
Serna et al., 2019 [52]	Spain	61 participants (M = 25; F = 36), age between 18 and 65 y/o, with tinnitus symptoms and TMD according to DC/TMD.	EG = Multimodal Manual therapy + Cervical and TMJ exercises + Self-massage + education—for 5 weeks CG = Cervical and TMJ exercises + Self-massage + education	Pain intensity (0–10 NRS); MMO (Adapted-Ruler); Disability (0–63 CF-PDI) Short and long-term

Table 1. Cont.

Study	Local	Participants	Intervention	Outcome Time-Points
Tuncer et al., 2012 [53]	Turkey	40 participants (M = 9; F = 31), age between 18–72 y/o, with TMD and disc displacement based on DC/TMD for ≥3 months.	EG = Soft tissue and joint mobilization + TMJ exercises and stretching + Education CG = TMJ exercises and stretching + Education	Pain intensity (0–100 VAS); MMO (Ruler) Short-term
Yoshida et al., 2005 [54]	Japan	305 participants (M = 76; F = 229), age between 18–74 y/o, with TMJ disc displacement.	EG = Jaw joint manipulation + NSAIDs CG = NSAIDs	MMO Immediate effects

TMD = Temporomandibular disorder; TMJ = Temporomandibular Joint; M = Male; F = Female; y/o = years old; DC/TMD = Diagnostic Criteria Temporomandibular Disorders; VAS = Visual Analogue Scale; NRS = Numerical Rating Scale; MMO = Maximum Mouth Opening (with or without pain); EG = Experimental Group; CG = Control Group; CBT = Cognitive-behavioural therapy; PNF = Proprioceptive Neuromuscular Facilitation; HVLAT= High-velocity, low amplitude technique; FPHI = Fonseca Patient History Index; NDI = Neck disability Index; MFIQ = Migraine Functional Impact Questionnaire; JFLS = Jaw Functional Limitation Scale; MRI = Magnetic Resonance Imaging; CF-PDI = Craniofacial Pain and Disability Inventory; NSAID = Nonsteroidal anti-inflammatory drug.

The PEDRO scores of the included trials ranged from 1 to 9 points out of 10 (median = 7 points). Fourteen trials (70%) were classified as low risk of bias (i.e., scores ≥ 7 points). The main reasons for increasing risk of bias were not blinding therapists (20 trials [100%]), not blinding participants (14 trials [70%]), not performing concealed allocation (7 trials [35%]) and not blinding assessors and not performing an intention-to-treat analysis (5 trials [25%]). Detailed risk of bias assessment is presented in Table 2.

Table 2. Risk of bias assessment—Pedro scale (n = 20).

Study	A	B	C	D	E	F	G	H	I	J	Score (0–10)
Alajbeg et al., 2015 [35]	Y	N	Y	N	N	Y	Y	Y	N	Y	6
Antunez et al., 2015 [36]	Y	N	Y	N	N	Y	Y	Y	N	Y	6
Blanco et al., 2015 [37]	Y	N	Y	Y	N	Y	Y	Y	Y	Y	8
Brochado et al., 2017 [38]	Y	N	Y	N	N	Y	N	Y	Y	Y	6
Devocht et al., 2013 [39]	Y	Y	Y	N	N	N	N	Y	Y	Y	6
Gomes et al., 2014 [40]	Y	Y	N	N	N	Y	Y	Y	Y	Y	7
Hernanz et al., 2018 [41]	Y	Y	Y	Y	N	N	Y	N	Y	Y	7
Kalamir et al., 2011 [42]	Y	Y	Y	N	N	Y	Y	Y	Y	N	7
Kanhachon et al., 2021 [43]	Y	Y	Y	N	N	Y	Y	Y	Y	Y	8
La Touche et al., 2013 [44]	Y	Y	Y	Y	N	Y	Y	Y	Y	Y	9
Leite et al., 2020 [45]	Y	N	Y	Y	N	Y	Y	Y	Y	Y	8
Lucas et al., 2017 [46]	Y	N	N	N	N	N	Y	N	N	N	2
Nagata et al., 2019 [47]	Y	Y	Y	N	N	N	Y	Y	Y	Y	7
Packer et al., 2015 [48]	Y	Y	Y	N	N	Y	Y	Y	N	Y	7
Reynolds et al., 2020 [49]	Y	Y	Y	Y	N	Y	Y	Y	Y	Y	9
Rezaie et al., 2022 [50]	Y	Y	Y	Y	N	Y	N	N	Y	Y	7
Sahin et al., 2020 [51]	Y	Y	Y	N	N	Y	Y	N	Y	Y	7
Serna et al., 2019 [52]	Y	Y	Y	N	N	Y	Y	Y	Y	Y	8
Tuncer et al., 2012 [53]	Y	Y	Y	N	N	Y	Y	Y	Y	Y	8
Yoshida et al., 2005 [54]	Y	N	N	N	N	N	N	N	N	N	1

Y = yes; N = no; A = Random allocation; B = Concealed allocation; C = Baseline Comparability; D = Blind subjects; E = Blind therapists; F = Blind assessors; G = Adequate follow-up; H = Intention-to-treat analysis; I = Between-group comparisons; J = Point estimates and variability.

3.2. Effects of Manual Therapy on Pain Intensity in People with Temporomandibular Disorders

Four trials [39,42,44,45] investigated the effects of manual therapy when compared with control (sham or waiting list) and twelve trials investigated the additional effects of manual therapy when combined with other active intervention on pain intensity [35,36,38,41,43,46,47,49–53]. Seven trials used the 0–10 NRS [39,42,46,47,49,50,52], five trials used the 0–10 VAS [36,38,41,43,51] and four trials used the 0–100 VAS [35,44,45,53]. For pooling, outcome data were converted to a common 0–10 points scale.

3.2.1. Manual Therapy versus Control on Pain Intensity

One trial [44] provided low quality evidence of an immediate effect of manual therapy on pain intensity (MD = −0.88 points on the 0–10 points scale, 95% CI −1.57 to −0.19; n = 32). Data from three trials [39,44,45] also provided low quality evidence of a potential short-term effect for manual therapy on pain intensity (95% CI −3.46 to −0.20; I^2 = 0.0; n = 111). Long-term, one trial [39] provided very-low quality evidence of no difference (95% CI −1.33 to 1.13; n = 39) (Figure 2). It was not possible to include one trial in the pooling due to skewed data [42]. In this trial, the author reported a statistically significant difference in favour of manual therapy versus control at short- and long-terms; however, no detailed information in regards to the between-group difference and variability was reported.

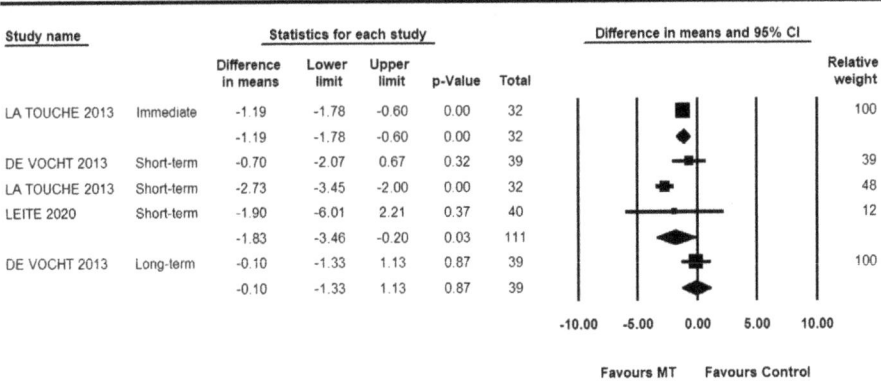

Figure 2. Forest plot of manual therapy versus control on pain intensity at immediate-, short- and long-term. Studies included were: Devocht et al., 2013 [39]; La Touche et al., 2013 [44]; Leite et al., 2020 [45].

3.2.2. Additional Effects of Manual Therapy on Pain Intensity

Five trials [36,43,46,47,49] investigated the immediate additional effects of manual therapy on pain intensity, and two of them were not pooled due to skewed data [36] and lack of standard deviation measures [46]. Pooled data provided moderate quality evidence for no immediate additional effect of manual therapy on pain intensity (95% CI −1.61 to 0.10; I^2 = 0.0; n = 149). One of the two trials not pooled [36] also showed no immediate additional effect for manual therapy (p = 0.53); however, the other trial [46] suggested an additional effect of manual therapy combined with exercise when compared with exercises alone (−2.9 points out of 10).

Short-term, high-quality evidence from 10 trials showed an additional effect of manual therapy on pain intensity (95% CI −2.12 to −0.82; I^2 = 10; n = 434). Publication bias was not found (Supplementary File S3: Funnel plot), and sensitivity analysis removing trials with a high risk of bias [35,38] did not detect any potential impact on the estimates (95% CI −2.41 to −1.00; 8 trials, n = 394). We also conducted a subgroup analysis exploring whether different modalities of manual therapy impacted on the estimates; no impact was found. Findings are available on Supplementary File S4: Manual therapy modalities subgroup analysis on pain intensity.

At long-term, moderate quality evidence from six trials supported an additional effect of manual therapy (95% CI −2.17 to −0.40; $I^2 = 0.0$; n = 342). Forest plots with estimates in the different time-points are shown in Figure 3.

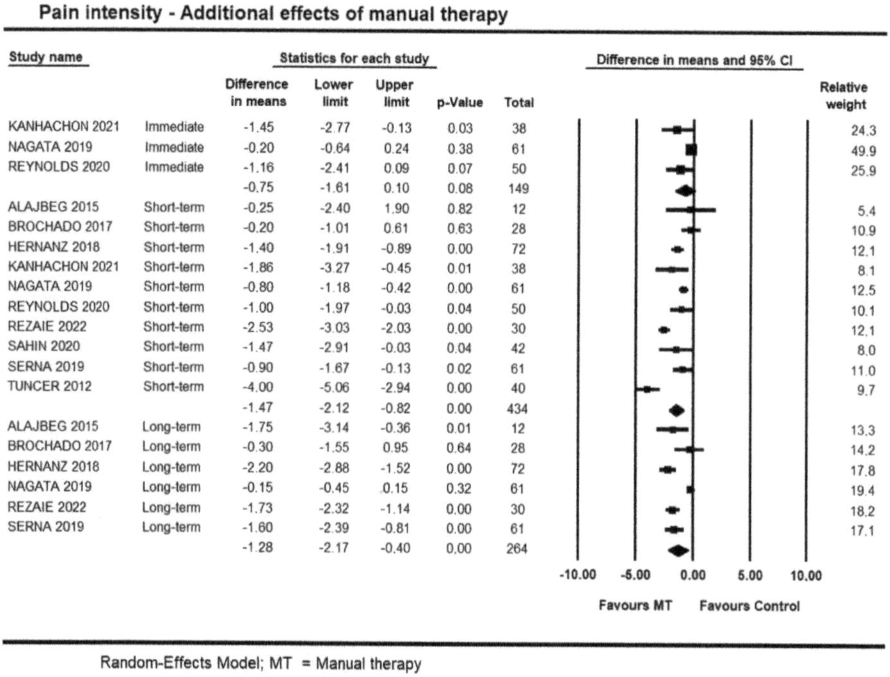
Pain intensity - Additional effects of manual therapy
Study name
Statistics for each study
Difference in means and 95% CI
Difference in means | Lower limit | Upper limit | p-Value | Total
Relative weight
KANHACHON 2021 | Immediate | -1.45 | -2.77 | -0.13 | 0.03 | 38 | 24.3
NAGATA 2019 | Immediate | -0.20 | -0.64 | 0.24 | 0.38 | 61 | 49.9
REYNOLDS 2020 | Immediate | -1.16 | -2.41 | 0.09 | 0.07 | 50 | 25.9
-0.75 | -1.61 | 0.10 | 0.08 | 149
ALAJBEG 2015 | Short-term | -0.25 | -2.40 | 1.90 | 0.82 | 12 | 5.4
BROCHADO 2017 | Short-term | -0.20 | -1.01 | 0.61 | 0.63 | 28 | 10.9
HERNANZ 2018 | Short-term | -1.40 | -1.91 | -0.89 | 0.00 | 72 | 12.1
KANHACHON 2021 | Short-term | -1.86 | -3.27 | -0.45 | 0.01 | 38 | 8.1
NAGATA 2019 | Short-term | -0.80 | -1.18 | -0.42 | 0.00 | 61 | 12.5
REYNOLDS 2020 | Short-term | -1.00 | -1.97 | -0.03 | 0.04 | 50 | 10.1
REZAIE 2022 | Short-term | -2.53 | -3.03 | -2.03 | 0.00 | 30 | 12.1
SAHIN 2020 | Short-term | -1.47 | -2.91 | -0.03 | 0.04 | 42 | 8.0
SERNA 2019 | Short-term | -0.90 | -1.67 | -0.13 | 0.02 | 61 | 11.0
TUNCER 2012 | Short-term | -4.00 | -5.06 | -2.94 | 0.00 | 40 | 9.7
-1.47 | -2.12 | -0.82 | 0.00 | 434
ALAJBEG 2015 | Long-term | -1.75 | -3.14 | -0.36 | 0.01 | 12 | 13.3
BROCHADO 2017 | Long-term | -0.30 | -1.55 | 0.95 | 0.64 | 28 | 14.2
HERNANZ 2018 | Long-term | -2.20 | -2.88 | -1.52 | 0.00 | 72 | 17.8
NAGATA 2019 | Long-term | -0.15 | -0.45 | 0.15 | 0.32 | 61 | 19.4
REZAIE 2022 | Long-term | -1.73 | -2.32 | -1.14 | 0.00 | 30 | 18.2
SERNA 2019 | Long-term | -1.60 | -2.39 | -0.81 | 0.00 | 61 | 17.1
-1.28 | -2.17 | -0.40 | 0.00 | 264
-10.00 -5.00 0.00 5.00 10.00
Favours MT
Favours Control
Random-Effects Model; MT = Manual therapy

Figure 3. Forest plot of the additional effects of manual therapy on pain intensity at immediate-, short- and long-term. Studies included were: Alajbeg et al., 2015 [35]; Brochado et al., 2017 [38]; Hernanz et al., 2018 [41]; Kanhachon et al., 2021 [43]; Nagata et al., 2019 [47]; Reynolds et al., 2020 [49]; Rezaie et al., 2022 [50]; Sahin et al., 2020 [51]; Serna et al., 2019 [52]; Tuncer et al., 2012.

3.3. *Effects of Manual Therapy on Maximum Mouth Opening in People with Temporomandibular Disorders*

Three trials [42,45,48] investigated the effects of manual therapy when compared with the control (sham or waiting list) and 13 trials investigated its additional effects on MMO [35–37,41,43,46,47,49–54]. MMO was assessed with Caliper in six trials [36,37,45,47,48,50], with Ruler in three trials [51–53], with other measurement tools in two trials [42,49] and four trials did not report the instrument used [35,41,46,54].

3.3.1. Manual Therapy versus Control on Maximum Mouth Opening

One trial [48] provided low quality evidence of no immediate effect of manual therapy on MMO (95% CI −4.64 to 8.64; n = 32). Short-term, moderate quality evidence from two trials [45,48] showed an effect on MMO (95% CI 0.01 to 7.30 mm; $I^2 = 0.0$; n = 72) (Figure 4). One trial [42] was not included in the pooling due to skewed data. A statistically significant difference was reported in favour of manual therapy versus control at the short- and long-term. No detailed information was available.

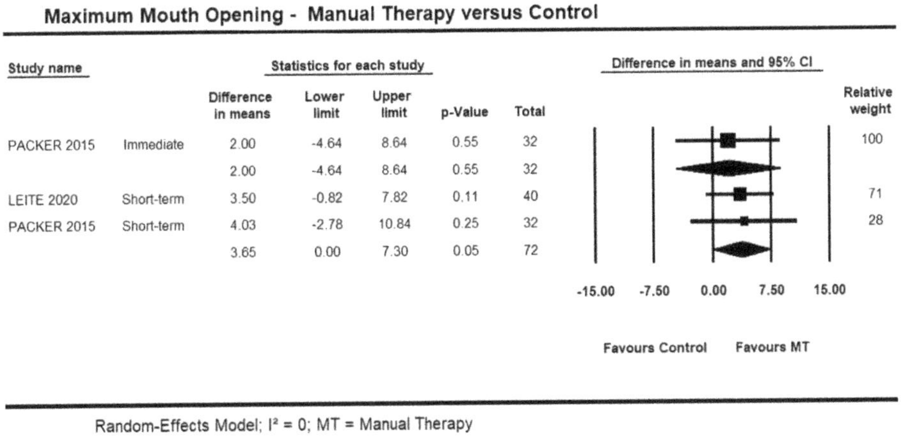

Maximum Mouth Opening - Manual Therapy versus Control

Study name		Statistics for each study					Difference in means and 95% CI	Relative weight
		Difference in means	Lower limit	Upper limit	p-Value	Total		
PACKER 2015	Immediate	2.00	-4.64	8.64	0.55	32		100
		2.00	-4.64	8.64	0.55	32		
LEITE 2020	Short-term	3.50	-0.82	7.82	0.11	40		71
PACKER 2015	Short-term	4.03	-2.78	10.84	0.25	32		28
		3.65	0.00	7.30	0.05	72		

-15.00   -7.50   0.00   7.50   15.00

Favours Control   Favours MT

Random-Effects Model; $I^2 = 0$; MT = Manual Therapy

Figure 4. Forest plot of manual therapy versus control on maximum mouth opening at immediate- and short-term. Studies included were: Leite et al., 2020 [45]; Packer et al., 2015.

3.3.2. Additional Effects of Manual Therapy on Maximum Mouth Opening

Seven trials [35,37,43,46,47,49,54] investigated the immediate additional effects of manual therapy on MMO. It was possible to pool data from five of them [35,37,43,47,49] due to a lack of standard deviations [46,54]. Moderate quality evidence demonstrated no between-group differences (95% CI −0.91 to 6.20 mm; $I^2 = 0.0$; n = 251). Contradictory findings were reported by the other two trials not included in the meta-analysis: Yoshida et al. [54] and Lucas et al. [46] found a between-group difference in favour of manual therapy on MMO.

Short-term, high-quality evidence from nine trials showed an additional effect of manual therapy on MMO (95% CI 1.58 to 3.58 mm; $I^2 = 0$; n = 494). Sensitivity analysis removing trials with high risk of bias [38] did not suggest an impact on the estimates (95% CI 1.43 to 3.88 mm; 8 trials, n = 394).

Long-term, moderate quality evidence from six trials showed an effect of manual therapy on MMO (95% CI 1.22 to 8.40 mm; $I^2 = 0.0$; n = 264). Sensitivity analysis removing trials with high risk of bias [35,38] did not suggest an impact on the estimates (95% CI 0.24 to 3.88; $I^2 = 0.0$; 4 trials, n = 224). Forest Plots with estimates at different time points are shown in Figure 5.

3.4. Effects of Manual Therapy on Disability in People with Temporomandibular Disorders

For disability, one trial [45] investigated the effects of manual therapy when compared with control (sham or wait list) and four trials investigated the additional effects of manual therapy [40,49,51,52]. The outcome measures used were the 0–68 MFIQ [45], the 0–100 Fonseca Patient History Index (FPHI) [40], the 0–8 points JFLS [51], the 0–20 points JFLS [49] and the 0–63 points Craniofacial Pain and Disability Inventory (CF-PDI) [52]. Due to the heterogeneity of measures, we reported SMD.

3.4.1. Manual Therapy versus Control on Disability

Short-term, one trial [45] suggested an effect of manual therapy on disability when compared with control. Post-intervention disability differed 6.5% in favour of manual therapy ($p = 0.01$).

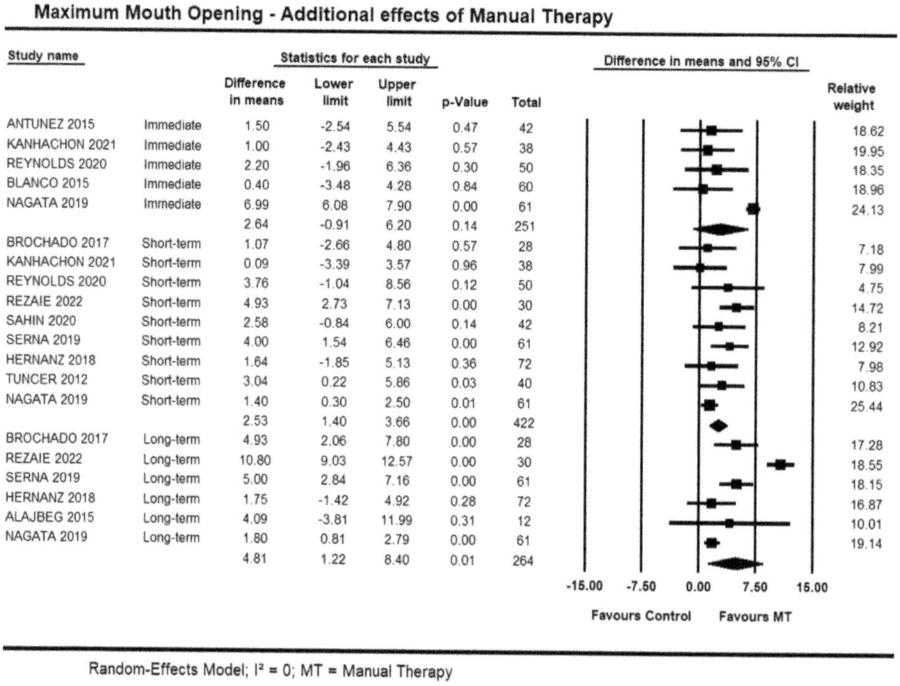

Maximum Mouth Opening - Additional effects of Manual Therapy

Study name		Difference in means	Lower limit	Upper limit	p-Value	Total	Relative weight
ANTUNEZ 2015	Immediate	1.50	-2.54	5.54	0.47	42	18.62
KANHACHON 2021	Immediate	1.00	-2.43	4.43	0.57	38	19.95
REYNOLDS 2020	Immediate	2.20	-1.96	6.36	0.30	50	18.35
BLANCO 2015	Immediate	0.40	-3.48	4.28	0.84	60	18.96
NAGATA 2019	Immediate	6.99	6.08	7.90	0.00	61	24.13
		2.64	-0.91	6.20	0.14	251	
BROCHADO 2017	Short-term	1.07	-2.66	4.80	0.57	28	7.18
KANHACHON 2021	Short-term	0.09	-3.39	3.57	0.96	38	7.99
REYNOLDS 2020	Short-term	3.76	-1.04	8.56	0.12	50	4.75
REZAIE 2022	Short-term	4.93	2.73	7.13	0.00	30	14.72
SAHIN 2020	Short-term	2.58	-0.84	6.00	0.14	42	8.21
SERNA 2019	Short-term	4.00	1.54	6.46	0.00	61	12.92
HERNANZ 2018	Short-term	1.64	-1.85	5.13	0.36	72	7.98
TUNCER 2012	Short-term	3.04	0.22	5.86	0.03	40	10.83
NAGATA 2019	Short-term	1.40	0.30	2.50	0.01	61	25.44
		2.53	1.40	3.66	0.00	422	
BROCHADO 2017	Long-term	4.93	2.06	7.80	0.00	28	17.28
REZAIE 2022	Long-term	10.80	9.03	12.57	0.00	30	18.55
SERNA 2019	Long-term	5.00	2.84	7.16	0.00	61	18.15
HERNANZ 2018	Long-term	1.75	-1.42	4.92	0.28	72	16.87
ALAJBEG 2015	Long-term	4.09	-3.81	11.99	0.31	12	10.01
NAGATA 2019	Long-term	1.80	0.81	2.79	0.00	61	19.14
		4.81	1.22	8.40	0.01	264	

Random-Effects Model; I² = 0; MT = Manual Therapy

Figure 5. Forest plot of the additional effects of manual therapy on maximum mouth opening at immediate-, short- and long-term. Studies included were: Alajbeg et al., 2015 [35]; Antunez et al., 2015 [36]; Blanco et al., 2015 [37]; Brochado et al., 2017 [38]; Hernanz et al., 2018 [41]; Kanhachon et al., 2021 [43]; Nagata et al., 2019 [47]; Reynolds et al., 2020 [49]; Rezaie et al., 2022 [50]; Sahin et al., 2020 [51]; Serna et al., 2019 [52]; Tuncer et al., 2012 [53].

3.4.2. Additional Effects of Manual Therapy on Disability

At short-term, moderate quality evidence from four trials showed an additional effect of manual therapy on disability (SMD = −0.51, 95% CI −0.87 to −0.14; n = 183). At long-term, one trial [52] provided low quality evidence for an additional effect of manual therapy on the disability (95% CI −7.01 to −1.39; I² = 8.17; n = 61) (Figure 6).

The overall quality of evidence in the systematic review ranged from very low to high. The summary of findings with the GRADE assessment is reported in Table 3.

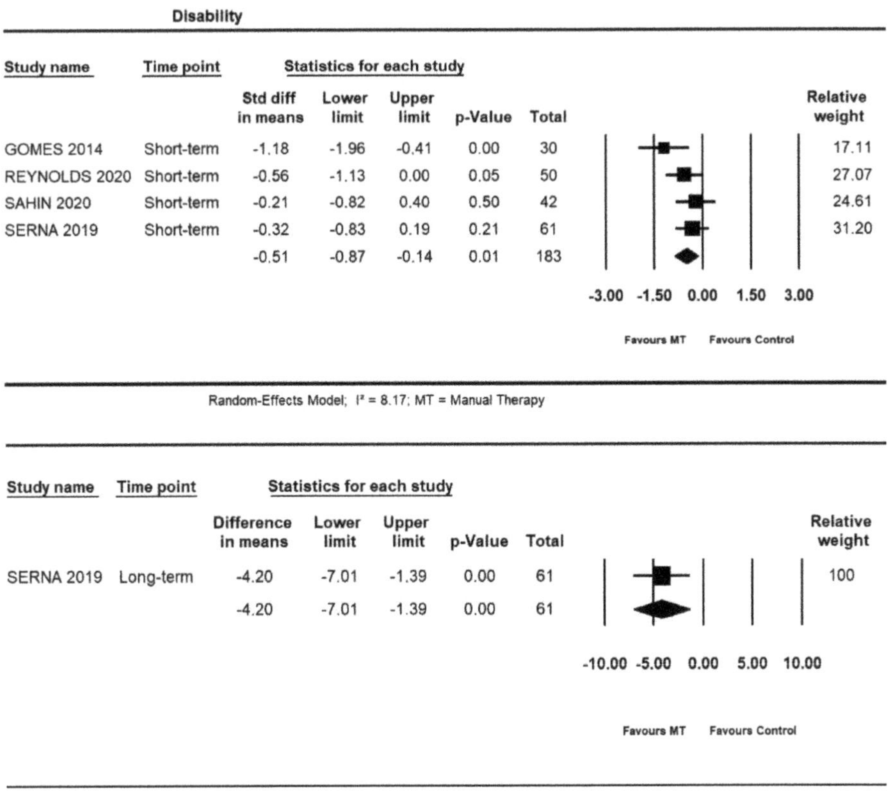
Disability
Study name
Time point
Statistics for each study
Std diff in means
Lower limit
Upper limit
p-Value
Total
Relative weight
GOMES 2014 Short-term -1.18 -1.96 -0.41 0.00 30 17.11
REYNOLDS 2020 Short-term -0.56 -1.13 0.00 0.05 50 27.07
SAHIN 2020 Short-term -0.21 -0.82 0.40 0.50 42 24.61
SERNA 2019 Short-term -0.32 -0.83 0.19 0.21 61 31.20
-0.51 -0.87 -0.14 0.01 183
-3.00 -1.50 0.00 1.50 3.00
Favours MT
Favours Control
Random-Effects Model; I² = 8.17; MT = Manual Therapy
Study name
Time point
Statistics for each study
Difference in means
Lower limit
Upper limit
p-Value
Total
Relative weight
SERNA 2019 Long-term -4.20 -7.01 -1.39 0.00 61 100
-4.20 -7.01 -1.39 0.00 61
-10.00 -5.00 0.00 5.00 10.00
Favours MT
Favours Control

Figure 6. Forest plot of the additional effects of manual therapy on disability short- and long-term. The studies included were: Gomes et al., 2014 [40]; Reynolds et al., 2020 [49]; Sahin et al., 2020 [51]; Serna et al., 2019 [52].

Table 3. Summary of findings with grade assessment (n = 20).

Population: People with Temporomandibular Disorder.
Intervention: Manual Pressure Release techniques (6 trials); Joint manipulation (4 trials); Joint mobilization (1 trial); Soft-tissue mobilization (1 trial); Stretching (1 trial); Instrumental-assisted techniques (2 trials); Massage (1 trial); MTs in combination (5 trials); Not specified (1 trial).
Comparison: No intervention (13 trials), sham (6 trials), wait-list (1 trial).
Outcome: Pain intensity (15 trials); MMO (15 trials); Disability (5 trials).
Setting: Spain (5 trials); Brazil (4 trials); Japan (2 trials); USA (2 trials); Turkey (2 trials); Australia (1 trial); Iran (1 trial); Portugal (1 trial); Thailand (1 trial); Croatia (1 trial).

Outcome Time-Point	MD or SMD (CI 95%)	Sample Size (No. of Studies)	GRADE Assessment	Comments
MT vs. Control 0–10 Pain intensity Immediate-effects	−0.88 (−1.57 to −0.19)	32 (1 study)	⊕⊕⊖⊖ LOW [a,b]	The difference is statistically significant but not clinically important based on a MCID = 2.
MT add effects 0–10 Pain intensity Immediate-effects	−0.75 (−1.61 to 0.10)	149 (3 studies)	⊕⊕⊕⊖ MODERATE [a]	The difference is not statistically significant.

Table 3. *Cont.*

Population: People with Temporomandibular Disorder.
Intervention: Manual Pressure Release techniques (6 trials); Joint manipulation (4 trials); Joint mobilization (1 trial); Soft-tissue mobilization (1 trial); Stretching (1 trial); Instrumental-assisted techniques (2 trials); Massage (1 trial); MTs in combination (5 trials); Not specified (1 trial).
Comparison: No intervention (13 trials), sham (6 trials), wait-list (1 trial).
Outcome: Pain intensity (15 trials); MMO (15 trials); Disability (5 trials).
Setting: Spain (5 trials); Brazil (4 trials); Japan (2 trials); USA (2 trials); Turkey (2 trials); Australia (1 trial); Iran (1 trial); Portugal (1 trial); Thailand (1 trial); Croatia (1 trial).

Outcome Time-Point	MD or SMD (CI 95%)	Sample Size (No. of Studies)	GRADE Assessment	Comments
MT vs. Control 0–10 Pain intensity Short-term	−1.83 (−3.46 to −0.20)	111 (3 studies)	⊕⊕⊖⊖ LOW [a,c]	The difference is statistically significant but may not be clinically important based on a MCID = 2.
MT add effects 0–10 Pain intensity Short-term	−1.47 (−2.12 to −0.82)	434 (10 studies)	⊕⊕⊕⊕ HIGH	The difference is statistically significant but may not be clinically important based on a MCID = 2.
MT vs. Control 0–10 Pain intensity Long-term	−0.10 (−1.33 to 1.13)	39 (1 study)	⊕⊖⊖⊖ VERY LOW [a,b,c]	The difference is not statistically significant.
MT add effects 0–10 Pain intensity Long-term	−1.28 (−2.17 to −0.40)	342 (6 studies)	⊕⊕⊕⊖ MODERATE [a]	The difference is statistically significant but may not be clinically important based on a MCID = 2.
Joint Manipulation 0–10 Pain intensity Short-term	−0.83 (−1.18 to −0.47)	111 (2 studies)	⊕⊕⊕⊖ MODERATE [a]	Subgroup analysis—MT modalities The difference is statistically significant but not clinically important based on a MCID = 2.
Manual Pressure 0–10 Pain intensity Short-term	−1.41 (−1.89 to −0.93)	114 (2 studies)	⊕⊕⊕⊖ MODERATE [a]	Subgroup analysis—MT modalities The difference is statistically significant but not clinically important based on a MCID of 2 points.
Multimodal 0–10 Pain intensity Short-term	−1.65 (−2.98 to −0.32)	171 (5 studies)	⊕⊕⊕⊖ MODERATE [a]	Subgroup analysis—MT modalities The difference is statistically significant but may not be clinically important based on a MCID = 2.
Stretching 0–10 Pain intensity Short-term	−1.86 (−3.27 to −0.45)	3 8(1 study)	⊕⊕⊖⊖ LOW [a,b]	Subgroup analysis—MT modalities The difference is statistically significant but may not be clinically important based on a MCID = 2.
MT vs. Control MMO—mm Immediate-effects	2.0 (−4.64 to 8.64)	32 (1 study)	⊕⊕⊖⊖ LOW [a,b]	The difference is not statistically significant.
MT add effects MMO—mm Immediate-effects	2.64 (−0.91 to 6.20)	251 (5 studies)	⊕⊕⊕⊖ MODERATE [a]	The difference is not statistically significant.
MT vs. Control MMO—mm Short-term	3.65 (0.00 to 7.30)	72 (2 studies)	⊕⊕⊕⊖ MODERATE [a]	The difference is statistically significant but may be not clinically important based on a MDC of 5 mm
MT add effects MMO—mm Short-term	2.5 8(1.58 to 3.58)	494 (9 studies)	⊕⊕⊕⊕ HIGH	The difference is statistically significant but not clinically important based on a MDC of 5 mm

Table 3. Cont.

Population: People with Temporomandibular Disorder.
Intervention: Manual Pressure Release techniques (6 trials); Joint manipulation (4 trials); Joint mobilization (1 trial); Soft-tissue mobilization (1 trial); Stretching (1 trial); Instrumental-assisted techniques (2 trials); Massage (1 trial); MTs in combination (5 trials); Not specified (1 trial).
Comparison: No intervention (13 trials), sham (6 trials), wait-list (1 trial).
Outcome: Pain intensity (15 trials); MMO (15 trials); Disability (5 trials).
Setting: Spain (5 trials); Brazil (4 trials); Japan (2 trials); USA (2 trials); Turkey (2 trials); Australia (1 trial); Iran (1 trial); Portugal (1 trial); Thailand (1 trial); Croatia (1 trial).

Outcome Time-Point	MD or SMD (CI 95%)	Sample Size (No. of Studies)	GRADE Assessment	Comments
MT add effects MMO—mm Long-term	4.81 (1.22 to 8.40)	264 (6 study)	⊕⊕⊕⊖ MODERATE [a]	The difference is statistically significant but may not be clinically important based on a MDC = 5 mm.
MT add effects Disability Short-term	−0.51 (−0.87 to −0.14) *	183 (4 studies)	⊕⊕⊕⊖ MODERATE [a]	The difference is statistically significant and may have a Moderate effect size based on the Hedges'g cut-off point of 0.5.
MT vs. Control Disability Long-term	−4.20 (−7.01 to −1.39)	61 (1 study)	⊕⊕⊖⊖ LOW [a,b]	The difference is statistically significant but not clinically important based on a MDC = 8.

GRADE Working Group grades of evidence
High certainty: We are very confident that the true effect lies close to that of the estimate of the effect;
Moderate certainty: We are moderately confident in the effect estimate: The true effect is likely to be close to the estimate of the effect, but there is a possibility that it is substantially different;
Low certainty: Confidence in the effect estimate is limited: The true effect may be substantially different from the estimated;
Very low certainty: We have very little confidence in the effect estimate: The true effect is likely to be substantially different from the estimate of effect.

Criteria for downgrade the certainty of evidence
[a] Downgraded owing to imprecision: Sample size < 400;
[b] Downgraded owing to inconsistence: When $I^2 > 50\%$ or when pooling was not possible;
[c] Downgraded owing to risk of bias: >25% of the participants were from studies with a high risk of bias.

MD = Mean difference; SMD = Standardized Mean Difference; * = SMD; MT = Manual Therapy; MT vs. Control = Comparison of manual therapy versus sham, placebo and wait-list; MT add effects = Comparison of manual therapy combined with other active intervention versus the active intervention alone; mm = millimetres; MCID = Minimum Clinically Important Difference; MDC = Minimal Detectable Change; MMO = Maximum Mouth Opening with or without pain; Instrumental MT = Use of devices to assist on manual therapy techniques; Manual Pressure = digital or manual pressure applied on a specific muscle area; Multimodal = Combination of two or more manual therapies.

4. Discussion

This systematic review and meta-analysis found that manual therapy may have positive effects in the management of pain intensity, MMO and disability related to TMD; however, the effects' sizes are small and may not be clinically relevant. Current quality of evidence ranged from very low to high, so future high quality RCTs are likely to change the estimates. Moderate quality of evidence supports joint manipulation, manual pressure, stretching and the combination of two or more manual therapies as additional therapies, with a similar small effect size. Therefore, the choice of the manual therapy technique should rely on the expertise of the health professional and preferences of the patient.

Our results corroborate with previous systematic reviews [17,19,55–59], which also found some positive effects in favour of manual therapy and other conservative interventions for pain intensity, MMO and disability, although the quality of the evidence has increased due to the inclusion of new trials. Among these, two recent systematic reviews [17,59] investigate the effects of conservative approaches in arthrogenic [17] and myogenic-related TMD [59]; however, manual therapy was considered as a general physical therapy approach and analysed together with other interventions such as exercises modalities, education and others. For that reason, our systematic review provides the most up-to-date evidence of manual therapy approaches for the management of TMD.

There are important issues to be addressed in order to improve the current state of the literature on this topic. The main reason to downgrade the level of evidence in our review was imprecision due to the sample size. Moreover, most of the included trials have a poor reporting quality and did not present data appropriately. Future high-quality RCTs should focus on recruit larger sample sizes and use the reporting checklist. Moreover, it is important to include economic evaluation and investigation of adverse events as outcomes to improve the decision-making process.

This systematic review was conducted with strong methodological rigor following recommendations. It updates and synthesizes all available evidence on the efficacy of manual therapy for pain intensity, MMO and disability in people with TMD. Estimating the effect sizes on critical outcomes for patients, assessing the certainty of evidence for each effect estimate and discussing the clinical relevance of the effect sizes across therapies informs patients and clinicians in their decision making. However, this review has some potential limitations. It included RCTs with patients with any diagnosis or type/classification (myogenic, arthrogenic or mixed) and also joint disorders. Subgroup analysis for the different classification of TMD was not possible due to the limited number of trials including specifics types of TMD. Future trials should explore the effects of manual therapy in the different TMD diagnosis. In addition, our investigation was restricted to three clinical outcomes. It could be valuable to investigate other important clinical outcomes such as a health-related quality of life, pain pressure threshold and most importantly, the costs and adverse effects of the intervention.

5. Conclusions

We found moderate to high quality evidence of the positive effects of manual therapy modalities for pain intensity, maximum mouth opening and disability in temporomandibular disorders. However, the effect sizes are small and may not be clinically important. Future high-quality RCTs with larger sample sizes should explore the effects of manual therapy in the different TMD diagnosis, clarify adverse effects and include an economic evaluation for a better decision-making process.

Supplementary Materials: The following supporting information can be downloaded at: https://www.mdpi.com/article/10.3390/life13020292/s1, Supplementary File S1: PRISMA Checklist; Supplementary File S2: Search Strategy; Supplementary File S3: Funnel plot; Supplementary File S4: Manual therapy modalities subgroup analysis on pain intensity.

Author Contributions: Conceptualization, V.C.O., J.P.M., L.S.V., P.R.M.P., F.S. and M.A.A.; Methodology, J.P.M., V.C.O. and L.A.S.; Analysis, J.P.M. and V.C.O.; Investigation, J.P.M., L.A.S. and V.C.O.; Resources, L.S.V. and F.S.; Writing—Original Draft Preparation, V.C.O., J.P.M., L.S.V., P.R.M.P., F.S. and M.A.A.; Writing—Review and Editing, V.C.O., J.P.M., L.S.V., P.R.M.P., F.S. and M.A.A. All authors have read and agreed to the published version of the manuscript.

Funding: This research received no external funding.

Acknowledgments: We thank the Universidade Federal dos Vales do Jequitinhonha e Mucuri (UFVJM) for institutional support and the CNPq, CAPES (Finance Code 001), and FAPEMIG for support and scholarships.

Conflicts of Interest: The authors declare no conflict of interest.

Abbreviations

Abbreviation	Definition
CF-PDI	Craniofacial pain and disability inventory
CIs	Confidence intervals
DC/TMD	The Diagnostic Criteria for Temporomandibular Disorders
FPHI	Fonseca Patient History Index
GRADE	Grading of Recommendations Assessment
JFLS	Jaw Functional Limitation Scale
MCID	Minimal clinical important difference
MDC	Minimal Detectable Change
MDs	Mean differences
MFIQ	Mandibular Function Impairment Questionnaire
MFIQ	Migraine Functional Impact Questionnaire
MMO	Maximum mouth opening
NRS	Numerical Rating Scale
PRISMA	Prospective Reporting Items for Systematic Review and Meta-Analyses
PROSPERO	Prospective Registry of Systematic Reviews
RCTs	Randomised controlled trials
SDs	Standard deviations
SMDs	Standardized mean differences
TMD	Temporomandibular disorders
VAS	Visual Analog Scale

References

1. Manfredini, D.; Chiappe, G.; Bosco, M. Research Diagnostic Criteria for Temporomandibular Disorders (RDC/TMD) axis I diagnoses in an Italian patient population. *J. Oral Rehabil.* **2006**, *33*, 551–558. [CrossRef]
2. Schiffman, E.; Ohrbach, R.; Truelove, E.; Look, J.; Anderson, G.; Goulet, J.-P.; List, T.; Svensson, P.; Gonzalez, Y.; Lobbezoo, F.; et al. Diagnostic Criteria for Temporomandibular Disorders (DC/TMD) for Clinical and Research Applications: Recommendations of the International RDC/TMD Consortium Network and Orofacial Pain Special Interest Group. *J. Oral Facial Pain Headache* **2014**, *28*, 6–27. [CrossRef]
3. Valesan, L.F.; Da-Cas, C.D.; Réus, J.C.; Denardin, A.C.S.; Garanhani, R.R.; Bonotto, D.; Januzzi, E.; de Souza, B.D.M. Prevalence of temporomandibular joint disorders: A systematic review and meta-analysis. *Clin. Oral Investig.* **2021**, *25*, 441–453. [CrossRef]
4. Minervini, G.; Mariani, P.; Fiorillo, L.; Cervino, G.; Cicciù, M.; Laino, L. Prevalence of temporomandibular disorders in people with multiple sclerosis: A systematic review and meta-analysis. *Cranio* **2022**, 1–9. [CrossRef]
5. Forssell, H.; Kauko, T.; Kotiranta, U.; Suvinen, T. Predictors for future clinically significant pain in patients with temporomandibular disorder: A prospective cohort study. *Eur. J. Pain* **2017**, *21*, 188–197. [CrossRef]
6. Ohrbach, R.; Dworkin, S.F. Five-year outcomes in TMD: Relationship of changes in pain to changes in physical and psychological variables. *Pain* **1998**, *74*, 315–326. [CrossRef]
7. Velly, A.M.; Elsaraj, S.M.; Botros, J.; Samim, F.; der Khatchadourian, Z.; Gornitsky, M. The contribution of pain and disability on the transition from acute to chronic pain-related TMD: A 3-month prospective cohort study. *Front. Pain Res.* **2022**, *3*, 956117. [CrossRef]
8. Nilsson, I.-M.; List, T. Does adolescent self-reported TMD pain persist into early adulthood? A longitudinal study. *Acta Odontol. Scand.* **2020**, *78*, 377–383. [CrossRef]
9. Barry, F.; Chai, F.; Chijcheapaza-Flores, H.; Garcia-Fernandez, M.J.; Blanchemain, N.; Nicot, R. Systematic review of studies on drug-delivery systems for management of temporomandibular-joint osteoarthritis. *J. Stomatol. Oral Maxillofac. Surg.* **2021**, *123*, e336–e341. [CrossRef]
10. Seo, H.; Jung, B.; Yeo, J.; Kim, K.-W.; Cho, J.-H.; Lee, Y.J.; Ha, I.-H. Healthcare utilisation and costs for temporomandibular disorders: A descriptive, cross-sectional study. *BMJ Open* **2020**, *10*, e036768. [CrossRef]
11. Riley, P.; Glenny, A.-M.; Worthington, H.V.; Jacobsen, E.; Robertson, C.; Durham, J.; Davies, S.; Petersen, H.; Boyers, D. Oral splints for patients with temporomandibular disorders or bruxism: A systematic review and economic evaluation. *Health Technol. Assess.* **2020**, *24*, 1–224. [CrossRef]
12. Prodoehl, J.; Kraus, S.; Stein, A.B. Predicting the number of physical therapy visits and patient satisfaction in individuals with temporomandibular disorder: A cohort study. *J. Oral Rehabil.* **2022**, *49*, 22–36. [CrossRef]
13. Kothari, K.; Jayakumar, N.; Razzaque, A. Multidisciplinary management of temporomandibular joint ankylosis in an adult: Journey from arthroplasty to oral rehabilitation. *BMJ Case Rep.* **2021**, *14*, e245120. [CrossRef]
14. Penlington, C.; Bowes, C.; Taylor, G.; Otemade, A.A.; Waterhouse, P.; Durham, J.; Ohrbach, R. Psychological therapies for temporomandibular disorders (TMDs). *Cochrane Database Syst. Rev.* **2022**, *2022*, CD013515. [CrossRef]

15. de Souza, R.F.; da Silva, C.H.L.; Nasser, M.; Fedorowicz, Z.; A Al-Muharraqi, M. Interventions for managing temporomandibular joint osteoarthritis. *Cochrane Database Syst. Rev.* **2012**, *2018*, CD007261. [CrossRef]
16. Mujakperuo, H.R.; Watson, M.; Morrison, R.; Macfarlane, T.V. Pharmacological interventions for pain in patients with temporomandibular disorders. *Cochrane Database Syst. Rev.* **2010**, *10*, CD004715. [CrossRef]
17. Ferrillo, M.; Nucci, L.; Giudice, A.; Calafiore, D.; Marotta, N.; Minervini, G.; D'Apuzzo, F.; Ammendolia, A.; Perillo, L.; de Sire, A. Efficacy of conservative approaches on pain relief in patients with temporomandibular joint disorders: A systematic review with network meta-analysis. *Cranio* **2022**, 1–17. [CrossRef]
18. Minervini, G.; Fiorillo, L.; Russo, D.; Lanza, A.; D'Amico, C.; Cervino, G.; Meto, A.; Di Francesco, F. Prosthodontic Treatment in Patients with Temporomandibular Disorders and Orofacial Pain and/or Bruxism: A Review of the Literature. *Prosthesis* **2022**, *4*, 253–262. [CrossRef]
19. Armijo-Olivo, S.; Pitance, L.; Singh, V.; Neto, F.; Thie, N.; Michelotti, A. Effectiveness of Manual Therapy and Therapeutic Exercise for Temporomandibular Disorders: Systematic Review and Meta-Analysis. *Phys. Ther.* **2016**, *96*, 9–25. [CrossRef]
20. Guyatt, G.H.; Oxman, A.D.; Schuenemann, H.J.; Tugwell, P.; Knottnerus, A. GRADE guidelines: A new series of articles in the Journal of Clinical Epidemiology. *J. Clin. Epidemiol.* **2011**, *64*, 380–382. [CrossRef]
21. Higgins, J.P.; Thomas, J.; Chandler, J.; Cumpston, M.; Li, T.; Page, M.J.; Welch, V.A. Cochrane Handbook for Systematic Reviews of Interventions. 2021. Available online: https://training.cochrane.org/cochrane-handbook-systematic-reviews-interventions (accessed on 7 December 2020).
22. Page, M.J.; McKenzie, J.E.; Bossuyt, P.M.; Boutron, I.; Hoffmann, T.C.; Mulrow, C.D.; Shamseer, L.; Tetzlaff, J.M.; Akl, E.A.; Brennan, S.E.; et al. The PRISMA 2020 Statement: An Updated Guideline for Reporting Systematic Reviews. *BMJ* **2021**, *372*, n71. [CrossRef]
23. Katz, J.; Melzack, R. Measurement of Pain. *Surg. Clin. North Am.* **1999**, *79*, 231–252. [CrossRef]
24. Wood, G.D.; A Branco, J. A comparison of three methods of measuring maximal opening of the mouth. *J. Oral Surg. (Am. Dent. Assoc. 1965)* **1979**, *37*, 175–177.
25. Ohrbach, R.; Larsson, P.; List, T. The jaw functional limitation scale: Development, reliability, and validity of 8-item and 20-item versions. *J. Orofac. Pain* **2008**, *22*, 219–230.
26. Stegenga, B.; De Bont, L.G.; De Leeuw, R.; Boering, G. Assessment of mandibular function impairment associated with temporomandibular joint osteoarthrosis and internal derangement. *J. Orofac. Pain* **1993**, *7*, 183–195.
27. Macedo, L.G.; Elkins, M.R.; Maher, C.G.; Moseley, A.M.; Herbert, R.D.; Sherrington, C. There was evidence of convergent and construct validity of Physiotherapy Evidence Database quality scale for physiotherapy trials. *J. Clin. Epidemiol.* **2010**, *63*, 920–925. [CrossRef]
28. Farrar, J.T.; Young, J.P., Jr.; LaMoreaux, L.; Werth, J.L.; Poole, R.M. Clinical importance of changes in chronic pain intensity measured on an 11-point numerical pain rating scale. *Pain* **2001**, *94*, 149–158. [CrossRef]
29. Kropmans, T.; Dijkstra, P.; Stegenga, B.; Stewart, R.; De Bont, L. Smallest detectable difference in outcome variables related to painful restriction of the temporomandibular joint. *J. Dent. Res.* **1999**, *78*, 784–789. [CrossRef]
30. Balshem, H.; Helfand, M.; Schünemann, H.J.; Oxman, A.D.; Kunz, R.; Brozek, J.; Vist, G.E.; Falck-Ytter, Y.; Meerpohl, J.; Norris, S.; et al. GRADE guidelines: 3. Rating the quality of evidence. *J. Clin. Epidemiol.* **2011**, *64*, 401–406. [CrossRef]
31. Guyatt, G.H.; Oxman, A.D.; Vist, G.E.; Kunz, R.; Falck-Ytter, Y.; Alonso-Coello, P.; Schünemann, H.J. GRADE: An emerging consensus on rating quality of evidence and strength of recommendations. *BMJ* **2008**, *336*, 924–926. [CrossRef]
32. Mueller, P.S.; Montori, V.; Bassler, D.; Koenig, B.A.; Guyatt, G.H. Ethical Issues in Stopping Randomized Trials Early Because of Apparent Benefit. *Ann. Intern. Med.* **2007**, *146*, 878–881. [CrossRef]
33. Foley, N.C.; Teasell, R.W.; Bhogal, S.K.; Speechley, M.R. Stroke Rehabilitation Evidence-Based Review: Methodology. *Top. Stroke Rehabil.* **2003**, *10*, 1–7. [CrossRef]
34. Ioannidis, J.P.; Trikalinos, T.A. The appropriateness of asymmetry tests for publication bias in meta-analyses: A large survey. *Can. Med. Assoc. J.* **2007**, *176*, 1091–1096. [CrossRef]
35. Alajbeg, I.; Gikić, M.; Peruzović, M.V. Mandibular Range of Movement and Pain Intensity in Patients with Anterior Disc Displacement without Reduction. *Acta Stomatol. Croat.* **2015**, *49*, 119–127. [CrossRef]
36. Espejo-Antúnez, L.; Castro-Valenzuela, E.; Ribeiro, F.; Albornoz-Cabello, M.; Silva, A.; Rodríguez-Mansilla, J. Immediate effects of hamstring stretching alone or combined with ischemic compression of the masseter muscle on hamstrings extensibility, active mouth opening and pain in athletes with temporomandibular dysfunction. *J. Bodyw. Mov. Ther.* **2016**, *20*, 579–587. [CrossRef]
37. Rodriguez-Blanco, C.; Cocera-Morata, F.M.; Heredia-Rizo, A.M.; Ricard, F.; Almazán-Campos, G.; Oliva-Pascual-Vaca, Á. Immediate Effects of Combining Local Techniques in the Craniomandibular Area and Hamstring Muscle Stretching in Subjects with Temporomandibular Disorders: A Randomized Controlled Study. *J. Altern. Complement. Med.* **2015**, *21*, 451–459. [CrossRef]
38. Brochado, F.T.; De Jesus, L.H.; Carrard, V.C.; Freddo, A.L.; Chaves, K.D.; Martins, M.D. Comparative effectiveness of photobiomodulation and manual therapy alone or combined in TMD patients: A randomized clinical trial. *Braz. Oral Res.* **2018**, *32*, e50. [CrossRef]
39. DeVocht, J.W.; Goertz, C.M.; Hondras, M.A.; Long, C.R.; Schaeffer, W.; Thomann, L.; Spector, M.; Stanford, C.M. A pilot study of a chiropractic intervention for management of chronic myofascial temporomandibular disorder. *J. Am. Dent. Assoc.* **2013**, *144*, 1154–1163. [CrossRef]

40. Gomes, C.A.F.D.P.; El Hage, Y.; Amaral, A.P.; Politti, F.; Biasotto-Gonzalez, D.A. Effects of massage therapy and occlusal splint therapy on electromyographic activity and the intensity of signs and symptoms in individuals with temporomandibular disorder and sleep bruxism: A randomized clinical trial. *Chiropr. Man. Ther.* **2014**, *22*, 43. [CrossRef]
41. Hernanz, G.S.; Angulo-Carrere, T.; Ardizone-García, I.; Svensson, P.; Álvarez-Méndez, A.M. Pressure Release Technique Versus Placebo Applied to Cervical and Masticatory Muscles in Patients with Chronic Painful Myofascial Temporomandibular Disorder. A Randomized Clinical Trial 2020, PREPRINT (Version 1) available at Research Square. Available online: https://www.researchsquare.com/article/rs-51085/v1 (accessed on 7 December 2020).
42. Kalamir, A.; Bonello, R.; Graham, P.; Vitiello, A.L.; Pollard, H. Intraoral Myofascial Therapy for Chronic Myogenous Temporomandibular Disorder: A Randomized Controlled Trial. *J. Manip. Physiol. Ther.* **2012**, *35*, 26–37. [CrossRef]
43. Kanhachon, W.; Boonprakob, Y. Modified-Active Release Therapy in Patients with Scapulocostal Syndrome and Masticatory Myofascial Pain: A Stratified-Randomized Controlled Trial. *Int. J. Environ. Res. Public Health* **2021**, *18*, 8533. [CrossRef]
44. La Touche, R.; Paris-Alemany, A.; Mannheimer, J.S.; Angulo-Díaz-Parreño, S.; Bishop, M.; Centeno, A.L.-V.; von Piekartz, H.; Fernandez-Carnero, J. Does Mobilization of the Upper Cervical Spine Affect Pain Sensitivity and Autonomic Nervous System Function in Patients With Cervico-craniofacial Pain? *Clin. J. Pain* **2013**, *29*, 205–215. [CrossRef] [PubMed]
45. Leite, W.B.; Oliveira, M.L.; Ferreira, I.C.; Anjos, C.F.; Barbosa, M.A.; Barbosa, A.C. Effects of 4-Week Diacutaneous Fibrolysis on Myalgia, Mouth Opening, and Level of Functional Severity in Women With Temporomandibular Disorders: A Randomized Controlled Trial. *J. Manip. Physiol. Ther.* **2020**, *43*, 806–815. [CrossRef]
46. Lucas, C.; Branco, I.; Silva, M.; Alves, P.; Pereira, Â.M. Benefits of manual therapy in temporomandibular joint dysfunction treatment. In *2nd International Congress of CiiEM-Translational Research and Innovation in Human and Health Science*; Campus Egas Moniz: Monte de Caparica, Portugal, 2017.
47. Nagata, K.; Hori, S.; Mizuhashi, R.; Yokoe, T.; Atsumi, Y.; Nagai, W.; Goto, M. Efficacy of mandibular manipulation technique for temporomandibular disorders patients with mouth opening limitation: A randomized controlled trial for comparison with improved multimodal therapy. *J. Prosthodont. Res.* **2019**, *63*, 202–209. [CrossRef] [PubMed]
48. Packer, A.C.; Pires, P.F.; Dibai-Filho, A.V.; Rodrigues-Bigaton, D. Effect of Upper Thoracic Manipulation on Mouth Opening and Electromyographic Activity of Masticatory Muscles in Women With Temporomandibular Disorder: A Randomized Clinical Trial. *J. Manip. Physiol. Ther.* **2015**, *38*, 253–261. [CrossRef] [PubMed]
49. Puentedura, E.J.; Kolber, M.J.; Cleland, J.A. Effectiveness of Cervical Spine High-Velocity, Low-Amplitude Thrust Added to Behavioral Education, Soft Tissue Mobilization, and Exercise for People With Temporomandibular Disorder With Myalgia: A Randomized Clinical Trial. *J. Orthop. Sport. Phys. Ther.* **2020**, *50*, 455–465. [CrossRef]
50. Rezaie, K.; Amiri, A.; Takamjani, E.E.; Shirani, G.; Salehi, S.; Alizadeh, L. The Efficacy of Neck and Temporomandibular Joint (TMJ) Manual Therapy in Comparison With a Multimodal Approach in the Patients with TMJ Dysfunction: A Blinded Randomized Controlled Trial. *Med. J. Islam. Repub. Iran* **2022**, *36*, 328–337. [CrossRef]
51. Şahin, D.; Mutlu, E.K.; Şakar, O.; Ateş, G.; Inan, Ş.; Taşkıran, H. The effect of the ischaemic compression technique on pain and functionality in temporomandibular disorders: A randomised clinical trial. *J. Oral Rehabil.* **2021**, *48*, 531–541. [CrossRef]
52. de la Serna, P.D.; Plaza-Manzano, G.; Cleland, J.; Fernández-De-Las-Peñas, C.; Martín-Casas, P.; Díaz-Arribas, M.J. Effects of Cervico-Mandibular Manual Therapy in Patients with Temporomandibular Pain Disorders and Associated Somatic Tinnitus: A Randomized Clinical Trial. *Pain Med.* **2020**, *21*, 613–624. [CrossRef]
53. Tuncer, A.; Ergun, N.; Tuncer, A.H.; Karahan, S. Effectiveness of manual therapy and home physical therapy in patients with temporomandibular disorders: A randomized controlled trial. *J. Bodyw. Mov. Ther.* **2013**, *17*, 302–308. [CrossRef]
54. Yoshida, H.; Fukumura, Y.; Suzuki, S.; Fujita, S.; Kenzo, O.; Yoshikado, R.; Nakagawa, M.; Inoue, A.; Sako, J.; Yamada, K.; et al. Simple manipulation therapy for temporomandibular joint internal derangement with closed lock. *J. Oral. Maxillofac. Surg.* **2005**, *17*, 256–260. [CrossRef]
55. Al-Moraissi, E.A.; Conti, P.C.R.; Alyahya, A.; Alkebsi, K.; Elsharkawy, A.; Christidis, N. The hierarchy of different treatments for myogenous temporomandibular disorders: A systematic review and network meta-analysis of randomized clinical trials. *Oral Maxillofac. Surg.* **2022**, *26*, 519–533. [CrossRef] [PubMed]
56. Dinsdale, A.; Costin, B.; Dharamdasani, S.; Page, R.; Purs, N.; Treleaven, J. What conservative interventions improve bite function in those with temporomandibular disorders? A systematic review using self-reported and physical measures. *J. Oral Rehabil.* **2022**, *49*, 456–475. [CrossRef] [PubMed]
57. Asquini, G.; Pitance, L.; Michelotti, A.; Falla, D. Effectiveness of manual therapy applied to craniomandibular structures in temporomandibular disorders: A systematic review. *J. Oral Rehabil.* **2022**, *49*, 442–455. [CrossRef]

58. Calixtre, L.B.; Moreira, R.F.C.; Franchini, G.H.; Alburquerque-Sendín, F.; Oliveira, A.B. Manual therapy for the management of pain and limited range of motion in subjects with signs and symptoms of temporomandibular disorder: A systematic review of randomised controlled trials. *J. Oral Rehabil.* **2015**, *42*, 847–861. [CrossRef]
59. Ferrillo, M.; Ammendolia, A.; Paduano, S.; Calafiore, D.; Marotta, N.; Migliario, M.; Fortunato, L.; Giudice, A.; Michelotti, A.; de Sire, A. Efficacy of rehabilitation on reducing pain in muscle-related temporomandibular disorders: A systematic review and meta-analysis of randomized controlled trials. *J. Back Musculoskelet. Rehabil.* **2022**, *35*, 921–936. [CrossRef]

Disclaimer/Publisher's Note: The statements, opinions and data contained in all publications are solely those of the individual author(s) and contributor(s) and not of MDPI and/or the editor(s). MDPI and/or the editor(s) disclaim responsibility for any injury to people or property resulting from any ideas, methods, instructions or products referred to in the content.

Systematic Review

Effectiveness of Manual Trigger Point Therapy in Patients with Myofascial Trigger Points in the Orofacial Region—A Systematic Review

Frauke Müggenborg [1,*], Ester Moreira de Castro Carletti [2], Liz Dennett [3], Ana Izabela Sobral de Oliveira-Souza [1,4], Norazlin Mohamad [5,6], Gunnar Licht [7], Harry von Piekartz [1] and Susan Armijo-Olivo [1,5,8,*]

1. Department of Physiotherapy, University of Applied Sciences Osnabrück, Faculty of Economics and Social Sciences Caprivistr. 30A, 49076 Osnabrück, Germany
2. Post Graduate Program in Human Movement Sciences, Methodist University of Piracicaba-UNIMEP, Piracicaba 13400-911, Brazil
3. Scott Health Sciences Library, University of Alberta, Edmonton, AB T6G 1C9, Canada
4. Graduate Program in Neuropsychiatry and Behavioral Sciences, Federal University of Pernambuco (UFPE), Av. Prof. Moraes Rego, 1235, Recife 50670-901, Brazil
5. Department of Physical Therapy, Faculty of Rehabilitation Medicine, Rehabilitation Research Center, University of Alberta, Edmonton, AB T6G 1C9, Canada
6. Centre of Physiotherapy, Faculty of Health Sciences, Universiti Teknologi MARA, Puncak Alam Campus, Shah Alam 42300, Malaysia
7. FOURBs-Specialist Medical Center for Orthopedics and Rehabilitation of the Locomotor System–Johannisstr. 19, 49074 Osnabrück, Germany
8. Faculty of Medicine and Dentistry, Department of Dentistry, University of Alberta, Edmonton, AB T6G 1C9, Canada
* Correspondence: frauke@hugenschuett.info (F.M.); sla4@ualberta.ca or susanarmijo@gmail.com (S.A.-O.)

Abstract: The objective was to compile, synthetize, and evaluate the quality of the evidence from randomized controlled trials (RCTs) regarding the effectiveness of manual trigger point therapy in the orofacial area in patients with or without orofacial pain. This project was registered in PROSPERO and follows the PRISMA guidelines. Searches (20 April 2021) were conducted in six databases for RCTs involving adults with active or latent myofascial trigger points (mTrPs) in the orofacial area. The data were extracted by two independent assessors. Four studies were included. According to the GRADE approach, the overall quality/certainty of the evidence was very low due to the high risk of bias of the studies included. Manual trigger point therapy showed no clear advantage over other conservative treatments. However, it was found to be an equally effective and safe therapy for individuals with myofascial trigger points in the orofacial region and better than control groups. This systematic review revealed a limited number of RCTs conducted with patients with mTrPs in the orofacial area and the methodological limitations of those RCTs. Rigorous, well-designed RCTs are still needed in this field.

Keywords: trigger points; myofascial pain; manual therapy; temporomandibular disorders; systematic review

1. Introduction

Myofascial trigger points (mTrPs) can be defined as hypersensitive or tender spots located within stretched muscle fibers (taut bands) of the skeletal muscles, which when compressed or stretched can cause referred or local pain [1]. Myofascial trigger points are associated with myofascial pain syndrome [1]. Myofascial pain can be defined as regional muscle pain that has increased pain sensitivity when palpated [2]. Myofascial pain and mTrP are commonly associated with orofacial pain and specifically associated with temporomandibular disorders (TMD), which are characterized by pain, reduced mouth opening, muscle or joint tenderness on palpation, limitation of mandibular movements, joint sounds, and otologic complaints such as tinnitus, vertigo or ear fullness among others. Orofacial pain (OFP) can be defined as pain originating below the orbitomeatal line, above the neck, and in front of the ears, including pain occurring in the mouth [3].

Pain disorders of the orofacial area are prevalent and can cause a significant personal and societal burden [4,5] The results of international epidemiological studies have shown that orofacial pain occurs in approximately 5–12% of the adult population, and young women are more affected by orofacial pain than men in a ratio of about 2:1 [5–7]. In fact, myofascial pain has been reported to play a major role in 45.3% of TMD diagnoses [8,9]. Myofascial pain is the second most common pain type of orofacial symptoms, and around 33% of the affected individuals have facial and masticatory musculoskeletal symptoms [9,10].

Due to the complexity of OFP and specifically TMD, their management has been interdisciplinary. Evidence-based treatments for these conditions, as stated by the guidelines of the American Academy of Orofacial Pain [10] include physical therapy (PT), patient education and self-management, behavioral therapy, pharmacologic management, orthopedic appliance therapy, dental and occlusal therapy, and surgery among others. Several systematic reviews [11–16] have looked at the effectiveness of these conservative therapies and have found them to be potentially effective at managing these disorders. However, the evidence is poor due to the high risk of bias and methodological issues in the primary studies.

Both non-invasive and invasive (such as manual trigger point therapy and dry needling) treatments exist for mTrPs. In the past few years, several studies have investigated the use of non-invasive therapies such as manual trigger point therapy [17], acupuncture [18], manual therapy [19], and laser [20], among others, to manage mTrPs. Manual trigger point therapy is a treatment method, which uses the hands of the therapist/doctor in a structured way to inactivate the mTrPs and to treat accompanying connective tissue changes, and movement restrictions [21]. The authors are not aware of any previous systematic review of the effectiveness of manual trigger point treatment, specifically in patients with myofascial trigger points, in the orofacial area. Based on our preliminary searches, previous reviews have included manual therapy in general, but they have not focused on manual trigger point therapy in particular and thus they have not exhaustively analyzed this specific literature and its effectiveness [13,14,22]. In addition, these reviews are already outdated since they were published almost seven years ago. The research in this area in the last couple of years has emphasized that there is a scarcity of available evidence in this field and therefore, there is an urgent need to fill this gap in the literature and provide focused and updated information regarding the effectiveness of manual trigger point therapy for the orofacial region [23–25].

Thus, the following objectives were set for this review: (1) To compile, synthesize, and evaluate the quality of the evidence from RCTs or clinical trials regarding the effectiveness of manual trigger point therapy compared with other treatment strategies, for managing mTrPs in the orofacial area in individuals with or without orofacial pain, and (2) To inform future practice and provide recommendations regarding manual trigger point therapy for people with mTrPs in the orofacial area.

2. Materials and Methods

This project was registered in PROSPERO (CRD42020169216) and reported based on the PRISMA guidelines [26].

Data Searches: This review was part of a large project looking at several interventions to manage orofacial pain; and manual trigger point therapy was one of them. The search (Appendix A) for all interventions was conducted at the same time and relevant keywords for manual trigger point therapy were included. A health sciences librarian (LD) conducted the searches in Medline (Ovid MEDLINE(R) ALL), Embase (Ovid interface), CINAHL PLUS with full text (EBSSCOhost interface), Cochrane Library Trials (Wiley Interface), Web of Science (Indexes=SCI-EXPANDED, SSCI, A&HCI, ESCI) and Scopus. The last search was conducted on 20 April 2021. The search included all relevant search terms from an earlier review [13] as well as new terms suggested by the research team. The search was limited to RCTs using a slightly modified version of Glanville et al.'s filter [27]. The date was limited to studies published after 2004 because of the earlier review [28]. No language limits were applied.

2.1. Eligibility Criteria

The eligibility criteria of this review used the PICOS format (population, intervention, comparison, outcome, and study design)

Population: This review considered studies that include adults (18+ years of age) diagnosed with active or latent TrPs in the orofacial region with or without orofacial pain. No limits were applied in terms of sex, ethnicity, or country of residence, but animal studies were excluded. Several diagnoses can be included in the umbrella term of orofacial pain (OFP), depending on the classification used. We included types of OFP diagnoses based on the International Classification of Orofacial Pain (ICOP) published in 2020 [3]: myofascial OFP (primary and secondary myofascial OFP), temporomandibular joint pain, OFP resembling presentations of primary headaches, and idiopathic OFP. A detailed description of these diagnoses can be found in Appendix B. The rest of the classifications stated in the ICOP were excluded due to the fact that they are most likely not associated with myofascial TrPs (e.g., dental pain (i.e., pulpal pain, periodontal pain, and gingival pain)).

Intervention(s)/Exposure(s): The intervention of interest in this review was manual trigger point therapy which included the following: ischemic compression [29], trigger point pressure release [30], myofascial release [31], manual pressure on taut bands [32], passive stretching [33,34], manual fascial techniques [35], manual intraoral or extraoral release [32], and strain–counterstrain technique [36,37]. The description of these techniques can be found in Appendix C.

Comparator(s)/Control: Manual trigger point therapy was compared with any medical or physiotherapeutic technique that included, but was not limited to, dry needling, electrotherapy, laser therapy, exercises, acupuncture, ultrasound, splint management, medication, placebo, no treatment (control) or sham-therapy.

Outcome: The primary outcome of this review was pain intensity, which is frequently measured with the following tools: visual analogue scale (VAS), numeric rating scale (NRS), verbal rating scales (VRS), or graphical scales.

The secondary outcomes for this review were: pain pressure threshold (PPT) [38,39], maximal mouth opening (MMO), and mandibular range of motion (ROM) (right and left lateral excursion, protrusion) [40] among others. This review collected all outcomes reported by the included studies.

All time-points reported from the primary and secondary outcomes were analyzed (i.e., immediate post-treatment, short-term, intermediate-term, and long-term follow-up).

Studies: This review included RCTs and controlled clinical trials (CCTs). All other types of studies were excluded. All therapeutic settings were included in this review.

2.2. Data Screening

Search results were compiled into an EndNote database and then imported into Covidence (www.covidence.org), which was used for the screening process. Two independent reviewers screened the titles and abstracts and full text. If disagreements occurred between the reviewers in the inclusion of an article, the reasons for the disagreement were discussed, and a consensus was reached.

2.3. Data Extraction

Data extraction was first performed independently by one reviewer using an electronic pilot-tested form created in Excel. A second reviewer checked the extracted information of each study. The data extraction contained qualitative and quantitative elements. The following qualitative elements were extracted: article information; main objective of the study, study design, type of interventions, study setting, population, diagnosis tools, data collection methods, RCT type, number of randomized groups; outcomes; data analysis, results, conclusions, limitations, among others. The quantitative elements for treatment effect estimates were extracted for outcomes at baseline and at different time points, including mean, standard deviation (SD), sample size, standard error (SE), and confidence intervals. Any disagreements on data extraction were resolved by consensus.

2.4. Risk of Bias (Quality Assessment)

Quality assessment (risk of bias—RoB) was conducted by two independent reviewers on all included studies using the new risk of bias tool (RoB2) recommended by the Cochrane Collaboration [41,42]. Two reviewers independently assessed the RoB in the primary studies [43]. For the overall assessment of the RoB for each study, studies were rated as follows: "high risk of bias" (if the study was rated high in at least one domain), "some concerns" (if the study was rated as "some concerns" in at least one domain and the other domains were low), or "low risk of bias" (if the study was rated as low risk in all individual domains). Similar decision rules have been used by previous studies when rating the overall risk of bias assessment of RCTs [44]. Disagreements in risk assessment ratings were resolved by consensus. In addition, we used a compiled set of items from seven scales used to evaluate the RoB in the physical therapy field [45]. This compiled set of items has been described previously and has been used in several systematic reviews of our team [12,13,46].

2.5. Data Synthesis

We summarized our findings using a narrative synthesis based on the type of intervention (e.g., ischemic compression, myofascial release, trigger point pressure release), type of diagnosis (e.g., latent or not latent masticatory mTrPs), and based on the type of outcome (e.g., pain intensity, maximum mouth opening, and pain pressure threshold). We presented the study results using evidence tables and forest plots when feasible. We used forest plots to visually show study results and direction of the treatment effects. Narrative and qualitative summaries were provided when possible. Revman 5.4 software was used to construct forest plots for all comparisons. Mean differences (MD) were used to analyze continuous outcomes and ordinal data were analyzed as continuous data. To interpret MD, the minimal important difference was used for each of the outcomes. To interpret the pain intensity, mouth opening, and tenderness, a mean difference of 1.9 cm [47], 5 mm [48], and 1.12 Kg/cm^2 [49], respectively, were considered a clinically significant finding for these outcomes.

Overall Quality of the Evidence: The evidence was classified as high, moderate, low, and very low based on the GRADE approach based on the outcomes of interest [50]. The evidence was downgraded by one or two points when serious or very serious limitations, respectively, were found in the following domains: risk of bias, consistency of results, indirectness (reproducible, targeted to the population of interest), imprecision (insufficient data), or publication bias [50]. The evidence was upgraded based on three factors when applicable: large effect (up to 2 points increase), dose–response gradient (1-point increase), and plausible confounding that would change the effect.

3. Results

3.1. Study Selection

A total number of 8483 studies were found in the databases. Twenty-four studies were selected for full-text screening; however, among those, 20 studies were excluded based on the reasons described in the PRISMA flowchart (Figure 1). A detailed list of excluded studies and reasons for exclusion can be obtained from the authors upon request. Four studies were selected for data extraction and risk of bias assessment and were included in this systematic review [17,51–53].

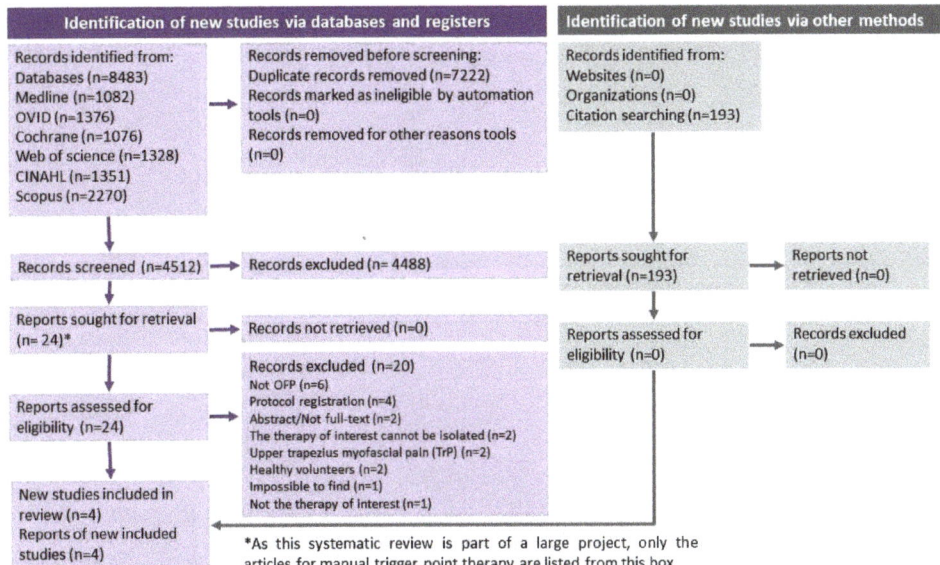

Figure 1. Flow diagram of included studies for this systematic review based on PRISMA guidelines.

3.2. Study Characteristics—Synthesis of Results

Table 1 summarizes the type of treatment, outcomes, results, and conclusions of each study. Regarding the diagnosis, two studies [17,53] included subjects with the diagnosis of trigger points and myogenic TMD using the RDC/TMD criteria [54] and two [51,52] included subjects with the diagnosis of latent mTrPs in the masseter muscles as stated by Simons et al. [2] but no OFP was identified by the authors.

Table 1. Summary of randomized controlled trials included in this systematic review.

Study (Year)	Intervention vs. Comparison Group(s)	Outcome Measure— Measure Tool	Results between Groups MD [95% CI]	Results between Groups p Value and Clinical Significance Assessment	Conclusion
Blanco et al. (2006) [51]	SC (masseter) vs.PIR (masseter) vs. Control: no therapy	MMO (mm)—NR	**MMO:** SC vs. PIR −1.80 mm [−5.12, 1.52] SC vs. CO 0.30 mm [−3.29, 3.89]	**MMO:** SC vs. PIR (p = 0.4090; no significant difference between groups; NCS) SC vs. CO (p = 0.84, no significant difference between groups; NCS)	For participants with latent mTrPs in the masseter muscle, the post-isometric relaxation technique showed a greater effect on active mouth opening than the strain/counterstrain technique.

Table 1. Cont.

Study (Year)	Intervention vs. Comparison Group(s)	Outcome Measure—Measure Tool	Results between Groups MD [95% CI]	Results between Groups p Value and Clinical Significance Assessment	Conclusion
Ibáñez-García et al. (2009) [52]	SC (masseter) vs. NT (masseter) vs. Control: no therapy	Pain intensity (0–10 cm)—VAS PPT (kg/cm^2)—mechanical pressure algometer MMO (mm)—NR	**Pain intensity:** SC vs. NT 0.40 cm [−0.54, 1.34] SC vs. CO 1.60 cm [0.77, 2.43] **PPT:** SC vs. NT 0.0 kg/cm^2 [−0.23, 0.23] SC vs. CO 0.70 kg/cm^2 [0.48, 0.92] **MMO:** SC vs. NT 0.00 mm [−3.30, 3.30] SC vs. CO 6.00 mm [1.97, 10.03]	**Pain intensity:** SC vs. NT (p = 0.9, no significant difference between groups; NCS) SC vs. CO (p <0.001, significant difference favoring SC; PCSR) **PPT:** SC vs. NT (p = 0.9, no significant difference between groups; NCS) SC vs. CO (p < 0.001, significant difference favoring SC; NCS) **MMO:** SC vs. NT (p = 0.9, no significant difference between groups; NCS) SC vs. CO (p < 0.001, significant difference favoring SC; CSR)	The neuromuscular or strain/counterstrain technique showed in the results' increased PPTs, increased active mouth opening, and decreased local pain by pressure over latent myofascial TrPs in the masseter muscle. For both intervention groups, the large effect sizes suggest a strong clinical effect, while the effect size of the control was small.
Espejo-Antúnez et al. (2016) [53]	IC (masseter) + HS (hamstrings) vs. HS (hamstrings)	Pain intensity (0–10 cm) – VAS PPT (kg/cm^2) – mechanical pressure algometer MMO/VMO (mm) – calibrated caliper ROM (degree °) – computer analysis of photographs	**Pain intensity:** HS vs. HS+IC_R 0.00 cm [−3.15, 3.15] HS vs. HS+IC_L 0.00 cm [−2.94, 2.94] **PPT:** HS vs. HS+IC_R −0.10 kg/cm^2 [−0.70, 0.50] HS vs. HS+IC_L 0.00 kg/cm^2 [−0.20, 0.20] **MMO/VMO:** HS vs. HS+IC 0.20 mm [−3.77, 4.17]	**Pain intensity:** HS vs. HS+IC_R (p = 1.0; no significant difference between groups; NCS) HS vs. HS+IC_L (p = 1.0; no significant difference between groups; NCS) **PPT:** HS vs. HS+IC_R (p = 0.7616; no significant difference between groups; NCS) HS vs. HS+IC_L (p = 1.0; no significant difference between groups; NCS) **MMO/VMO:** HS vs. HS+IC (p = 0.4708; no significant difference between groups; NCS)	Both groups showed an increased hamstrings extensibility, active mouth opening, and pressure pain threshold, as well as decreased pain intensity. Adding ischemic compression did not result in further improvements in hamstrings extensibility or clinical features of TMD.

Table 1. Cont.

Study (Year)	Intervention vs. Comparison Group(s)	Outcome Measure—Measure Tool	Results between Groups MD [95% CI]	Results between Groups p Value and Clinical Significance Assessment	Conclusion
Lietz-Kijak et al. (2018) [17]	IC (masseter) vs. KT (masseter)	Pain intensity (0–10 cm) – VAS	Pain intensity: KT vs. IC −1.30 cm [−2.05, −0.55]	Pain intensity: KT vs. IC ($p < 0.001$; significant difference favoring KT; PCSR)	Significant analgesic effects were achieved by kinesiotaping (KT) and TrP inactivation for the treatment of painful forms of functional disorders of the masticatory muscles; however, more beneficial results were observed in the KT group.

CSR: clinically significant result; CO: Control group; d: days; F: female; HS: Hamstring-stretching; IC: Ischemic compression; SC: Strain/Counterstrain technique; KT: Kinesiotaping; L: left side; M: male; MTT: Manual TrP therapy; MMO: Maximal mouth opening; MD: Mean difference; m: months; NA: Not applicable; NCS: not clinically significant; NR: not reported; NT: Neuromuscular technique; PIR: Post-isometric relaxation; PCSR: potentially clinically significant result; PPT: Pressure pain threshold; ROM: Range of motion (knee extension); R: right side; TT: time of treatment of mTrP; T: treatment; w: week; VMO: vertical mouth opening.

In terms of manual trigger points techniques, two studies [51,52] used the strain/counterstrain technique to treat latent mTrPs, and two studies [37,55] used ischemic compression to treat patients with myogenic TMD.

The duration of the sessions and exposure times, as well as the duration of the whole treatment (in weeks) were poorly described in all studies. No adverse effects were described in any of the included studies. No other outcome was used besides the ones presented in Table 1 (i.e., pain intensity, pressure pain threshold, maximum/active mouth opening, and range of motion for active knee extension). The timing of outcome measurements was carried out immediately after each intervention in all four studies. No follow-up analysis was performed.

The results and characteristics of the studies are shown in detail in Appendix D. Meta-analysis was not possible due to the low number of studies and heterogeneity among the protocols.

3.3. Pain Intensity

Comparison of manual trigger point therapy vs. control group: Only one study [52] evaluated the effect of a manual trigger point technique (strain/counterstrain technique) compared to a control group. The qualitative comparison presented in the forest plot (Figure 2) and Table 2 (effect sizes), showed that the results favored the manual trigger point therapy (strain/counterstrain technique) when compared to the control group (MD [95% CI] 1.60 cm [0.77, 2.43]). The MD between groups was potentially clinically significant based on the minimally important difference of pain intensity reported (Figure 2) [47].

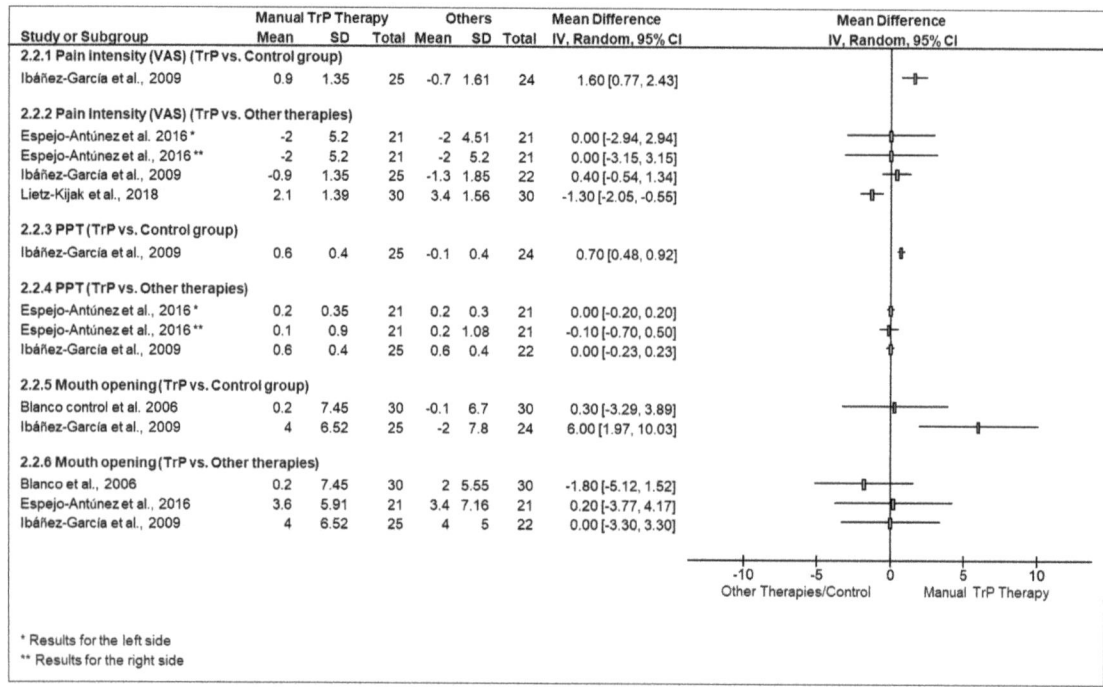

Figure 2. Forest plot for qualitative comparison of manual TrP therapy vs. any other therapy or controls used in the analyzed studies. Pain is reported in cm, pressure pain thresholds (PPT) in kg/cm^2, and mouth opening in mm).

Comparison of manual trigger point therapy vs. other therapies: Three of the studies [17,52,53] evaluated the effect of manual trigger point techniques (strain/counterstrain technique and ischemic compression) versus other interventions such as neuromuscular technique, [52] ischemic compression plus stretching of the hamstring, [53] kinesiotaping [17] to reduce pain provoked by TrPs. Based on the qualitative analyses, no significant differences in pain intensity favoring manual trigger point therapies versus other passive treatments were found. Kinesiotaping was found to be potentially clinically relevant based on the minimal important difference found between groups (MD [95% CI] −1.30 cm [−2.05, −0.55]) [47] (Figure 2 and Table 2 (Effect size)).

3.4. Pressure Pain Threshold

Comparison of manual trigger point therapy vs. control group: One study [52] evaluated the effect of a manual trigger point technique (strain/counterstrain technique) compared to a control group (i.e., no treatment). The forest plot (Figure 2) and Table 2 (effect sizes) showed that the results favored manual trigger point therapy (MD [95%]: 0.70 kg/cm^2 [0.48, 0.92]). However, this difference was not clinically relevant (Figure 2) [49].

Comparison of manual trigger point therapy vs. other therapies: Two studies [52,53] evaluated the effect of manual trigger point techniques (strain/counterstrain technique, ischemic compression) versus other intervention methods such as neuromuscular technique [52], or hamstring stretching [53]. There were no significant differences between groups for pressure pain threshold values in both studies (Table 1 and Figure 2) [49].

Table 2. Quality of evidence (GRADE) between manual TrP therapy versus other interventions.

Comparisons	No. of Studies (Design; Time of measurement)	Quality Assessment					No. of Patients		Summary of Findings	
		Risk of Bias	Inconsistency	Indirectness	Imprecision	Publication Bias	Patients in Tx group	Patients in Comparison/Control Group	Estimate (MD) [95% CI]	Quality
Pain Intensity (assessed with VAS: scale from 0 – 10 cm)—Manual TrP therapy vs. Control										
Strain/Counterstrain technique vs. Control (no treatment)	1 RCT [52]; right-after treatment	Very Serious [a]	NA	Serious [d]	Serious [e]	Undetected [f]	25	24	MD = 1.60 cm [0.77, 2.43]	Low
Pain Intensity (assessed with VAS: scale from 0 – 10 cm)—Manual TrP therapy vs. Other therapies										
Hamstring stretching + Ischemic compression vs. Hamstring stretching (left)	1 RCT [53]; right-after treatment	Very Serious [a]	NA	No serious [c]	Serious [e]	Undetected [f]	21	21	MD = 0.00 cm [−2.94, 2.94]	Low
Hamstring stretching + Ischemic compression vs. Hamstring stretching (right)	1 RCT [53]; right-after treatment	Very Serious [a]	NA	No serious [c]	Serious [e]	Undetected [f]	21	21	MD = 0.00 cm [−3.15, 3.15]	Low
Strain/Counterstrain technique vs. Neuromuscular technique	1 RCT [52]; right-after treatment	Very Serious [a]	NA	Serious [d]	Serious [e]	Undetected [f]	22	22	MD = 0.40 cm [−0.54, 1.34]	Low
Ischemic compression vs. Kinesio taping	1 RCT [17]; right-after treatment	Very Serious [a]	NA	No serious [c]	Serious [e]	Undetected [f]	30	30	MD = −1.30 cm [−2.05, −0.55]	Low
Pressure Pain Threshold (assessed with pressure algometer: kg/cm^2)—Manual TrP therapy vs. Control										
Strain/Counterstrain technique vs. Control (no treatment)	1 RCT [52]; right-after treatment	Very Serious [a]	NA	Serious [d]	Serious [e]	Undetected [f]	25	24	MD = 0.70 kg/cm^2 [0.48, 0.92]	Low

Table 2. Cont.

Comparisons	No. of Studies (Design; Time of measurement)	Quality Assessment					No. of Patients		Summary of Findings	
		Risk of Bias	Inconsistency	Indirectness	Imprecision	Publication Bias	Patients in Tx group	Patients in Comparison/Control Group	Effect Estimate (MD) [95% CI]	Quality
Pressure Pain Threshold (assessed with pressure algometer: kg/cm^2)—Manual TrP therapy vs. Other therapies										
Hamstring stretching + Ischemic compression vs. Hamstring stretching (left)	1 RCT [53]; right after treatment	Very Serious [a]	NA	No Serious [c]	Serious [e]	Undetected [f]	21	21	MD = 0.00 kg/cm^2 [−0.20, 0.20]	Low
Hamstring stretching + Ischemic compression vs. Hamstring stretching (right)	1 RCT [53]; right after treatment	Very Serious [a]	NA	No Serious [c]	Serious [e]	Undetected [f]	21	21	MD = −0.10 kg/cm^2 [−0.70, 0.50]	Low
Strain/Counterstrain technique vs. Neuromuscular technique	1 RCT [52]; right after treatment	Very Serious [a]	NA	Serious [d]	Serious [e]	Undetected [f]	25	22	MD = 0.00 kg/cm^2 [−0.23, 0.23]	Low
Mouth Opening (assessed with calibrated caliper (Blanco et al.): scale in mm; in Ibáñez-García: NR: scale in mm) – Manual TrP therapy vs. Control										
Strain/Counterstrain technique vs. Control (no treatment)	1 RCT [51]; right after treatment	Very Serious [a]	Very serious [b]	Serious [d]	Serious [e]	Undetected [f]	30	30	Total MD = 0.30 mm [−3.29, 3.89]	Very Low
Strain/Counterstrain technique vs. Control (no treatment)	1 RCT [52]; right after treatment	Very Serious [a]	Very serious [b]	Serious [d]	Serious [e]	Undetected [f]	30	30	Total MD = 6.00 mm [1.97, 10.03]	Very Low
Mouth Opening (assessed with calibrated caliper (Espejo-Antúnez et al.): scale in mm; in Ibáñez-García: NR: scale in mm)—Manual TrP therapy vs. Other therapies										
Strain/Counterstrain technique vs. post-isometric relax.	1 RCT [51]; right after treatment	Very Serious [a]	NA	Serious [d]	Serious [e]	Undetected [f]	30	30	MD = −1.80 mm [−5.12, 1.52]	Very Low

Table 2. Cont.

Comparisons	Quality Assessment						Summary of Findings			
	No. of Studies (Design; Time of measurement)	Risk of Bias	Inconsistency	Indirectness	Imprecision	Publication Bias	No. of Patients		Effect	Quality
							Patients in Tx group	Patients in Comparison/Control Group	Estimate (MD) [95% CI]	
Hamstring stretching + Ischemic comp. vs. Hamstring stretching	1 RCT [53]; right after treatment	Very Serious [a]	NA	No serious [c]	Serious [e]	Undetected [f]	21	21	MD = 0.20 mm [−3.77, 4.17]	Low
Strain/Counterstrain technique vs. Neuromuscular technique	1 RCT [52]; right after treatment	Very Serious [a]	NA	Serious [d]	Serious [e]	Undetected [f]	25	22	MD = 0.00 mm [−3.30, 3.30]	Very Low

CI: Confidence Interval; MD: Mean difference; NA: Not applicable. **Explanations:** [a] Allocation concealment unclear in two studies ([17,51], performance bias and co-interventions are unclear, and incomplete outcome data have a high risk of bias for all four studies. Three studies with unclear intention to treat [17,51,53]. All studies were considered to have high risk of bias overall. [b] Both studies used control groups without receiving any treatment, and the same treatment method for manual TrP therapy (strain/ counterstrain technique). Both studies investigated the effect of manual TrP on patients with latent myofascial TrPs in the masseter muscle. However, a high heterogeneity was obtained in the effect estimates. [c] No serious indirectness, as these studies match the PICO format of this systematic review. [d] Serious indirectness, as these studies do not match with all aspects of PICO format; population with latent myofascial TrPs. [e] All the studies have a wide confidence interval (CI) and unclear or inadequate sample sizes. [f] Undetected publication bias due to the precise literature search performed by an experienced scientific librarian.

3.5. Maximum or Vertical Mouth Opening

Comparison of manual trigger point therapy vs. control group: Two studies [51,52] evaluated the effect of the manual trigger point technique (strain/counterstrain technique) compared to a control group (Figure 2, 2.3.6). Results of these studies were mixed; one study [51] found no statistical difference between groups and the other [52] found significant results favoring the manual trigger point therapy group. This study showed a clinically relevant increase on maximal mouth opening in the manual trigger point therapy group compared to the control group (MD [95% CI]: 6.00 mm [1.97, 10.03]) (Figure 2).

Comparison of manual trigger point therapy vs. other therapies: Three studies [51–53] evaluated the effect of strain/counterstrain technique or ischemic compression versus other intervention methods such as post-isometric relaxation [51], neuromuscular technique [52], or hamstring stretching [53]. None of the studies showed a clear and significant difference between manual trigger point therapy and any of the other techniques analyzed (Figure 2 and Table 1).

3.6. Risk of Bias of Analyzed Studies

The risk of bias (RoB) is summarized in detail in Appendix E and Figure 3. All the included studies for this systematic review used a random sequence generation, provided well defined inclusion and exclusion criteria for their populations, and gave a detailed description of the protocols used for treatment. However, all of them had some methodological flaws (Appendix E). Questions regarding the interventions revealed that the treatment protocol was inadequately described by all included studies, as some details of exposure were not reported. Therefore, the reproducibility of these interventions is not possible.

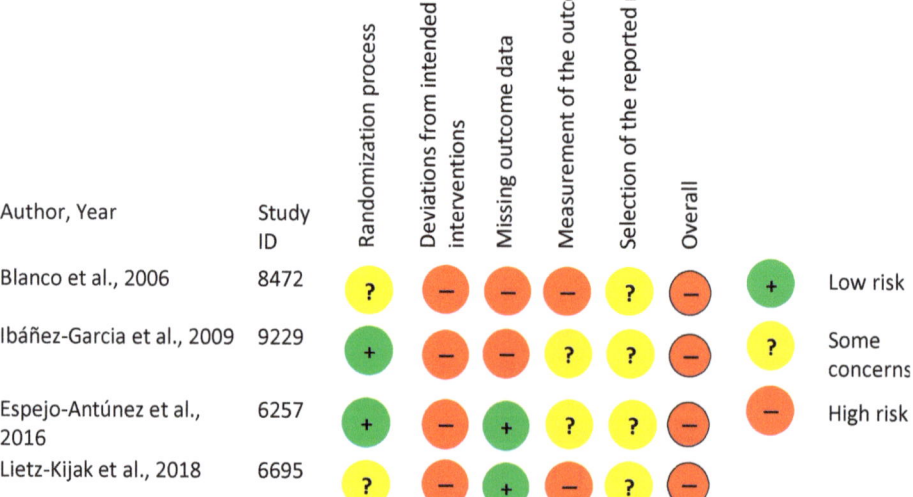

Figure 3. Risk of bias summary performed using the Cochrane Risk of Bias tool to evaluate the quality of the RCTs.

Regarding all aspects of the compiled set of items and the RoB assessment tool, the four studies included in this systematic review were considered to have an overall high risk RoB (Figures 3 and 4, and Appendix E).

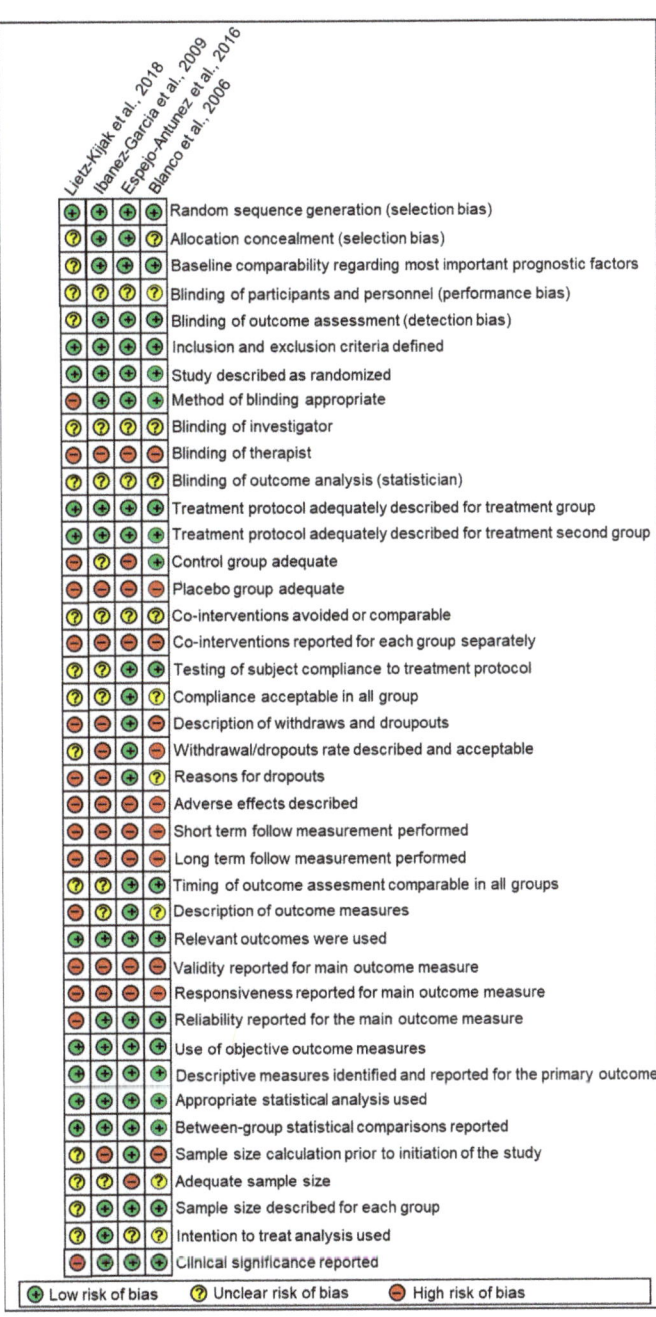

Figure 4. Risk of bias summary performed using the compiled set of items to evaluate the quality of the RCTs.

3.7. Quality of Evidence

The study quality was assessed using the GRADE approach [50]. The overall quality of evidence was very low (Table 2) due to the high RoB of all included studies and due to the indirectness in some of the comparisons in this systematic review. The evidence was generally downgraded for three reasons including RoB, imprecision, and indirectness of the reported results.

4. Discussion

The findings from this systematic review show that manual trigger point therapy could potentially be beneficial for patients with mTrPs in the orofacial area. Even though manual trigger point therapy did not show a clear advantage over other conservative treatments, it was found to be an effective therapy for patients with mTrPs in the orofacial area and better than control groups. However, the number of studies was limited, the RoB was high, and the certainty of evidence was low. Despite the poor quality of the evidence, the non-invasive nature of the manual myofascial techniques can be an attractive complement or even alternative to other interventions. In addition, although we aimed to pool studies, this was not possible due to the heterogeneity of the results of the included studies.

4.1. Effectiveness of Manual Trigger Point Therapy in Comparison with Other Reviews

This systematic review results are in agreement with other systematic reviews focusing on other regions of the body, such as headache or neck pain, and myofascial pain syndromes [24,25,56]. All reviews agree that treatment with manual trigger point therapy techniques leads to a significant or promising improvement in several outcomes when compared with home exercises [57], physical therapy modalities (i.e., hot packs, transcutaneous electric nerve stimulation (TENS), stretch with spray, and others) [58], or transverse friction massage [59], but the level of evidence remains low to very low. Although previous reviews on this topic are available, they are already outdated (in the view of the Cochrane collaboration), as they were published more than 5 years ago, their conclusions can be maintained as their results agree with ours, which provides an updated analysis of this literature.

One finding of clinical importance from these reviews is that the included trials in these reviews had a low number of sessions or they did not implement follow-ups of the manual therapy treatment, similar to the findings of this systematic review. It is unlikely that short treatment exposure from these manual TrPs techniques (i.e., a limited number of sessions) can produce a significant and long-lasting effect as highlighted by our review.

4.2. Methodological Biases and Evidence Quality

As shown previously, all the included studies were considered to have a high risk of bias (Figure 3). These common biases in the included studies could have impacted the results of this review and are shown in Figure 4. The lack of blinding might have influenced the results of the analyzed studies, but due to the nature of the treatment methods used, blinding might not have been possible in all cases. There are some strategies that have been suggested to overcome lack of blinding in this type of studies that could be used in future research in this area [60]. Even though the studies reported the interventions they used adequately for their treatment groups, they did not report on co-interventions, adverse effects, or adequate adherence to the treatments. In addition, it is unclear whether the participants received all scheduled treatment sessions and whether they received a sufficient dose of treatments, especially since some of the included studies [51,53] used only one session of manual trigger point therapy (Tables 1 and 2). Furthermore, none of the trials investigated any short-term or long-term effects of the interventions (no follow-ups). All these shortcomings make the evidence from these studies uncertain and poor.

4.3. Future Directions

This review shows that there is a paucity of studies looking at the effectiveness of manual trigger point therapy in individuals with myofascial trigger points in the orofacial region. In addition, from the few studies included, no high-quality evidence could be found, which indicates that there is great uncertainty about the effectiveness of manual trigger point therapy in comparison with other therapies in this area. There is a great need for well-designed RCTs considering the limitations highlighted by this review (see section above) to specifically investigate manual trigger point therapy for patients with mTrPs in the orofacial area [23–25].

4.4. Clinical and Research Implications

One of the striking results of this systematic review was that manual trigger point therapy techniques were only applied in a few sessions and were not followed up. Further studies are needed to examine the effect of manual trigger point therapy involving a longer period (more sessions) and measure the long-term effects of these interventions, especially the ischemic compression and strain/counterstrain techniques.

Surprisingly, none of the studies included in this systematic review used a placebo group. Thus, it is unclear, whether manual trigger point therapy was better than a placebo treatment. Future studies evaluating the effect of manual trigger point therapy techniques might need a stronger study design including a placebo intervention.

4.5. Strengths and Limitations of This Review

This systematic review has some strengths and limitations that need to be addressed at this point. The literature searches were performed by an experienced health sciences librarian. This enabled accurate identification of possible studies from the respective databases. In addition, our systematic review did not limit on the basis of language and we searched from 1946 to April 2021 (i.e., database inception to date of last search). Our inclusion criteria were also broad since our objective was to include all studies looking at manual trigger point therapies. Despite these broad criteria and the thorough search conducted, only four studies were found that met our criteria for inclusion. Furthermore, this review was the first to specifically investigate manual trigger point therapy in patients with latent mTrPs in muscles of the orofacial region. Nevertheless, the most common condition reported on was TMD.

In addition, it is important to note that a high risk of bias was found across all included studies, which limits the confidence of the effect of manual trigger point therapies. In addition, due to the paucity of the evidence (i.e., limited number of studies) as well as the heterogeneity of the literature (i.e., not used standardized protocols in the studies), no meta-analysis of the effect estimates could be performed. In addition, we could not explore publication biases through a funnel plot due to the limited number of studies. However, due to the comprehensive searches performed, we do not believe this is a concern.

5. Conclusions

The results from this systematic review support that strain/counterstrain therapy was superior to control groups for patients with mTrPs in the orofacial area to improve pain intensity, pain pressure threshold and mouth opening. However, manual trigger point therapy was equivalent to other active treatment techniques. Overall, the quality of evidence was very low and the risk of bias was high. Therefore, manual trigger point techniques could potentially be used as a complementary technique in the treatment of patients with mTrP in the orofacial area. In addition, there is a paucity of well conducted RCTs in patients with mTrPs in the orofacial region. Rigorous, well-designed RCTs are still needed in this field.

Author Contributions: Conceptualization: S.A.-O. and H.v.P.; methodology: S.A.-O. and L.D.; data search: L.D.; data screening: F.M., E.M.d.C.C., A.I.S.d.O.-S. and N.M. formal analysis: F.M. and E.M.d.C.C.; writing—original draft preparation: F.M.; writing—review and editing: E.M.d.C.C., S.A.-O., H.v.P., L.D. and G.L.; supervision: S.A.-O.; project administration: S.A.-O. All authors have read and agreed to the published version of the manuscript.

Funding: The authors declare that no financial support was used to write this paper.

Data Availability Statement: Data can be made available upon request to the authors.

Acknowledgments: Sincere thanks to the entire team who put so much time and effort into this project.

Conflicts of Interest: The authors declare that there were no conflict of interest.

Appendix A. Search Strategies

Appendix A.1. Ovid MEDLINE(R) ALL 1946 to 20 April 2021

Search date: 20 April 2021
1. exp Temporomandibular Joint/
2. craniomandibular disorders/ or exp temporomandibular joint disorders/
3. (((temporomandibular or craniomandibular) adj4 (disorder* or disease* or syndrome* or pain*)) or tmj or tmd or costen*).mp.
4. Facial Pain/
5. exp Myofascial Pain Syndromes/
6. ((myofascial or facial or orofacial or craniofacial or jaw) adj2 pain*).mp.
7. exp Masticatory Muscles/
8. (Masticatory or Masseter or pterygoid or (Temporal adj2 Muscl*)).mp.
9. or/1–8
10. exp cryotherapy/ or exp electric stimulation therapy/ or exp diathermy/ or acupuncture/ or exp acupuncture therapy/ or exp phototherapy/
11. exp Biofeedback, Psychology/
12. Iontophoresis/
13. exp Electrophoresis/
14. exp lasers/ or laser therapy/ or low-level light therapy/
15. (Ultrasound or ultrasonic therap* or ultrasonograph* or TENS or ((transcutaneous or electric* or intramuscular) adj3 stimulation) or Electrostimulation or electroanalges* or electrotherap* or ((electric* or percutaneous) adj3 neuromodulation*) or (Interferential adj2 (current or therapy or treatment)) or microcurrent* or russian-current or (burst-modulat* adj3 alternating-current*) or pulsed-radio-frequency-energy or pulsed-radiofrequency-energy or Biofeedback or laser* or photobiomodulation* or phototherap* or Shortwave or short-wave or Electromagnetic-fields or Iontophores* or Electrophores* or acupuncture or Electroacupuncture or acupressure or needling or myofascial-release or (trigger-point* adj4 (therap* or treatment* or massage or release)) or ((manual or ischemic) adj3 compression) or diathermy or ice or heat or cold or cryotherap* or Cryogenic-therap* or cryotreatment or cryothermy).mp.
16. or/10–15
17. exp Clinical trial/ or randomized.tw. or placebo.tw. or randomly.tw. or trial.tw. or groups.tw.
18. 9 and 16 and 17
19. limit 18 to yr = "2004—Current"
20. limit 19 to animals
21. limit 20 to humans
22. 19 not 20 not 21

Appendix A.2. Embase 1974 to April 2021 (OVID Interface)

Search date: 20 April 2021
1. exp temporomandibular joint/
2. temporomandibular joint disorder/
3. face pain/
4. myofascial pain/
5. exp masticatory muscle/
6. (((temporomandibular or craniomandibular) adj4 (disorder* or disease* or syndrome* or pain*)) or tmj or tmd or costen* or (pain adj2 (myofascial or facial or orofa-

cial or jaw or craniofacial)) or ((masticatory or masseter or pterygoid or temporal) adj2 muscl*)).mp.

7. or/1–6
8. cryotherapy/
9. exp electrotherapy/
10. exp ultrasound therapy/
11. exp diathermy/
12. exp acupuncture/
13. exp phototherapy/
14. exp biofeedback/
15. exp electrophoresis/
16. exp laser/
17. (Ultrasound or ultrasonic therap* or ultrasonograph* or TENS or ((transcutaneous or electric* or intramuscular) adj3 stimulation) or Electrostimulation or electroanalges* or electrotherap* or ((electric* or percutaneous) adj3 neuromodulation*) or (Interferential adj2 (current or therapy or treatment)) or microcurrent* or russian-current or (burst-modulat* adj3 alternating-current*) or pulsed-radio-frequency-energy or pulsed-radiofrequency-energy or Biofeedback or laser* or photobiomodulation* or phototherap* or Shortwave or short-wave or Electromagnetic-fields or Iontophores* or Electrophores* or acupuncture or Electroacupuncture or acupressure or needling or myofascial-release or (trigger-point* adj4 (therap* or treatment* or massage or release)) or ((manual or ischemic) adj3 compression) or diathermy or ice or heat or cold or cryotherap* or Cryogenic-therap* or cryotreatment or cryothermy).mp.
18. or/8–17
19. exp clinical trial/
20. (randomized or placebo or randomly or trial or groups).tw.
21. 19 or 20
22. 7 and 18 and 21
23. limit 22 to animals
24. 22 not 23
25. limit 24 to yr ="2004—Current"
26. limit 25 to conference abstract status
27. 25 not 26

Appendix A.3. Wiley Cochrane Library Trials Database

Search date: 20 April 2021

#1 [mh "Temporomandibular Joint"] or [mh ^"craniomandibular disorders"] or [mh "temporomandibular joint disorders"] or [mh ^"Facial Pain"] or [mh "Myofascial Pain Syndromes"] or [mh "Masticatory Muscles"]
#2 ((((temporomandibular or craniomandibular) near/4 (disorder* or disease* or syndrome* or pain*)) or tmj or tmd or costen*):ti,ab,kw
#3 ((myofascial or facial or orofacial or craniofacial or jaw) near/2 pain*):ti,ab,kw
#4 (Masticatory or masseter or pterygoid or (temporal near/2 muscl*)):ti,ab,kw
#5 #1 OR #2 OR #3 OR #4
#6 [mh "cryotherapy"] or [mh "electric stimulation therapy"] or [mh "diathermy"] or [mh ^"acupuncture"] or [mh "acupuncture therapy"] or [mh "phototherapy"]
#7 [mh "Biofeedback, Psychology"] or [mh ^"Iontophoresis"] or [mh "Electrophoresis"] or [mh "lasers"] or [mh ^"laser therapy"]
#8 [mh ^"low-level light therapy"]
#9 (Ultrasound or (ultrasonic NEXT therap*) or ultrasonograph* or TENS or ((transcutaneous or electric* or intramuscular) near/3 stimulation) or Electrostimulation or electroanalges* or electrotherap* or ((electric* or percutaneous) near/3 neuromodulation*) or (Interferential near/2 (current or therapy or treatment)) or microcurrent* or

russian-current or (burst-modulat* near/3 alternating-current*) or pulsed-radio-frequency-energy or pulsed-radiofrequency-energy or Biofeedback or laser* or photobiomodulation* or phototherap* or Shortwave or short-wave or Electromagnetic-fields or Iontophores* or Electrophores* or acupuncture or Electroacupuncture or acupressure or needling or myofacial-release or ((trigger NEXT point*) near/4 (therap* or treatment* or massage or release)) or ((manual or ischemic) near/3 compression) or diathermy or ice or heat or cold or cryotherap* or (Cryogenic NEXT (therap* or treatment)) or cryotreatment or cryothermy):ti,ab,kw

#10   #6 OR #7 OR #8 OR #9
#11   [mh "Clinical trial"] or randomized:ab or placebo:ab or randomly:ab or trial:ab or groups:ab
#12   #5 AND #10 AND #11
(Must limit to year specifically for TRIALS 2004–2019)

Appendix A.4. Web of Science (Indexes=SCI-EXPANDED, SSCI, A&HCI, ESCI)

Search date: 20 April 2021

#1 TS=(((temporomandibular or craniomandibular) NEAR/4 (disorder* or disease* or syndrome* or pain*)) or tmj or tmd or costen* or ((myofascial or facial or orofacial or craniofacial or jaw) NEAR/2 pain*) or ((masticatory or masseter or pterygoid or temporal) NEAR/2 muscl*))

#2 TS=(Ultrasound or ultrasonic-therap* or ultrasonograph* or TENS or ((transcutaneous or electric* or intramuscular) NEAR/3 stimulation) or Electrostimulation or electroanalges* or electrotherap* or ((electric* or percutaneous) NEAR/3 neuromodulation*) or (Interferential NEAR/2 (current or therapy or treatment)) or microcurrent* or russian-current or (burst-modulat* NEAR/3 alternating-current*) or pulsed-radio-frequency-energy or pulsed-radiofrequency-energy or Biofeedback or laser* or photobiomodulation* or phototherap* or Shortwave or short-wave or Electromagnetic-fields or Iontophores* or Electrophores* or acupuncture or Electroacupuncture or acupressure or needling or myofascial-release or (trigger-point* NEAR/4 (therap* or treatment* or massage or release)) or ((manual or ischemic) NEAR/3 compression) or diathermy or ice or heat or cold or cryotherap* or Cryogenic-therap* or cryogenic-treatment* or cryotreatment or cryothermy)

#3 TS= (Clinical-trial or randomized or placebo or randomly or trial or groups) OR TI=(rct)

#4 #1 AND #2 AND #3

#5 #4 NOT TI= (rat or rats or pig or pigs or porcine or mouse or mice or rabbit* or hamster or hamsters or animal or animals or bovine or sheep or murine or primate* or animal or pain-model*)

Indexes=SCI-EXPANDED, SSCI, A&HCI, ESCI Timespan=2004–2019

Appendix A.5. CINAHL Plus with Full Text

Date searched: 20 April 2021

Mode: Boolean Phrase (deselect "Apply equivalent subjects")

S1. ((MH "Temporomandibular Joint") OR (MH "Myofascial Pain Syndromes+") OR (MH "Craniomandibular Disorders+") OR (MH "Masticatory Muscles+") OR (MH "Facial Pain")) OR (((temporomandibular or craniomandibular) N4 (disorder* or disease* or syndrome* or pain*)) or tmj or tmd or costen* or ((facial or orofacial or myofascial or jaw or craniofacial) N2 pain*) or Masticatory or Masseter or pterygoid or (Temporal N2 Muscl*))

S2 (MH "Diathermy+") OR (MH "Electric Stimulation+") OR (MH "Cryotherapy") OR (MH "Electrotherapy+") OR (MH "Heat-Cold Application") OR (MH "Laser Therapy") OR (MH "Lasers") OR (MH "Biofeedback") OR (MH "Phototherapy") OR (MH "Electrophoresis+")) OR (Ultrasound or ultrasonic-therap* or ultrasonograph* or TENS or ((transcutaneous or electric* or intramuscular) N3 stimulation) or Electrostimulation or electroanalges* or electrotherap* or ((electric* or percutaneous) N3 neuromodulation*) or

(Interferential N2 (current or therapy or treatment)) or microcurrent* or russian-current or (burst-modulat* N3 alternating-current*) or pulsed-radio-frequency-energy or pulsed-radiofrequency-energy or Biofeedback or laser* or photobiomodulation* or phototherap* or Shortwave or short-wave or Electromagnetic-fields or Iontophores* or Electrophores* or acupuncture or Electroacupuncture or acupressure or needling or myofacial-release or (trigger-point* N4 (therap* or treatment* or massage or release)) or ((manual or ischemic) N3 compression) or diathermy or ice or heat or cold or cryotherap* or Cryogenic-therap* or cryogenic-treatment* or cryotreatment or cryothermy)

S3 (MH "Clinical Trials+") OR (randomized or placebo or randomly or trial or groups)
Limiters—Published Date: 20040101–20191231

Appendix A.6. SCOPUS

Date searched: 20 April 2021

(((TITLE-ABS-KEY (((temporomandibular OR craniomandibular) W/4 (disorder* OR disease* OR syndrome* OR pain*)) OR tmj OR costen* OR ((myofascial OR facial OR orofacial OR craniofacial OR jaw) W/2 pain*) OR ((masticatory OR masseter OR pterygoid OR temporal) W/2 muscl*))) AND (TITLE-ABS-KEY (ultrasound OR ultrasonic-therap* OR ultrasonograph* OR tens OR ((transcutaneous OR electric*OR intramuscular) W/3 stimulation) OR electrostimulation OR electroanalges* OR electrotherap* OR ((electric* OR percutaneous) W/3 neuromodulation*) OR (interferential W/2 (current OR therapy OR treatment)) OR microcurrent* OR russian-current OR (burst-modulat* W/3 alternating-current*) or pulsed-radio-frequency-energy or pulsed-radiofrequency-energy or biofeedback OR laser* OR photobiomodulation* OR phototherap* OR shortwave OR short-wave OR electromagnetic-fields OR iontophores* OR electrophores* OR acupuncture OR electroacupuncture OR acupressure or needling or myofacial-release or (trigger-point* W/4 (therap* or treatment* or massage or release)) or ((manual or ischemic) W/3 compression) OR diathermy OR ice OR heat OR cold OR cryotherap* OR cryogenic-therap* OR cryogenic-treatment* OR cryotreatment OR cryothermy)) AND (TITLE-ABS-KEY (Clinical trial OR randomized OR placebo OR randomly OR trial OR groups) OR TITLE (rct))) AND NOT (TITLE (rat OR rats OR pig OR pigs OR porcine OR mouse OR mice OR rabbit* OR hamster OR hamsters OR animal OR animals OR bovine OR sheep OR murine OR primate* OR animal OR pain-model*)) AND PUBYEAR > 2003) AND (EXCLUDE (DOCTYPE, "cp"))

Appendix B. Description of the Orofacial Pain Diagnosis

Following the orofacial pain diagnosis included in this systematic review, it can be defined as:

1. **Orofacial pain associated with regional muscles:** painful and nonpainful disorders affecting masticatory muscles, temporomandibular joint, and contiguous structures. These are specified according to the items below:

    (a) **Primary myofascial pain:** Pain in jaw, temple, ear or in front of ear, modified with jaw movement, function, or parafunction. It should present a familiar pain in the temporal or masseter muscles and the pain can also be referred.

    (b) **Secondary myofascial pain:** Persistent inflammation, structural changes, injury, or diseases of the nervous system. This pain can be developed, become worse or improve, according to the presumed causative disorder.

2. **Orofacial pain associated with disorders of the temporomandibular joint (TMJ):** condition attributed to arthralgia in the temporomandibular joint; classified as:

    (a) **Primary TMJ arthralgia:** Familiar pain in front of the ear, or in the ear confirmed by the palpation of the lateral pole or around the lateral pole, which modified with jaw movement, function, or parafunction.

    (b) **Secondary TMJ arthralgia:** TMJ pain related to inflammation, sensitization of the tissues, injury diseases of the nervous system, or structural changes.

3. **Orofacial pain resembling presentations of primary headaches:** pain exclusively in the facial area resembling primary headaches but without head pain; classified as:
   (a) **Orofacial migraine:** Unilateral pulsating pain with moderate or severe intensity. It can be aggravated by routine physical activity and present association with nausea and/or photophobia and phonophobia.
   (b) **Tension-type orofacial pain:** Facial muscle tension that occurs during rest and improves with voluntary muscle activity (e.g., mastication).
4. **Idiopathic orofacial pain:** pain without a clear causative disorder. Specified as:
   (a) **Burning mouth syndrome:** Intraoral sensation of burning and felt superficially in the oral mucosa, but the oral mucosa has a normal appearance.
   (b) **Persistent idiopathic facial pain:** Facial pain dull, aching or nagging, poorly located and without following the peripheral nerve distribution.

Appendix C. Trigger Point Therapy—Description of Techniques

The manual trigger point therapy techniques targeted in this review will be the following:

Ischemic compression: A manual therapeutic technique used in physical therapy, where blood is deliberately blocked in an area of the body, so that a resurgence of local blood flow will occur upon release. (1)

Trigger point pressure release: Applying sustained pressure on a trigger point without inducing additional ischemia in trigger point zone. The amount of pressure applied should be enough to produce gradual relaxation of the tension within the trigger point zone, without causing pain. (2)

Myofascial release: Myofascial release is a therapeutic method for stimulating connective tissue fibers. The treatment usually takes place locally on altered fascial structures and involves an application of a low load and long duration stretch. Myofascial release can be used to treat and especially decrease pain, restore optimal length of tissue and to improve the function. (3)

Manual pressure on taut bands: Pressure, applied manually, on a myofascial trigger point, which is defined as a hyperirritable spot, usually within a taut band of skeletal muscle which is painful on compression. (4)

Passive stretching: A passive stretch is one where the patient is asked to assume a position and hold it with the assistance of a therapist to stretch a determined muscle. The stretch is held until the stretched muscle tissue starts to relax. Passive stretch reduces muscle tissue stiffness, most likely by signaling connective tissue remodeling via fibroblasts (5, 6).

Manual fascial techniques: The technique involves deep manual friction over specific points on the deep muscular fascia that are always at a distance from the actual site of pain (7).

Manual intraoral or extraoral release: The intraoral techniques usually involve applying digital pressure (known variously as ischemic compression, pressure release, myotherapy, or acupressure) into masticatory muscle trigger points, origins, or insertions, using intra-oral contact points. The extraoral technique applies the same digital pressure into the masticatory muscles but using extra-oral contact points (4).

Strain/counterstrain technique: This technique attempts to achieve the most comfortable position possible to relax muscle spasm by reducing abnormal afferent flow from the muscle spindle. If a myofascial trigger point is located in a muscle, a therapist applies gradually increasing pressure on that point until the feeling of pressure becomes a feeling of pressure and pain. Then there is a passive change of position of the patient performed by the therapist, until the tension under the palpating fingers and the pain reduces in intensity (8, 9).

Appendix D. Detailed Study Characteristics

Table A1. The results from the data extraction, showing the qualitative elements concerning article and study information.

Study Details	Population Details	Treatment Details	Statistical Analysis Description	Limitation, Comments and Recommendations
First author: Cleofás Rodríguez Blanco, 2006 [51] **Country:** Spain **Language:** English **Trial registered:** Unclear **Study Design:** RCT **Study setting:** Unclear **RCT Type:** Parallel **Objective:** To emphasize the immediate effect on MMO in performing a single treatment of latent mTrPs in the masseter muscle using a post-isometric relaxation, and the strain/counterstrain technique. **Ethical approval:** Yes	**Population age:** 25 ± 4.3 years **Population sex:** Mixed **Population diagnosis:** Latent mTrPs in the masseter muscle, either left or right side **Diagnosis tool used:** Clinical Diagnoses; Simons diagnostic criteria **Sampling method used:** Convenience **Sample size calculation:** NR **Total sample size:** 90; 42 male, 48 female **Recruitment period (start–end):** NR **No. of randomized groups:** 3	**T1:** Post-isometric relaxation technique **T1 combined:** Alone **Duration of T1 (weeks):** 0 weeks **Duration of session/exposure (min):** 0.55 min **No. of sessions:** 1 (3x exposure) **Percentage of compliance:** NR **Compliance with treatment:** Yes **Application area (T1):** Masseter muscles; Mouth **T2:** Strain/counterstrain technique **T2 combined:** Alone **Duration T2 (weeks):** unclear **Duration of session/exposure (min):** ~1.5 min, but more time was used to apply pressure on mTrP **No. of sessions:** 1 **Application area (T2):** Masseter muscles, Cervical region **Manual TrP therapy concept (T2):** Strain/counterstrain technique **T3:** Control **T3 combined:** Alone **Duration of T3 (weeks):** 0 weeks **Duration of session/exposure (min):** 5 min	**Data Analysis description:** • Between the groups: ANOVA test for continuous data, and for categorical data, the χ^2 test; • Within-group: Dependent t-test for the differences and for the effect sizes, the Cohen's d coefficient • Between changes produced by the three interventions: One-way ANOVA test (the Bonferroni correction was used as post hoc analysis); Statistical analysis was conducted as a 95% confidence level and a P-value less than 0.05 was considered as statistically significant.	**Limitations/Comments:** • Immediate effect of the techniques; • Participants had no symptoms that might be typical for the population seeking manual therapy treatment; • The only outcome was active mouth opening. **Recommendations:** • Evaluate long-term effect of the interventions; • Include a placebo group; • Include participants with symptoms and complaints caused by myofascial TrPs; • Evaluate the pain sensitivity as an outcome.

Table A1. Cont.

Study Details	Population Details	Treatment Details	Statistical Analysis Description	Limitation, Comments and Recommendations
First author: Jordi Ibáñez-García,2009 [52] **Country:** Spain **Language:** English **Trial registered:** Unclear **Study Design:** RCT **Study setting:** Unclear **RCT Type:** Parallel **Objective:** To compare the immediate effects on MMO and pressure pain sensitivity as a result of the treatment of latent mTrPs in the masseter muscle by treating with neuromuscular or strain/counterstrain technique. **Ethical approval:** Yes	**Population age:** 36 ± 14.7 years **Population sex:** Mixed **Population diagnosis:** Latent mTrPs in the masseter muscle, either left or right sides. **Diagnosis tool used:** Clinical Diagnoses; Simons diagnostic criteria **Sampling method used:** Convenience **Sample size calculation:** NR **Total sample size:** 71; 34 male, 37 female **Recruitment period (start-end):** NR **No. of randomized groups:** 3	**T1:** Strain/counterstrain technique **T1 combined:** Alone **Duration of T1 (weeks):** 3 weeks **Duration of session/exposure (min):** 1.5 min **No. of sessions:** 3 **Percentage of compliance:** NR **Compliance with treatment:** NR **Application area (T1):** Masseter muscles, Cervical region **Manual TrP therapy concept (T1):** Strain/counterstrain technique **T2:** Neuromuscular technique **T2 combined:** Alone **Duration of T2 (weeks):** 3 weeks **Duration of session/exposure (min):** max. 0.666 min **No. of sessions:** 3 **Application area (T2):** Masseter muscles **Manual TrP therapy concept (T2):** Neuromuscular technique **T3:** Control **T3 combined:** Alone **Duration of T3 (weeks):** Unclear **Duration of session/exposure (min):** 5 min **No. of sessions:** 3	**Data Analysis description:** • Data expressed as mean and standard deviations or 95% confidence interval; • ANOVA test was used for continuous data to compare baseline values, and for categorical data, the X^2 tests were performed; • To evaluate changes after the interventions: Two-way mixed analysis of variance (ANOVA), using the time (pre-post test measurements) as the within-subject variable and group as between-subject variable; • The intention-to-treat analysis was used to analyze the subjects in the group to which they were allocated Within groups: The effect sizes were calculated using the Cohen d coefficient; • The statistical analysis was conducted at a 95% confidence level and a p-value less than 0.05 was considered as statistically significant.	**Limitations/Comments:** Immediate effect of neuromuscular or strain/counterstrain techniques; Participants had no symptoms and might not be typical for the population seeking manual therapy treatment. **Recommendations:** Evaluate the long-term effect of the technique; Include a placebo group; Include participants with symptoms and complaints caused by myofascial TrPs.

Table A1. Cont.

Study Details	Population Details	Treatment Details	Statistical Analysis Description	Limitation, Comments and Recommendations
First author: Luis Espejo-Antúnez, 2016 [61] **Country:** Spain **Language:** English **Trial registered:** No **Study Design:** RCT **Study setting:** Unclear **RCT Type:** Parallel **Objective:** This study aimed to assess the immediate effects on MMO, pain and hamstrings extensibility by treating athletes diagnosed with TMD and hamstring shortening with either hamstring stretching alone or combined with ischemic compression of the masseter muscle. **Ethical approval:** Yes	**Population age:** 21.2 ± 1.6 years **Population sex:** Mixed **Population diagnosis:** Myogenic TMD and trigger points **Diagnosis tool used:** RDC/TMD, Clinical Diagnoses **Duration of diagnosis:** 6 months chronicity of pain **Population other conditions:** Hamstring shortening **Population other characteristics:** Participants with regular sports practice (≥5 h per week), without previous hamstrings injury **Sampling method used:** Convenience **Sample size calculation:** Yes **Total sample size:** 42; 14 male, 28 female **Total sample size start-finish:** NR **Recruitment period (start-end):** NR **No. of randomized groups:** 2	**T1:** Proprioceptive neuromuscular facilitation technique **T1 combined:** Alone **Duration of T1 (weeks):** 0 weeks **Duration of session/exposure (min):** 1.6 min **No. of sessions:** 1 **Percentage of compliance:** 100% **Compliance with treatment:** Yes **Application area (T1):** Hamstrings **T2:** Hamstring stretching + ischemic compression technique **T2 combined:** Combined **T2 how many therapies combined:** 2 **T2 which therapies are combined:** Ischemic compression and proprioceptive neuromuscular facilitation technique **Duration of T2 (weeks):** 0 weeks **Duration of session/exposure (min):** 3.1 min **No. of sessions:** 1 **Percentage of compliance:** 100% **Compliance with treatment:** Yes **Application area (T2):** Masseter muscles and hamstrings **Manual TrP therapy concept (T2):** Ischemic compression	**Data Analysis description:** • Data are reported as mean ± SD or median (interquartile range). • Association tests (between gender and active mouth opening, hamstrings extensibility, pressure pain threshold or pain intensity): Pearson Correlation or Spearman's test • Within groups (for normally and not normally distributed data): Student's paired t-test and the Wilcoxon signed-rank test; • Between groups (normally distributed, not distributed, and nominal data): Student's in dependent t-test, the Mann–Whitney U test and the χ^2 test; • Effect size between groups: Cohen's d coefficient; • The significance level was established at $p < 0.05$.	**Limitations/Comments:** • Participants included were amateur athletes; • Evaluation of the acute effects; • Unimplemented follow-up; • The treatments were not well described. **Recommendations:** • Include of a follow-up (medium and long-term); • Include athlete's performance level as participants.

Table A1. *Cont.*

Study Details	Population Details	Treatment Details	Statistical Analysis Description	Limitation, Comments and Recommendations
First author: Danuta Lietz-Kijak, 2018 [17] **Country:** Poland **Language:** English **Trial registered:** No **Study Design:** RCT **Study setting:** NR **RCT Type:** Parallel **Objective:** This study aimed at the evaluation of the effect on pain in patients diagnosed with TMD by treatment with kinesiotaping and trigger points inactivation. **Ethical approval:** Yes **Trial registered:** No	**Population age:** 25.87 ± 4.86 years **Population sex:** Mixed **Population diagnosis:** Latent trigger points and myogenic TMD **Diagnosis tool used:** RDC/TMD **Population other characteristics:** Diagnosed with an excessive strain of masseter muscles and muscular pain, without limitations in the movements of the mandible and disc derangement and joint pain **Sampling method used:** Convenience **Sample size calculation:** No **Total sample size:** 60; 29 male, 31 female **Recruitment period (start-end):** 2015–2016 **No. of randomized groups:** 2	**T1:** Kinesiotaping **T1 combined:** Alone **Duration of T1 (weeks):** 0.71 weeks **Duration of session/exposure (min):** 7.200 min **No. of sessions:** 1 **Percentage of compliance:** NR **Compliance with treatment:** NR **Application area (T1):** Masseter muscles **T2:** Ischemic compression **T2 combined:** Alone **Duration of T2 (weeks):** 0.71 weeks **No. of sessions:** 3 (on the first, third and fifth day of treatment) **Application area (T2):** Masseter muscles **Manual TrP therapy concept (T2):** Ischemic compression	**Data Analysis Description:** • Within groups: Paired sample Welch t-test; • To test the influence of gender and age on treatment efficacy: linear regression models; • Between groups: Welch t-test for unpaired samples.	**Limitations/Comments:** • Do not have a control group; • Randomization and blinding process not very well described; • Withdrawals and dropouts were not described; • Methods not very well described; • Does not have a follow-up analysis; • Short time of treatment. **Recommendations:** • Implement a control group; • Describe methods better; • Provide information about the randomization and blinding methods; • Describe the withdrawals and dropouts; • Increase the time of treatment and include a follow-up analysis.

T1: Treatment arm 1; T2: Treatment arm 2; T3: Treatment arm 3.

Appendix E. Risk of Bias—Compiled Set of Items Table

Table A2. Summary of the compiled set of items used to evaluate the risk of bias of the studies included in this systematic review.

Items	Blanco et al., 2006 [51]	Ibáñez García et al., 2009 [52]	Espejo Antúnez et al., 2016 [53]	Lietz et al., 2018 [17]	Total	
	Consensus	Consensus	Consensus	Consensus		
Inclusion and exclusion criteria clearly defined consensus	Yes	Yes	Yes	Yes	4	100%
Study described as randomized consensus	Yes	Yes	Yes	Yes	4	100%
Method of randomization described and appropriate consensus	Yes	Yes	Yes	Unclear	3	75%
Method of randomization concealed Consensus	Unclear	Yes	Yes	Unclear	2	50%
Baseline comparability regarding the most important prognostic indicators consensus	Yes	Yes	Yes	Unclear	3	75%
Study described as double-blind consensus	No	No	No	Unclear	0	0%
Method of blinding appropriate consensus	Yes	Yes	Yes	No	3	75%
Blinding investigator consensus	Unclear	Unclear	Unclear	Unclear	0	0%
Blinding of assessors' consensus	Yes	Yes	Yes	Unclear	3	75%
Blinding of participants consensus	Unclear	Unclear	Unclear	Unclear	0	0%
Blinding of therapist consensus	No	No	No	No	0	0%
Blinding of outcomes analysis (statistician) consensus	Unclear	Unclear	Unclear	Unclear	0	0%
Treatment protocol adequately described for treatment group consensus	Yes	Yes	Yes	Yes	4	100%
Treatment protocol adequately described for treatment second group consensus	Yes	Yes	Yes	Yes	4	100%
Control group adequate consensus	Yes	Unclear	No	No	1	25%
Placebo group adequate consensus	No	No	No	No	0	0%
Co-interventions avoided or comparable consensus	Unclear	Unclear	Unclear	Unclear	0	0%
Co-interventions reported for each group separately consensus	No	No	No	No	0	0%
Testing of subject compliance to treatment protocol consensus	Yes	Unclear	Yes	Unclear	2	50%
Compliance acceptable in all group consensus	Unclear	Unclear	Yes	Unclear	1	25%
Description of withdraws and dropout's consensus	No	No	Yes	No	1	25%
Withdrawal/dropouts rate described and acceptable consensus	No	No	Yes	Unclear	1	25%
Reasons for dropouts consensus	Unclear	No	Yes	No	1	25%
Adverse effects described consensus	No	No	No	No	0	0%
Short term follow measurement performed consensus	No	No	No	No	0	0%
Long term follow measurement performed consensus	No	No	No	No	0	0%
The timing of the outcome assessment was comparable in all group's consensus	Yes	Unclear	Yes	Unclear	2	50%
Description of outcome measures consensus	Unclear	Unclear	Yes	No	1	25%
Relevant outcomes were used consensus	Yes	Yes	Yes	Yes	4	100%
Validity reported for the main outcome measure consensus	No	No	No	No	0	0%
Responsiveness reported for the main outcome measure consensus	No	No	No	No	0	0%
Reliability reported for the main outcome measure consensus	Yes	Yes	Yes	No	3	75%
Use of objective outcome measures consensus	Yes	Yes	Yes	Yes	4	100%

Table A2. Cont.

Items	Blanco et al., 2006 [51]	Ibáñez García et al., 2009 [52]	Espejo Antúnez et al., 2016 [53]	Lietz et al., 2018 [17]	Total	
	Consensus	Consensus	Consensus	Consensus		
Descriptive measures identified and reported for the primary outcome consensus	Yes	Yes	Yes	Yes	4	100%
Appropriate statistical analysis used consensus	Yes	Yes	Yes	Yes	4	100%
Between-group statistical comparisons reported Consensus	Yes	Yes	Yes	Yes	4	100%
Sample size calculation prior to initiation of the study consensus	No	No	Yes	Unclear	1	25%
Adequate sample size consensus	Unclear	Unclear	No	Unclear	0	0%
Sample size described for each group consensus	Yes	Yes	Yes	Unclear	3	75%
Intention to treat analysis used consensus	Unclear	Yes	Unclear	Unclear	1	25%
Clinical significance reported consensus	Yes	Yes	Yes	No	3	75%
Number of items accomplished/total of applicable items	18/40	17/40	24/40	8/40		
Number of items applicable	40	40	40	40		
% of items accomplished	45%	42.50%	60%	20%		
Risk of Bias Tool Assessment	High	High	High	High		

References

1. Li, L.; Stoop, R.; Clijsen, R.; Hohenauer, E.; Fernández-de-Las-Peñas, C.; Huang, Q.; Barbero, M. Criteria Used for the Diagnosis of Myofascial Trigger Points in Clinical Trials on Physical Therapy: Updated Systematic Review. *Clin. J. Pain* **2020**, *36*, 955–967. [CrossRef]
2. Travell, J.G.; Simons, D.G.; Simons, L.S. *Myofascial Pain and Dysfunction: The Trigger Point Manual: Vol. 1: Upper Half of Body*; Williams & Wilkins: Baltimore, MD, USA, 1999.
3. International Classification of Orofacial Pain, 1st edition (ICOP). *Cephalalgia* **2020**, *40*, 129–221. [CrossRef] [PubMed]
4. Romero-Reyes, M.; Uyanik, J. Orofacial pain management: Current perspectives. *J. Pain Res.* **2014**, *7*, 99. [CrossRef] [PubMed]
5. Jin, L.J.; Lamster, I.; Greenspan, J.; Pitts, N.; Scully, C.; Warnakulasuriya, S. Global burden of oral diseases: Emerging concepts, management and interplay with systemic health. *Oral Dis.* **2016**, *22*, 609–619. [CrossRef]
6. LeResche, L. Epidemiology of temporomandibular disorders: Implications for the investigation of etiologic factors. *Crit. Rev. Oral Biol. Med.* **1997**, *8*, 291–305. [CrossRef] [PubMed]
7. Kohlmann, T. Epidemiologie orofazialer Schmerzen. *Der Schmerz* **2002**, *16*, 339–345. [CrossRef]
8. Manfredini, D.; Guarda-Nardini, L.; Winocur, E.; Piccotti, F.; Ahlberg, J.; Lobbezoo, F. Research diagnostic criteria for temporomandibular disorders: A systematic review of axis I epidemiologic findings. *Oral Surg. Oral Med. Oral Pathol. Oral Radiol. Endodontol.* **2011**, *112*, 453–462. [CrossRef]
9. Vier, C.; de Almeida, M.B.; Neves, M.L.; Dos Santos AR, S.; Bracht, M.A. The effectiveness of dry needling for patients with orofacial pain associated with temporomandibular dysfunction: A systematic review and meta-analysis. *Braz. J. Phys. Ther.* **2019**, *23*, 3–11. [CrossRef]
10. Leeuw, R.D.; Klasser, G.D.; American Academy of Orofacial, P. *Orofacial Pain: Guidelines for Assessment, Diagnosis, and Management*; Quintessence Publishing: Batavia, IL, USA, 2018.
11. Ferrillo, M.; Ammendolia, A.; Paduano, S.; Calafiore, D.; Marotta, N.; Migliario, M.; Fortunato, L.; Giudice, A.; Michelotti, A.; de Sire, A. Efficacy of rehabilitation on reducing pain in muscle-related temporomandibular disorders: A systematic review and meta-analysis of randomized controlled trials. *J. Back Musculoskelet. Rehabil.* **2022**, *35*, 921–936. [CrossRef]
12. Armijo-Olivo, S.; Magee, D.; Gross, D. Effects of exercise therapy on endogenous pain-relieving peptides in musculoskeletal pain: A systematic review. *Clin. J. Pain* **2011**, *27*, 365–374.
13. Armijo-Olivo, S.; Pitance, L.; Singh, V.; Neto, F.; Thie, N.; Michelotti, A. Effectiveness of manual therapy and therapeutic exercise for temporomandibular disorders: Systematic review and meta-analysis. *Phys. Ther.* **2016**, *96*, 9–25. [CrossRef] [PubMed]
14. Calixtre, L.; Moreira, R.F.C.; Franchini, G.H.; Alburquerque-Sendín, F.; Oliveira, A.B. Manual therapy for the management of pain and limited range of motion in subjects with signs and symptoms of temporomandibular disorder: A systematic review of randomised controlled trials. *J. Oral Rehabil.* **2015**, *42*, 847–861. [CrossRef] [PubMed]

15. Brantingham, J.W.; Cassa, T.K.; Bonnefin, D.; Pribicevic, M.; Robb, A.; Pollard, H.; Tong, V.; Korporaal, C. Manipulative and multimodal therapy for upper extremity and temporomandibular disorders: A systematic review. *J. Manip. Physiol.* **2013**, *36*, 143–201. [CrossRef]
16. Paço, M.; Peleteiro, B.; Duarte, J.; Pinho, T. The Effectiveness of Physiotherapy in the Management of Temporomandibular Disorders: A Systematic Review and Meta-analysis. *J. Oral Facial Pain Headache* **2016**, *30*, 210–220. [CrossRef] [PubMed]
17. Lietz-Kijak, D.; Kopacz, Ł.; Ardan, R.; Grzegocka, M.; Kijak, E. Assessment of the short-term effectiveness of kinesiotaping and trigger points release used in functional disorders of the masticatory muscles. *Pain Res. Manag.* **2018**, *2018*, 5464985. [CrossRef] [PubMed]
18. Fernandes, A.C.; Duarte Moura, D.M.; Da Silva, L.G.D.; De Almeida, E.O.; Barbosa, G.A.S. Acupuncture in Temporomandibular Disorder Myofascial Pain Treatment: A Systematic Review. *J. Oral Facial Pain Headache* **2017**, *31*, 225–232. [CrossRef]
19. Díaz-Sáez, M.; Sáenz-Jiménez, C.; Villafañe, J.H.; Paris-Alemany, A.; La Touche, R. Hypoalgesic and Motor Effects of Neural Mobilisation versus Soft-Tissue Interventions in Experimental Craniofacial Hyperalgesia: A Single-Blinded Randomised Controlled Trial. *J. Clin. Med.* **2021**, *10*, 4334. [CrossRef]
20. Sajedi, S.M.; Abbasi, F.; Asnaashari, M.; Jafarian, A.A. Comparative Efficacy of Low-Level Laser Acupuncture and Cupping for Treatment of Patients with Myofascial Pain Dysfunction Syndrome: A Double-blinded, Randomized Clinical Trial: Comparison of the Effects of LLL Acupuncture and Cupping. *Galen Med. J.* **2022**, *11*, 1–13. [CrossRef]
21. Gautschi, R.; Böhni, U. Das myofasziale Schmerzsyndrom. *Man. Med.* **2014**, *52*, 203–213. [CrossRef]
22. Martins, W.R.; Blasczyk, J.C.; de Oliveira, M.A.F.; Gonçalves, K.F.L.; Bonini-Rocha, A.C.; Dugailly, P.-M.; de Oliveira, R.J. Efficacy of musculoskeletal manual approach in the treatment of temporomandibular joint disorder: A systematic review with meta-analysis. *Man. Ther.* **2016**, *21*, 10–17. [CrossRef]
23. Denneny, D.; Frawley, H.C.; Petersen, K.; McLoughlin, R.; Brook, S.; Hassan, S.; Williams, A.C. Trigger point manual therapy for the treatment of chronic noncancer pain in adults: A systematic review and meta-analysis. *Arch. Phys. Med. Rehabil.* **2019**, *100*, 562–577. [CrossRef]
24. de las Peñas, C.F.; Campo, M.S.; Fernandez-Carnero, J.; Palge, J.C.M. Manual therapies in myofascial trigger point treatment: A systematic review. *J. Bodyw. Mov. Ther.* **2005**, *9*, 27–34. [CrossRef]
25. Falsiroli Maistrello, L.; Geri, T.; Gianola, S.; Zaninetti, M.; Testa, M. Effectiveness of trigger point manual treatment on the frequency, intensity and duration of attacks in primary headaches: A systematic review and meta-analysis of randomized controlled trials. *Front. Neurol.* **2018**, *9*, 254. [CrossRef]
26. Moher, D.; Liberati, A.; Tetzlaff, J.; Altman, D.G.; PRISMA Group. Preferred reporting items for systematic reviews and meta-analyses: The PRISMA statement. *Ann. Intern. Med.* **2009**, *151*, 264–269. [CrossRef]
27. Glanville, J.M.; Lefebvre, C.; Miles, J.N.V.; Camosso-Stefinovic, J. How to identify randomized controlled trials in MEDLINE: Ten years on. *J. Med. Libr. Assoc.* **2006**, *94*, 130.
28. McNeely, M.L.; Olivo, S.A.; Magee, D. A systematic review of the effectiveness of physical therapy interventions for temporomandibular disorders. *Phys. Ther.* **2006**, *86*, 710–725. [CrossRef]
29. Travell, J.G.; Simons, D.G. *Myofascial Pain and Dysfunction. The Trigger Point Manual*; Williams & Wilkins: Baltimore, MD, USA, 1983; Volume 1.
30. Simons, D.G. Understanding effective treatments of myofascial trigger points. *J. Bodyw. Mov. Ther.* **2002**, *6*, 81–88. [CrossRef]
31. Ajimsha, M.; Al-Mudahka, N.; Al-Madzhar, J. Effectiveness of myofascial release: Systematic review of randomized controlled trials. *J. Bodyw. Mov. Ther.* **2015**, *19*, 102–112. [CrossRef] [PubMed]
32. Gautschi, R. *Manuelle Triggerpunkt-Therapie: Myofasziale Schmerzen und Funktionsstörungen Erkennen, Verstehen und Behandeln*; Thalia: Berlin, Germany, 2016.
33. Page, P. Current concepts in muscle stretching for exercise and rehabilitation. *Int. J. Sport. Phys. Ther.* **2012**, *7*, 109.
34. Mandroukas, A.; Vamvakoudis, E.; Metaxas, T.; Papadopoulos, P.; Kotoglou, K.; Stefanidis, P.; Christoulas, K.; Kyparos, A.; Mandroukas, K. Acute partial passive stretching increases range of motion and muscle strength. *J. Sport. Med. Phys. Fit.* **2014**, *54*, 289–297.
35. Bordoni, B.; Marelli, F. The fascial system and exercise intolerance in patients with chronic heart failure: Hypothesis of osteopathic treatment. *J. Multidiscip. Healthc.* **2015**, *8*, 489. [CrossRef]
36. Dardzinski, J.; Ostrov, B.; Hamann, L. Successful Use of a Strain and Counterstrain Technique with Physical Therapy: Myofascial Pain Unresponsive to Standard Treatment. *JCR J. Clin. Rheumatol.* **2000**, *6*, 169–174. [CrossRef]
37. Jones, L.N. *Strain and Counterstrain*; American Academy of Osteopathy: Newark, OH, USA, 1981.
38. Maquet, D.; Croisier, J.-L.; Demoulin, C.; Crielaard, J.-M. Pressure pain thresholds of tender point sites in patients with fibromyalgia and in healthy controls. *Eur. J. Pain* **2004**, *8*, 111–117. [CrossRef]
39. Hong, C.-Z. Algometry in evaluation of trigger points and referred pain. *J. Musculoskelet. Pain* **1998**, *6*, 47–59. [CrossRef]
40. Svechtarov, V.; Croisier, J.-L.; Demoulin, C.; Crielaard, J.-M. Mandibular range of motion and its relation to temporomandibular disorders. *Scr. Sci. Med. Dent.* **2015**, *1*, 21–26. [CrossRef]
41. Higgins, J.P.; Sterne, J.A.; Savovic, J.; Page, M.J.; Hróbjartsson, A.; Boutron, I.; Reeves, B.; Eldridge, S. A revised tool for assessing risk of bias in randomized trials. *Cochrane Database Syst. Rev.* **2016**, *10*, 29–31.
42. Sterne, J.A.; Savović, J.; Page, M.J.; Elbers, R.G.; Blencowe, N.S.; Boutron, I.; Cates, C.J.; Cheng, H.Y.; Corbett, M.S.; Eldridge, S.M.; et al. RoB 2: A revised tool for assessing risk of bias in randomised trials. *BMJ* **2019**. [CrossRef] [PubMed]

43. Higgins, J.P.; Thomas, J.; Chandler, J.; Cumpston, M.; Li, T.; Page, M.J.; Welch, V.A. *Cochrane Handbook for Systematic Reviews of Interventions*; John Wiley & Sons: Hoboken, NJ, USA, 2019.
44. Armijo-Olivo, S.; Ospina, M.; da Costa, B.R.; Egger, M.; Saltaji, H.; Fuentes, J.; Ha, C.; Cummings, G.G. Poor reliability between Cochrane reviewers and blinded external reviewers when applying the Cochrane risk of bias tool in physical therapy trials. *PloS ONE* **2014**, *9*, e96920. [CrossRef]
45. Olivo, S.A.; Macedo, L.; Gadotti, I.C.; Fuentes, J.; Stanton, T.; Magee, D.J. Scales to assess the quality of randomized controlled trials: A systematic review. *Phys. Ther.* **2008**, *88*, 156–175. [CrossRef] [PubMed]
46. Fuentes, J.P.; Olivo, S.A.; Magee, D.J.; Gross, D.P. Effectiveness of interferential current therapy in the management of musculoskeletal pain: A systematic review and meta-analysis. *Phys. Ther.* **2010**, *90*, 1219–1238. [CrossRef]
47. Calixtre, L.B.; Olivetira, A.B.; Alburquerque-Sendín, F.; Armijo-Olivo, S. What is the minimal important difference of pain intensity, mandibular function, and headache impact in patients with temporomandibular disorders? Clinical significance analysis of a randomized controlled trial. *Musculoskelet. Sci. Pract.* **2020**, *46*, 102108. [CrossRef] [PubMed]
48. Kropmans, T.J.; Dijkstra, P.U.; Stegenga, B.; Stewart, R.; De Bont LG, M. Smallest detectable difference in outcome variables related to painful restriction of the temporomandibular joint. *J. Dent. Res.* **1999**, *78*, 784–789. [CrossRef]
49. Fuentes, C.J.; Armijo-Olivo, S.; Magee, D.J.; Gross, D.P. A preliminary investigation into the effects of active interferential current therapy and placebo on pressure pain sensitivity: A random crossover placebo controlled study. *Physiotherapy* **2011**, *97*, 291–301. [CrossRef] [PubMed]
50. Guyatt, G.H.; Oxman, A.D.; Vist, G.E.; Kunz, R.; Falck-Ytter, Y.; Alonso-Coello, P.; Schünemann, H.J. GRADE: An emerging consensus on rating quality of evidence and strength of recommendations. *BMJ* **2008**, *336*, 924–926. [CrossRef]
51. Blanco, C.R.; Peñas, C.F.D.L.; Xumet, J.E.H.; Algaba, C.P.; Rabadán, M.F.; de la Quintana, M.C.L. Changes in active mouth opening following a single treatment of latent myofascial trigger points in the masseter muscle involving post-isometric relaxation or strain/counterstrain. *J. Bodyw. Mov. Ther.* **2006**, *10*, 197–205. [CrossRef]
52. Ibáñez-García, J.; Alburquerque-Sendín, F.; Rodríguez-Blanco, C.; Girao, D.; Atienza-Meseguer, A.; Planella-Abella, S.; Fernández-de-Las Peñas, C. Changes in masseter muscle trigger points following strain-counterstrain or neuro-muscular technique. *J. Bodyw. Mov. Ther.* **2009**, *13*, 2–10. [CrossRef]
53. Espejo-Antúnez, L.; Castro-Valenzuela, E.; Ribeiro, F.; Albornoz-Cabello, M.; Silva, A.; Rodríguez-Mansilla, J. Immediate effects of hamstring stretching alone or combined with ischemic compression of the masseter muscle on hamstrings extensibility, active mouth opening and pain in athletes with temporomandibular dysfunction. *J. Bodyw. Mov. Ther.* **2016**, *20*, 579–587. [CrossRef]
54. Dworkin, S.F. Research diagnostic criteria for temporomandibular disorders: Review, criteria, examinations and classification, critique. *J. Orofac. Pain* **1992**, *6*, 302–355.
55. D'Ambrogio, K.J.; Roth, G.B. *Positional Release Therapy: Assessment & Treatment of Musculoskeletal Dysfunction*; Mosby Incorporated: Maryland Heights, MI, USA, 1997.
56. Vernon, H.; Schneider, M. Chiropractic management of myofascial trigger points and myofascial pain syndrome: A systematic review of the literature. *J. Manip. Physiol. Ther.* **2009**, *32*, 14–24. [CrossRef]
57. Hanten, W.P.; Olson, S.L.; Butts, N.L.; Nowicki, A.L. Effectiveness of a home program of ischemic pressure followed by sustained stretch for treatment of myofascial trigger points. *Phys. Ther.* **2000**, *80*, 997–1003. [CrossRef]
58. Hou, C.-R.; Tsai, L.-C.; Cheng, K.-F.; Chung, K.-C.; Hong, C.-Z. Immediate effects of various physical therapeutic modalities on cervical myofascial pain and trigger-point sensitivity. *Arch. Phys. Med. Rehabil.* **2002**, *83*, 1406–1414. [CrossRef]
59. Fernández-de-las-Peñas, C.; Alonso-Blanco, C.; Fernández-Carnero, J.; Miangolarra-Page, J.C. The immediate effect of ischemic compression technique and transverse friction massage on tenderness of active and latent myofascial trigger points: A pilot study. *J. Bodyw. Mov. Ther.* **2006**, *10*, 3–9. [CrossRef]
60. Armijo-Olivo, S.; Mohamad, N.; de Oliveira-Souza AI, S.; de Castro-Carletti, E.M.; Ballenberger, N.; Fuentes, J. Performance, Detection, Contamination, Compliance, and Cointervention Biases in Rehabilitation Research: What Are They and How Can They Affect the Results of Randomized Controlled Trials? Basic Information for Junior Researchers and Clinicians. *Am. J. Phys. Med. Rehabil.* **2022**, *101*, 864–878. [CrossRef] [PubMed]
61. Espejo-Antúnez, L.; Tejeda, J.F.-H.; Albornoz-Cabello, M.; Rodríguez-Mansilla, J.; De-La-Cruz-Torres, B.; Ribeiro, F.; Silva, A.G. Dry needling in the management of myofascial trigger points: A systematic review of randomized controlled trials. *Complement. Ther. Med.* **2017**, *33*, 46–57. [CrossRef]

Disclaimer/Publisher's Note: The statements, opinions and data contained in all publications are solely those of the individual author(s) and contributor(s) and not of MDPI and/or the editor(s). MDPI and/or the editor(s) disclaim responsibility for any injury to people or property resulting from any ideas, methods, instructions or products referred to in the content.

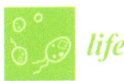

Article

Functioning of the Masticatory System in Patients with an Alloplastic Total Temporomandibular Joint Prostheses Compared with Healthy Individuals: A Pilot Study

Caroline M. Speksnijder [1,2,*], Nadiya E. A. Mutsaers [1,2] and Sajjad Walji [1]

1 University Medical Center Utrecht, Department of Oral and Maxillofacial Surgery and Special Dental Care, Utrecht University, 3584 CX Utrecht, The Netherlands
2 Department of Oral and Maxillofacial Surgery, Jeroen Bosch Hospital, 5223 GZ 's-Hertogenbosch, The Netherlands
* Correspondence: c.m.speksnijder@umcutrecht.nl

Abstract: Background: Most patients with temporomandibular joint (TMJ) issues are successfully treated with nonsurgical methods. However, when end-stage TMJ pathologies occur, invasive management can be required, such as a total TMJ replacement. This cross-sectional pilot study aimed to provide insight into the functioning of the masticatory system, pain, and patient satisfaction in patients treated with a total joint replacement (TJR). Methods: A cross-sectional pilot study was conducted to determine the postoperative clinical results of an alloplastic TJR TMJ. Masticatory performance and also insight into maximum voluntary bite force (MVBF), active and passive maximum mouth opening (aMMO/pMMO), pain, and patient satisfaction were measured. Masticatory performance, MVBF, and aMMO of patients with a TJR TMJ were compared with healthy individuals. Results: Masticatory performance is equal between patients with a TJR TMJ and healthy individuals, but both MVBF and aMMO were significantly smaller in patients with a TJR TMJ. However, patients had almost no pain and were very satisfied with the TJR TMJ treatment. Conclusion: This study revealed that most patients with an alloplastic TJR TMJ were able to function without pain, showed good masticatory performance, and were highly satisfied with their alloplastic TJR TMJ. However, MVBF and aMMO were lower than in healthy individuals.

Keywords: mastication; bite force; alloplastic total joint replacement; temporomandibular joint

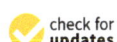

Citation: Speksnijder, C.M.; Mutsaers, N.E.A.; Walji, S. Functioning of the Masticatory System in Patients with an Alloplastic Total Temporomandibular Joint Prostheses Compared with Healthy Individuals: A Pilot Study. *Life* **2022**, *12*, 2073. https://doi.org/10.3390/life12122073

Academic Editors: Zuzanna Nowak and Aleksandra Nitecka-Buchta

Received: 15 October 2022
Accepted: 8 December 2022
Published: 10 December 2022

Publisher's Note: MDPI stays neutral with regard to jurisdictional claims in published maps and institutional affiliations.

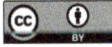

Copyright: © 2022 by the authors. Licensee MDPI, Basel, Switzerland. This article is an open access article distributed under the terms and conditions of the Creative Commons Attribution (CC BY) license (https://creativecommons.org/licenses/by/4.0/).

1. Introduction

The temporomandibular joint (TMJ) is a complex articulation in the human body, supporting functions such as mastication and mouth opening [1]. When oral functions are impaired by issues with the TMJ, temporomandibular dysfunction (TMD) can occur [1–3]. The prevalence of TMD pain complaints in the Dutch general population ranges between 7.2 and 8.0% and is more reported in women [4,5]. In most cases, patients with TMJ issues are successfully treated with nonsurgical methods, such as physiotherapy, splint therapy, behavioral therapy, and pharmacological treatment [6]. However, between 3 and 5% of the population who seek help for their TMJ issues are not successfully treated with nonsurgical methods and require invasive management [7]. When end-stage TMJ pathologies occur, such as severe osteoarthritis, inflammatory arthrosis, fibrous and bony ankyloses, deformities such as excessive condylar resorption, autoimmune disease, certain congenital disorders, trauma, chronic pain, and multiple failed prior TMJ surgeries [2,8,9], invasive management can be required by a total joint replacement (TJR) of the TMJ [10–12]. Important goals of this joint replacement are the optimization of mandibular function, such as mastication, and a reduction in pain [13].

Surgical replacement by an alloplastic TJR TMJ has shown to significantly increase maximum voluntary bite force (MVBF), maximum mouth opening (MMO), and masticatory functioning and reduces pain and diet restriction due to these [2,8,14,15]. To our knowledge, masticatory functioning is only obtained by patient-reported outcomes (PROs) in patients with a TJR TMJ. With such a PRO, the patient's own perception of mastication can be measured, which is defined as masticatory ability. However, with the mixing ability test (MAT), mastication can be measured objectively, which is defined as masticatory performance. This MAT assesses the comminution of a bolus by a standard number of chewing cycles [16–20]. Measuring masticatory performance will complement the knowledge of masticatory ability in patients with an alloplastic TJR TMJ [20,21]. Therefore, the first aim of this cross-sectional pilot study was to provide insight into masticatory performance, but also insight into MVBF, active MMO (aMMO), passive MMO (pMMO), pain, patient satisfaction related to their alloplastic TJR TMJ, and masticatory ability in patients who received an alloplastic TJR TMJ. The second aim was to compare masticatory performance, MVBF, and aMMO between patients who received an alloplastic TJR TMJ and matched healthy individuals.

2. Materials and Methods

A cross-sectional pilot study was conducted to determine the postoperative clinical results of an alloplastic TJR TMJ. Patients who received an alloplastic TJR TMJ during the period January 2013 to April 2018 at the Jeroen Bosch Hospital ('s-Hertogenbosch; The Netherlands) were contacted for recruitment and examination. In- and exclusion criteria for patients are depicted in Table 1. All patients received a letter by email including information about the study. Within 2 weeks, the patients were contacted by telephone to ask whether they were willing to participate in this study and to provide more information about the study when needed. Patients who were willing to participate were invited to Jeroen Bosch Hospital for screening. Approval was obtained from the Medical Ethics Committee Brabant (file no. NL65072.028.18).

Table 1. In- and exclusion criteria for patients treated with a TMJ TJR.

Inclusion Criteria	Exclusion Criteria
Unilateral or bilateral stock total TMJ reconstruction	Edentulous and had no denture prosthesis
Minimal 3 months postsurgery	TJR TMJ surgery-related complication
	Not able to speak or understand Dutch or English

TMJ: temporomandibular joint; TJR: temporomandibular joint replacement. Surgical and postsurgical procedures.

We matched the included patients in this study with healthy individuals on age, gender, and dental state. These healthy individuals had no temporomandibular deficits and were part of a former study in which the mixing ability test (MAT) was validated [18]. Approval was obtained from the Medical Ethics Committee of the University Medical Center Utrecht (file no. NL12006.041.06). All participants received a written and verbal explanation of the study. Written informed consent was obtained from each participating subject before starting the study.

The alloplastic TJR TMJ involves the reconstruction of both the mandibular condyle and temporal bone fossa, such as a ball and socket similar to the hip prosthesis. This includes a resection of the diseased joint, detachment of several masticatory muscles, and replacement with one of these alloplastic TMJ devices [22,23]. Indications for an alloplastic TJR TMJ combined with one of the end-stage pathologies are ongoing intermittent pain, more than 5 cm on a visual analog scale (VAS) (no pain = 0 cm, severe pain = 10 cm), a restricted mouth opening (<35 mm), low dietary scores (VAS < 5 cm, liquid score = 0 cm, full diet score = 10 cm), and/or occlusal collapse [8]. For the alloplastic TJR TMJ, the Stock Biomet microfixation system (Jacksonville, FL, USA) was used in patients treated in the Jeroen Bosch Hospital. The surgical approach in each patient was through a preauricular and submandibular/retromandibular incision. Both the native mandibular condyle and the coronoid process were removed with loss of attachment of the temporal and lateral pterygoid muscle. The masseter muscle was stripped at its aponeurotic insertion and reconstructed again at closing. The alloplastic fossa component was attached to the zygomatic arch, and the mandibular component was attached to the ramus of the mandible. After the reconstruction was completed, patients were allowed to function immediately. This included the freedom to choose any diet.

2.1. Measurements

Age, gender, dental state, preoperative variables (TMJ diagnosis, number of prior TMJ surgeries), operative variables (number, side, time since surgery), and postoperative reports, including postsurgical complications, were collected and taken from the clinical records of the included patients. Masticatory performance, MVBF, active MMO (aMMO), passive MMO (pMMO), pain, patient satisfaction related to their alloplastic TJR TMJ, and masticatory ability were measured in these patients. Of the healthy individuals in this study, age, gender, dental state, masticatory performance, MVBF, and aMMO were collected.

For the objective measurements, the participants were asked to keep their buttocks and lower back against the back of the chair and their knees flexed in a 90-degree flexion, with their feet flat on the floor and no armrest. Their head was kept in a neutral position; the head was considered neutral if the tragus of the ear was in line with the shoulder. To maintain this head position, the participants were asked to focus on a point directly in front of them.

2.2. Masticatory Performance

Masticatory performance was measured by the mixing ability test (MAT). The MAT is a valid and reliable test for masticatory performance and is highly suitable when masticatory performance is compromised [16–20]. This test evaluates the capacity of the participants to mix and knead a food bolus after a fixed number of chewing cycles. The tablet consists of two layers of red and blue wax (plasticine modeling wax, nontoxic DIN EN-71, art. no. crimson 52801 and blue 52809, Stockmar, Kalten Kirchen, Germany). The diameter of the tablet is 20 mm. Both layers of red and blue wax are 3 mm thick. When the tablet is chewed on, the colors mix; when the tablet is not chewed on, the colors do not mix, and the intensity of both colors is maximal. The measure of mixing is the spread of the color intensities of both sides.

The wax tablets were offered at room temperature (20°). Each participant masticated twenty times on the tablet. After the participants masticated twenty times on the tablet, the tablet was washed and dried. The chewed tablets were flattened, and both sides were photographed using a high-quality scanner (Epson V750, Long Beach, CA, USA). After that, the spread of the color intensity was measured by computer analysis of the digital images using Photoshop CS3 (Adobe, San Jose, CA, USA). The spread of the color intensities of both images was used as a measure of mixing. This is termed the mixing ability index (MAI). A lower MAI score represents a better-mixed tablet and, thus, better masticatory performance.

2.3. Maximum Voluntary Bite Force

MVBF was measured with the unilateral strain-gauge bite force transducer. It has been documented that both unilateral and bilateral bite force transducers can be used as valid and reliable measures [24,25]. The reliability of the results has been reported to depend on the position of the transducer within the dental arch. It has been documented that MVBF recorded posteriorly, both unilateral and bilateral, were notably higher than those recorded anteriorly [26]. Therefore, in this study, MVBF was recorded with the strain-gauge mouthpiece placed on the first molar region. The design consists of a unilateral strain gauge mounted on a mouthpiece. It has a surface area of 100 mm^2 and a vertical height of 2.8 mm.

To build confidence, the participants were allowed to become familiar with the force transducer by producing several test bites without producing their maximum force. The strain-gauge mouthpiece was placed on the first molar region. The mouthpiece was protected from humidity with a plastic film. After several test bites, the participants were asked to bite as hard as possible for a few seconds. The participants clenched twice on the left side of the jaw and twice on the right side of the jaw with an interval of 10 s in between. The mean of the highest bite force of the left side and the highest bite force of the right side was the MVBF used in this study.

2.4. Maximum Mouth Opening

To measure aMMO, participants who routinely used a dental prosthesis were instructed to wear their prosthesis during the measurements. Then, participants were asked to open their mouth as wide as possible to measure aMMO. In patients with an alloplastic TMJ TJR, at first, the overbite of participants was measured. After that, these patients were asked to open their mouth as wide as possible whilst maintaining the head position, and then the distance between the interincisors was measured from the upper right central incisor to the lower right central incisor.

To measure pMMO in patients, the examiner gave a slight overpressure on the edges of the upper and lower front teeth. Then, the distance between the interincisors was measured from the upper right central incisor to the lower right central incisor. The interincisal distance plus the vertical overbite was used in this study to determine the MMO.

In healthy individuals, aMMO was measured extraorally [27]. Two fixed points were marked with a pencil; one point was on the lower side of the chin, and the other was on the tip of the nose. The distance between the two points was measured using a digital slide gauge with the mouth at rest and at its maximum open position. For the resting position measurement, patients were instructed to close their mouth without their teeth making contact. For the maximum open position measurement, patients were instructed to open their mouth as wide as possible.

Each MMO measurement in patients and healthy individuals was performed twice, and the highest outcome was used in the subsequent analyses. Both ways of measuring MMO are reliable and do not differ in their result [28].

2.5. Masticatory Ability

To evaluate patients' masticatory ability, the Dutch version of the Mandibular Function Impairment Questionnaire (MFIQ) was used [29]. This PRO of mandibular function focuses on limitations in chewing various foods, drinking, yawning, impairment of normal activities, and speech. The Dutch MFIQ has 17 items assessing perceived difficulties in mandibular functioning; each item presents a 5-point Likert scale on which patients can indicate the experienced level of difficulty while performing particular mandibular movements or tasks (e.g., speech, daily activities, drinking, laughing, yawning, eating different types of food). The scores are: 0 = no difficulty, 1 = a little difficulty, 2 = quite a bit of difficulty, 3 = much difficulty, and 4 = very difficult or impossible without help. A total score ranging from 0 to 68 is possible, where 0 indicates no mandibular function impairment and 68 a poor functional outcome and very great difficulty.

2.6. Pain

Pain was in this study measured by a visual analog scale (VAS_{pain}) [30,31] consisting of a horizontal line, with 'no pain' (0 cm) on the left end, and on the right end 'worst pain imaginable' (10 cm), indicating no pain (0–0.4 cm), mild pain (0.5–4.4 cm), moderate pain (4.5–7.4 cm), and severe pain (7.5–10 cm) [32]. Patients were asked to fill in a VAS_{pain} related to perceived pain during the last week before further measurements took place. Patients also filled in a VAS_{pain} after each measurement (i.e., MAT, MVBF, aMMO, and pMMO).

2.7. Patient Satisfaction

$VAS_{satisfaction}$ was used to measure present satisfaction with the alloplastic TJR TMJ [33] consisting of a horizontal line, with 'no satisfaction' (0 cm) on the left end and on the right end, 'extreme satisfaction' (10 cm).

2.8. Statistical Analysis

The presentation of results is primarily descriptive, with frequency and percentages for categorical data, means and standard deviations (SDs) for continuous data, and medians and interquartile ranges (IQRs) for ordinal and non-normally distributed continuous data.

Differences between the alloplastic TMJ TJR group and the healthy group were analyzed by Fisher's exact test for categorical data, the independent t-test for continuous data, and the Mann–Whitney U test when continuous data were non-normally distributed. Statistical analyses were regarded as significant if the p-value was equal to or lower than 0.05. Data were evaluated using SPSS (IBM version 27.0).

3. Results

In total, 15 patients were treated with an alloplastic TMJ TJR in the period from January 2013 to April 2018 at the Jeroen Bosch Hospital. However, one patient was in hospital for a different disease, one patient was not able to speak or understand Dutch or English, and one patient was not willing to participate. Therefore, 12 patients (10 women) were included in this study after TMJ TJR with a unilateral Biomet Microfixation stock prosthesis (Inc., Jacksonville, FL, USA). The mean age at the time of the measurements was 61.69 years ($\pm$6.77), and the mean time after surgery on the day the measurements took place was 2.54 years ($\pm$1.26). Four patients had their natural teeth, two patients had implant-retained overdentures in the upper and lower jaw, and three patients had complete dentures (Table 2). The patients had an MAI of 19.56 ($\pm$2.45), an MVBF of 201.04 ($\pm$159.72), an aMMO of 42.50 ($\pm$7.93), a pMMO of 44.50 ($\pm$6.72), and an MFIQ outcome of 33.42 ($\pm$15.72), as depicted in Table 3.

Table 2. Demographic and clinical characteristics of patients treated with a TMJ TJR and matched healthy individuals.

Patient Number	Sex	Age at Measurement Moment (Years)	Time after Surgery (Years)	Dental State	Diagnoses	TJR Side	Prior TMJ Surgery at TJR Side	Healthy Individual Number	Sex	Age at Measurement Moment (Years)	Dental State
1	Female	59.79	2.30	Natural dentition	Arthrosis	Left	0	1	Female	58.35	Natural dentition
2	Male	70.34	2.66	Implant-retained overdenture in upper and lower jaw	Arthrosis	Right	1	2	Male	68.98	Implant-retained overdenture in lower jaw and natural dentition in upper jaw
3	Female	71.90	2.12	Complete denture	Arthrosis	Left	0	3	Female	61.74	Complete denture
4	Female	59.76	2.43	Natural dentition	Condylar resorption	Right	1	4	Female	55.96	Natural dentition
5	Female	60.58	2.84	Implant-retained overdenture in upper and lower jaw	Ankyloses	Right	0	5	Female	60.03	Implant-retained overdenture in lower jaw and natural dentition in upper jaw
6	Female	56.96	0.52	Complete denture	Osteoarthritis	Left	0	6	Female	56.62	Complete denture
7	Female	50.68	3.63	Natural dentition	Arthrosis	Right	1	7	Female	50.56	Natural dentition
8	Female	51.12	3.82	Natural dentition	Arthrosis	Right	1	8	Female	50.89	Natural dentition
9	Female	67.18	0.39	Natural dentition	Osteoarthritis	Right	1	9	Female	64.66	Natural dentition
10	Male	66.55	4.27	Complete denture	Osteoarthritis	Left	0	10	Male	69.05	Complete denture
11	Female	64.37	1.68	Complete denture	Osteoarthritis	Left	1	11	Female	61.48	Complete denture
12	Female	61.01	3.86	Natural dentition	Ankyloses	Right	0	12	Female	61.83	Natural dentition

TMJ: temporomandibular joint; TJR, temporomandibular joint replacement.

The Shapiro–Wilk test showed that all VAS$_{pain}$ and VAS$_{satisfaction}$ outcomes in patients were not normally distributed. VAS$_{pain}$ during last week, pain during MAT, pain during MVBF, and pain during aMMO had a median of 0.00, indicating that the patients had no pain. Patients' pain during pMMO had a median of 1.75, indicating mild pain. Patients were very satisfied with their TMJ TJR (Table 3).

A total of 12 matched healthy individuals (10 women) aged 60 (±6.0) years were included in this study. Four healthy individuals had their natural teeth, two healthy individuals had implant-retained overdentures in the lower jaw and natural teeth in the upper jaw, and three healthy individuals had complete dentures (Table 2). The healthy individuals had an MAI of 18.21 (±1.89), MVBF of 463.88 (±301.16), and aMMO of 51.79 (±6.96), as depicted in Table 3.

Table 3. Comparison of characteristics and outcomes of patients treated with an alloplastic total temporomandibular joint prostheses and healthy individuals.

	Patients with TMJ TJR N = 12	Healthy Individuals (N = 12)	p-Value
Sex (N (%))			1.000 ‡
Female	10 (83%)	10 (83%)	
Male	2 (17%)	2 (17%)	
Age (years) (mean (SD))	61.69 (6.77)	60.01 (6.00)	0.528 †
Time after surgery (mean (SD))	2.54 (1.26)	-	-
Prior TMJ surgery at TJR side			
Yes	6 (50%)	-	-
No	6 (50%)	-	-
Dental state (N (%))			0.456 ‡
Natural dentition	6 (50%)	6 (50%)	
Implant-retained overdenture in lower jaw and natural dentition in upper jaw	0 (0%)	2 (17%)	
Implant-retained overdenture in lower and upper jaw	2 (17%)	0 (0%)	
Complete denture	4 (33%)	4 (33%)	
Mixing ability index (mean (SD))	19.56 (2.45)	18.21 (1.89)	0.145 †
Maximum voluntary bite force (mean (SD))	201.04 (159.7)	463.88 (301.16)	0.014 *†
Active maximum mouth opening (mean (SD))	42.50 (7.93)	51.79 (6.96)	0.006 **†
Passive maximum mouth opening (mean (SD))	44.50 (6.72)	-	-
Pain during last week (median (IQR))	0.00 (0.00–0.23)	-	-
Pain during mastication of Mixing Ability Test (median (IQR))	0.00 (0.00–0.30)	-	-
Pain during maximum bite force at the non-operative site (median (IQR))	0.00 (0.00–0.00)	-	-
Pain during maximum bite force at the operative site (median (IQR))	0.00 (0.00–2.85)	-	-
Pain during active maximum mouth opening (median (IQR))	0.00 (0.00–3.53)	-	-
Pain during passive maximum mouth opening (median (IQR))	1.75 (0.00–3.53)	-	-
Satisfaction (median (IQR))	10.00 (9.80–10.00)	-	-
Mandibular Functional Index Questionnaire; total (mean (SD))	33.42 (15.72)	-	-
1. Social activities (median (IQR))	0.00 (0.00–1.00)	-	-
2. Speaking (median (IQR))	0.00 (0.00–1.00)	-	-
3. Biting something big (median (IQR))	1.00 (0.00–3.75)	-	-
4. Eating hard food (median (IQR))	1.00 (0.00–2.00)	-	-
5. Eating soft food (median (IQR))	0.00 (0.00–0.00)	-	-
6. Daily activities (median (IQR))	0.00 (0.00–0.75)	-	-
7. Drinking (median (IQR))	0.00 (0.00–0.00)	-	-
8. Laughing (median (IQR))	0.00 (0.00–0.00)	-	-
9. Chewing resistant food (median (IQR))	1.50 (0.00–3.75)	-	-
10. Yawning (median (IQR))	1.00 (0.00–1.75)	-	-
11. Kissing (median (IQR))	0.00 (0.00–0.00)	-	-
12. Eating hard cookies (median (IQR))	0.50 (0.00–1.00)	-	-
13. Eating meat (median (IQR))	0.50 (0.00–1.00)	-	-
14. Eating raw carrot (median (IQR))	1.50 (0.00–4.00)	-	-
15. Eating French bread (median (IQR))	0.50 (0.00–2.75)	-	-
16. Eating peanuts (median (IQR))	0.50 (0.00–3.75)	-	-
17. Eating whole apple (median (IQR))	1.50 (0.00–4.00)	-	-

*, $p < 0.05$; **, $p < 0.01$; ‡, Fisher's exact test; †, independent t-test; IQR, interquartile range; SD, standard deviation; TMJ, temporomandibular joint; TJR, temporomandibular joint replacement.

Statistical comparison of patients with an alloplastic TMJ TJR and healthy individuals showed that patients with an alloplastic TMJ TJR had a significantly lower MVBF ($p = 0.014$) and aMMO ($p = 0.006$) compared with healthy individuals. There was no significant difference in MAI ($p = 0.145$) between patients with an alloplastic TMJ TJR and healthy individuals. Individual outcomes for MAI, MVBF, and aMMO can be found in Figure 1 for both patients with an alloplastic TMJ TJR and healthy individuals.

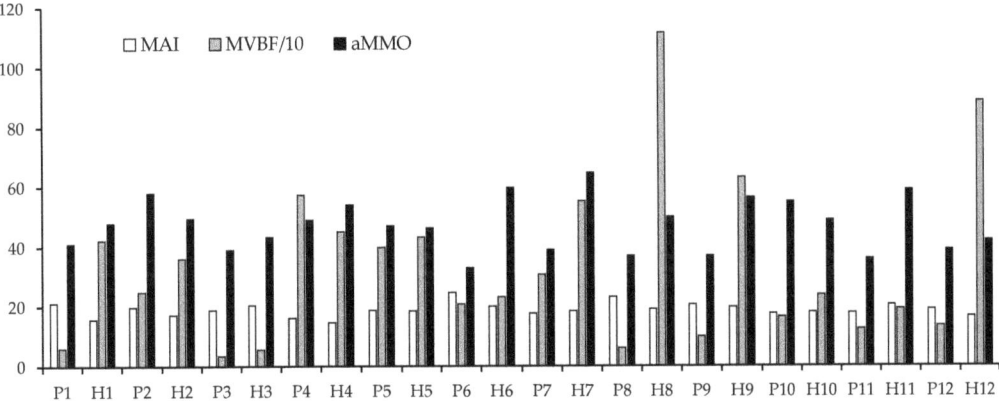

Figure 1. Individual outcomes of patients and healthy individuals: P1, patient 1 of Table 2; H2, healthy individual 2 of Table 2; MAI, mixing ability index; MVBF/10, maximum voluntary bite force divided by 10; aMMO: active maximum mouth opening.

4. Discussion

The masticatory performance in patients with a TJR TMJ showed to be equal to the healthy individuals matched on age and dental state. However, maximum voluntary bite force and active maximum mouth opening were significantly lower. Looking at MFIQ masticatory outcomes, patients with a TJR TMJ experienced limitations with eating hard and tough food and biting something big; however, these deficits were still very little (median: 0.5–1.5). These masticatory ability outcomes are comparable with the masticatory ability found in patients with a TJR TMJ in two other observational studies [34,35].

In this study, MVBF was significantly lower in patients with TMJ TJR than in healthy individuals. A possible explanation could be that removal of the temporal and lateral pterygoid muscle leads to a loss in muscle action and neuromuscular control. Moreover, the masseter muscle is stripped at its aponeurotic insertion; even though this muscle is reconstructed at closing, it still has an impact on power and neuromuscular control [13,36]. An additional explanation could be the lack of a postoperative rehabilitation protocol. The patients in this study had no physiotherapeutic support after the replacement of an alloplastic TJR TMJ. However, it has been reported in the literature that functions are not optimized after the replacement of an alloplastic TJR TMJ when patients do not follow a rehabilitation protocol [37]. While there is growing interest in this surgical intervention, there is still a paucity of data about postoperative protocols for physiotherapy and functional rehabilitation in patients with an alloplastic TJR TMJ. It has been stated that by the year 2030, there will be an increasing demand for the use of TJR TMJ prostheses in the United States of America [38]. In addition, in Europe, there is an increasing demand for the use of TJR TMJ prostheses [39]. Future research into the influence of rehabilitation interventions in patients with an alloplastic TJR TMJ, such as orofacial physiotherapy, is crucial since important goals of this surgery include functional improvement in the masticatory system [13]. Furthermore, we observed great interindividual differences in MVBF. In a prospective study, substantial interindividual differences were also observed in MVBF in patients with an alloplastic TJR TMJ [13]. An attempt to explain this wide interindividual variance is the voluntary influence of the measurement. The willingness and courage to bite as hard as possible are known to be influenced by the mental attitude of the patient and also by the comfort of the patient's teeth [1,14].

aMMO was also significantly lower in patients with a TJR TMJ than in healthy individuals. Patients with a TJR TMJ experienced only a little restriction with yawning. Thereby, the patient results showed an aMMO ranging from 33 to 58 mm and a pMMO ranging from 35 to 59 mm, which demonstrates that these patients had a satisfactory mandibular range of motion. In most other studies, lower MMO results were found postoperatively [35,40–52]. Only one prospective cohort study showed similar MMO results at the 12-month follow-up and thereafter [53]. This difference cannot be explained by the use of the Biomet prosthesis because the MMO results of other studies using the Biomet found lower as well as equal MMO results [35,43,51,53].

Our study demonstrated that pain scores in most patients were very low. These findings are consistent with the findings of previous studies [15,47,54]. Another interesting observation is that in our study, patients reported being extremely satisfied with their alloplastic TJR TMJ. In previous studies, patients also reported being satisfied with their TJR TMJ, but were, on average, not as highly satisfied compared with the patient-reported outcomes in our study [55,56]. In an 8-year longitudinal follow-up study, it was reported that patient satisfaction was positive even when pain and poor mandibular function were reported in these patients. They assumed that the effort made to inform patients what to expect had contributed to treatment satisfaction [56]. In our study, one patient reported experiencing moderate pain during all measurements and during the last week. This patient also scored the lowest on the satisfaction rating scale. Therefore, in our study, the patients were extremely satisfied even when MVBF was impaired because they reported experiencing almost no pain, and the most important reason patients first seek treatment is TMJ pain [57].

The strength of this study is that, to our knowledge, no other studies have reported on masticatory performance in patients treated with an alloplastic TJR TMJ. Therefore, this study may add knowledge about masticatory functioning in patients with a TJR TMJ. Thereby, this study contributes to a better understanding of the results after replacing the temporomandibular joint. However, limitations also need to be taken into consideration. A limitation of this study is the limited number of participants. In addition, the findings are based on postoperative measurements and cannot be compared with preoperative findings. Despite these limitations, the findings of this study can provide a basis for future research into measuring the masticatory functioning outcomes of this surgical option in a larger number of patients.

In conclusion, this study revealed that most patients with an alloplastic TJR TMJ were able to function without pain, showed good masticatory performance, and were highly satisfied with their alloplastic TJR TMJ. However, MVBF and aMMO were lower than in healthy individuals. Despite the fact that the success of alloplastic TJR TMJ has been established in the literature, research has to be continued to optimize rehabilitation care in patients with an alloplastic TJR TMJ.

Author Contributions: Conceptualization, C.M.S.; methodology, C.M.S.; formal analysis, C.M.S.; investigation, C.M.S. and N.E.A.M.; resources, C.M.S. and S.W.; data curation, C.M.S. and N.E.A.M.; writing—original draft preparation, C.M.S. and N.E.A.M.; writing—review and editing, S.W.; supervision, C.M.S.; project administration, N.E.A.M. All authors have read and agreed to the published version of the manuscript.

Funding: This research received no external funding.

Institutional Review Board Statement: The study was conducted in accordance with the Declaration of Helsinki, and approved by the Medical Ethics Committee Brabant (file no. NL65072.028.18; 24 April 2018) and Medical Ethics Committee of the University Medical Center Utrecht (file no. NL12006.041.06; 27 April 2007).

Informed Consent Statement: Informed consent was obtained from all subjects involved in the study.

Data Availability Statement: The data in this study are available on request.

Conflicts of Interest: The authors declare no conflict of interest.

References

1. van der Bilt, A. Assessment of mastication with implications for oral rehabilitation: A review. *J. Oral Rehabil.* **2011**, *38*, 754–780. [CrossRef] [PubMed]
2. Guarda-Nardini, L.; Manfredini, D.; Ferronato, G. Temporomandibular joint total replacement prosthesis: Current knowledge and considerations for the future. *Int. J. Oral Maxillofac. Surg.* **2008**, *37*, 103–110. [CrossRef] [PubMed]
3. Harrison, A.L.; Thorp, J.N.; Ritzline, P.D. A proposed diagnostic classification of patients with temporomandibular disorders: Implications for physical therapists. *J. Orthop. Sport Phys. Ther.* **2014**, *44*, 182–198. [CrossRef] [PubMed]
4. Visscher, C.M.; Ligthart, L.; Schuller, A.; Lobbezoo, F.; de Jongh, A.; van Houtem, C.M.; Boomsma, D.I. Comorbid disorders and sociodemographic variables in temporomandibular pain in the general Dutch population. *J. Oral Facial Pain Headache* **2015**, *29*, 51–59. [CrossRef]
5. Oral, K.; Küçük, B.B.; Ebeoğlu, B.; Dinçer, S. Etiology of temporomandibular disorder pain. *Agri* **2009**, *21*, 89–94.
6. Wieckiewicz, M.; Boening, K.; Wiland, P.; Shiau, Y.Y.; Paradowska-Stolarz, A. Reported concepts for the treatment modalities and pain management of temporomandibular disorders. *J. Headache Pain* **2015**, *16*, 1–12. [CrossRef]
7. Mesnard, M.; Ramos, A.; Ballu, A.; Morlier, J.; Cid, M.; Simoes, J.A. Biomechanical analysis comparing natural and alloplastic temporomandibular joint replacement using a finite element model. *J. Oral Maxillofac. Surg.* **2011**, *69*, 1008–1017. [CrossRef]
8. Johnson, N.R.; Roberts, M.J.; Doi, S.A.; Batstone, M.D. Total temporomandibular joint replacement prostheses: A systematic review and bias-adjusted meta-analysis. *Int. J. Oral Maxillofac. Surg.* **2017**, *46*, 86–92. [CrossRef]
9. Niezen, E.T.; van Minnen, B.; Bos, R.R.M.; Dijkstra, P.U. Temporomandibular joint prosthesis as treatment option for mandibular condyle fractures: A systematic review and meta-analysis. *Int. J. Oral Maxillofac. Surg.* **2022**, *23*, S0901-5027(22)00227-2. [CrossRef]
10. Gauer, R.L.; Semidey, M.J. Diagnosis and treatment of temporomandibular disorders. *Am. Fam. Physician* **2015**, *91*, 378–386.
11. Dimitroulis, G. Management of temporomandibular joint disorders: A surgeon's perspective. *Aust. Dent. J.* **2018**, *63*, 79–90. [CrossRef] [PubMed]
12. Sidebottom, A.J. Guidelines for the replacement of temporomandibular joints in the United Kingdom. *Br. J. Oral Maxillofac. Surg.* **2008**, *46*, 146–147. [CrossRef] [PubMed]
13. Mercuri, L.G. The use of alloplastic prostheses for temporomandibular joint reconstruction. *J. Oral Maxillofac. Surg.* **2000**, *58*, 70–75. [CrossRef]
14. Linsen, S.S.; Reich, R.H.; Teschke, M. Maximum voluntary bite force in patients with alloplastic total TMJ replacement: A prospective study. *J. Cranio-Maxillofac. Surg.* **2013**, *41*, 423–428. [CrossRef] [PubMed]
15. Giannakopoulos, H.E.; Sinn Douglas, P.; Quinn, P.D. Temporomandibular joint replacement system: A 3-year follow-up study of patients treated during 1995 to 2005. *J. Oral Maxillofac. Surg.* **2012**, *70*, 787–794. [CrossRef] [PubMed]
16. Vermaire, J.A.; Weinberg, F.M.; Raaijmakers, C.P.J.; Verdonck-de Leeuw, I.M.; Terhaard, C.H.J.; Speksnijder, C.M. Reliability of the mixing ability test testing masticatory performance in patients with head and neck cancer and healthy controls. *J. Oral Rehabil.* **2020**, *47*, 961–966. [CrossRef]
17. Remijn, L.; Vermaire, J.A.; der Sanden, M.W.G.N.-V.; Groen, B.E.; Speksnijder, C.M. Validity and reliability of the mixing ability test as masticatory performance outcome in children with spastic cerebral palsy and children with typical development: A pilot study. *J. Oral Rehabil.* **2018**, *45*, 790–797. [CrossRef]
18. Speksnijder, C.M.; Abbink, J.H.; Van Der Glas, H.W.; Janssen, N.G.; Van Der Bilt, A. Mixing ability test compared with a comminution test in persons with normal and compromised masticatory performance. *Eur. J. Oral Sci.* **2009**, *117*, 580–586. [CrossRef]
19. van der Bilt, A.; Speksnijder, C.M.; de Liz Pocztaruk, R.; Abbink, J.H. Digital image processing versus visual assessment of chewed two-colour wax in mixing ability tests. *J. Oral Rehabil.* **2012**, *39*, 11–17. [CrossRef]
20. Weinberg, F.M.; Vermaire, J.A.; Forouzanfar, T.; Rosenberg, A.J.W.P.; Speksnijder, C.M. Reproducibility and construct validity of the utrecht mixing ability test to obtain masticatory performance outcome in patients with condylar mandibular fractures. *J. Oral Rehabil.* **2020**, *47*, 460–466. [CrossRef]
21. Vermaire, J.A.; Raaijmakers, C.P.J.; Leeuw, I.M.V.-D.; Jansen, F.; Leemans, C.R.; Terhaard, C.H.J.; Speksnijder, C.M. Mastication, swallowing, and salivary flow in patients with head and neck cancer: Objective tests versus patient-reported outcomes. *Support Care Cancer* **2021**, *29*, 7793–7803. [CrossRef] [PubMed]
22. Westermark, A. Total reconstruction of the temporomandibular joint. Up to 8 years of follow-up of patients treated with Biomet total joint prostheses. *Int. J. Oral Maxillofac. Surg.* **2010**, *39*, 951–955. [CrossRef] [PubMed]
23. Gerbino, G.; Zavattero, E.; Bosco, G.; Berrone, S.; Ramieri, G. Temporomandibular joint reconstruction with stock and custom-made devices: Indications and results of a 14-year experience. *J. Cranio-Maxillofac. Surg.* **2017**, *45*, 7–12. [CrossRef]
24. Koc, D.; Dogan, A.; Bek, B. Bite force and influential factors on bite force measurements: A literature review. *Eur. J. Dent.* **2010**, *4*, 223–232. [CrossRef]
25. Fontijn-Tekamp, F.A.; Slagter, A.P.; van't Hof, M.A.; Geertman, M.E.; Kalk, W. Bite forces with mandibular implant-retained overdentures. *J. Dent. Res.* **1998**, *77*, 1832–1839. [CrossRef] [PubMed]

26. Tortopidis, D.; Lyons, M.F.; Baxendale, R.H.; Gilmour, W.H. The variability of bite force measurement between sessions, in different positions within the dental arch. *J. Oral Rehabil.* **1998**, *25*, 681–686. [CrossRef]
27. McCord, J.F.; Grant, A.A. Registration: Stage II—Intermaxillary relations. *Br. Dent. J.* **2000**, *188*, 601–606.
28. van Hinte, G.; Leijendekkers, R.A.; Molder, B.T.; Jansen, L.; Bol, C.; Merkx, M.A.W.; Takes, R.; der Sanden, M.W.G.N.-V.; Speksnijder, C.M. Reproducibility of measurements on physical performance in head and neck cancer survivors; measurements on maximum mouth opening, shoulder and neck function, upper and lower body strength, level of physical mobility, and walking ability. *PLoS ONE* **2020**, *15*, e0233271. [CrossRef]
29. Kropmans, T.; Dijkstra, P.; Stegenga, B.; van Veen, A.; de Bont, L. The smallest detectable difference of mandibular function impairment in patients with a painfully restricted temporomandibular joint. *J. Dent. Res.* **1999**, *78*, 1445–1449. [CrossRef]
30. Boonstra, A.M.; Schiphorst Preuper, H.R.; Reneman, M.F.; Posthumus, J.B.; Stewart, R.E. Reliability and validity of the visual analogue scale for disability in patients with chronic musculoskeletal pain. *Int. J. Rehabil. Res.* **2008**, *31*, 165–169. [CrossRef]
31. Price, D.D.; Mcgrath, P.A.; Rafii, A.; Buckingham, B. The validation of visual analogue scales as ratio scale measures for chronic and experimental pain. *Pain* **1983**, *17*, 45–56. [CrossRef] [PubMed]
32. Hawker, G.; Mian, S.; Kendzerska, T.; French, M. Measures of adult pain. *Arthritis Care Res.* **2011**, *63*, 240–252. [CrossRef] [PubMed]
33. Brokelman, R.B.G.; Haverkamp, D.; Veth, R. The validation of the visual analogue scale for patient satisfaction after total hip arthroplasty. *Eur. Orthop. Traumatol.* **2012**, *3*, 101–105. [CrossRef] [PubMed]
34. Zumbrunn Wojczyńska, A.; Steiger, B.; Leiggener, C.S.; Ettlin, D.A.; Gallo, L.M. Quality of life, chronic pain, insomnia, and jaw malfunction in patients after alloplastic temporomandibular joint replacement: A questionnaire-based pilot study. *Int. J. Oral Maxillofac. Surg.* **2021**, *50*, 948–955. [CrossRef] [PubMed]
35. Kunjur, J.; Niziol, R.; Matthews, N.S. Quality of life: Patient-reported outcomes after total replacement of the temporomandibular joint. *Br. J. Oral Maxillofac. Surg.* **2016**, *54*, 762–766. [CrossRef]
36. Singh, A.; Roychoudhury, A.; Bhutia, O.; Yadav, R.; Bhatia, R.; Yadav, P. Longitudinal changes in electromyographic activity of masseter and anterior temporalis muscles before and after allo-plastic total joint replacement in patients with temporomandibular ankylosis: A prospective study. *Br. J. Oral Maxillofac. Surg.* **2022**, *60*, 896–903. [CrossRef]
37. Guarda-nardini, L.; Manfredini, D.; Ferronato, G. Total temporomandibular joint replacement: A clinical case with a proposal for post-surgical rehabilitation. *J. Cranio-Maxillofac. Surg.* **2008**, *36*, 403–409. [CrossRef]
38. Onoriobe, U.; Miloro, M.; Sukotjo, C.; Mercuri, L.G.; Lotesto, A.; Eke, R. How many temporomandibular joint total joint alloplastic implants will be placed in the United States in 2030? *J. Oral Maxillofac. Surg.* **2016**, *74*, 1531–1538. [CrossRef]
39. Rajapakse, S.; Ahmed, N.; Sidebottom, A.J. Current thinking about the management of dysfunction of the temporomandibular joint: A review. *Br. J. Oral Maxillofac. Surg.* **2017**, *55*, 351–356. [CrossRef]
40. Gerbino, G.; Zavattero, E.; Berrone, S.; Ramieri, G. One stage treatment of temporomandibular joint complete bony ankylosis using total joint replacement. *J. Cranio-Maxillofac. Surg.* **2016**, *44*, 487–492. [CrossRef]
41. Mercuri, L.G.; Ali, F.A.; Woolson, R. Outcomes of total alloplastic replacement with periarticular autogenous fat grafting for management of reankylosis of the temporomandibular joint. *J. Oral Maxillofac. Surg.* **2008**, *66*, 1794–1803. [CrossRef] [PubMed]
42. Kanatas, A.N.; Needs, C.; Smith, A.B.; Moran, A.; Jenkins, G.; Worrall, S.F. Short-term outcomes using the Christensen patient-specific temporomandibular joint implant system: A prospective study. *Br. J. Oral Maxillofac. Surg.* **2012**, *50*, 149–153. [CrossRef] [PubMed]
43. MacHon, V.; Hirjak, D.; Beno, M.; Foltan, R. Total alloplastic temporomandibular joint replacement: The Czech-Slovak initial experience. *Int. J. Oral Maxillofac. Surg.* **2012**, *20*, 515–526. [CrossRef] [PubMed]
44. Neuhaus, M.T.; Zeller, A.N.; Jehn, P.; Lethaus, B.; Gellrich, N.C.; Zimmerer, R.M. Intraoperative real-time navigation and intraoperative three-dimensional imaging for patient-specific total temporomandibular joint replacement. *Int. J. Oral Maxillofac. Surg.* **2021**, *50*, 1342–1350. [CrossRef]
45. Zou, L.; He, D.; Yang, C.; Lu, C.; Zhao, J.; Zhu, H. Preliminary study of standard artificial temporomandibular joint replacement with preservation of muscle attachment. *J. Oral Maxillofac. Surg.* **2021**, *79*, 1009–1018. [CrossRef]
46. Mercuri, L.G.; Wolford, L.M.; Sanders, B.; Dean White, R.; Giobbie-Hurder, A. Long-term follow-up of the CAD/CAM patient fitted total temporomandibular joint reconstruction system. *J. Oral Maxillofac. Surg.* **2002**, *60*, 1440–1448. [CrossRef]
47. Mercuri, L.G.; Edibam, N.R.; Giobbie-Hurder, A. Fourteen-year follow-up of a patient-fitted total temporomandibular joint reconstruction system. *J. Oral Maxillofac. Surg.* **2007**, *65*, 1140–1148. [CrossRef]
48. Mercuri, L.G.; Wolford, L.M.; Sanders, B.; White, R.D.; Hurder, A.; Henderson, W. Custom CAD/CAM total temporomandibular joint reconstruction system. Preliminary multicenter report. *J. Oral Maxillofac. Surg.* **1995**, *53*, 106–115. [CrossRef]
49. Gruber, E.A.; McCullough, J.; Sidebottom, A.J. Medium-term outcomes and complications after total replacement of the temporomandibular joint. Prospective outcome analysis after 3 and 5 years. *Br. J. Oral Maxillofac. Surg.* **2015**, *53*, 412–415. [CrossRef] [PubMed]
50. Sidebottom, A.J.; Gruber, E. One-year prospective outcome analysis and complications following total replacement of the temporomandibular joint with the TMJ Concepts system. *Br. J. Oral Maxillofac. Surg.* **2013**, *51*, 620–624. [CrossRef]
51. Aagaard, E.; Thygesen, T. A prospective, single-centre study on patient outcomes following temporomandibular joint replacement using a custom-made Biomet TMJ prosthesis. *Int. J. Oral Maxillofac. Surg.* **2014**, *43*, 1229–1235. [CrossRef] [PubMed]

52. Mani, B.; Balasubramaniam, S.; Balasubramanian, S.; Jayara-man, B.; Thirunavukkarasu, R. Role of custom-made prosthesis for temporomandibular joint replacement in unilateral ankylosis: An evaluative study. *Ann. Maxillofac. Surg.* **2020**, *10*, 344–352. [PubMed]
53. Gonzalez-Perez, L.; Gonzalez-Perez-Somarriba, B.; Centeno, G.; Vallellano, C.; Montes-Carmona, J.; Torres-Carranza, E.; Ambrosiani-Fernandez, J.; Infante-Cossio, P. Prospective study of five-year outcomes and postoperative complications after total temporomandibular joint replacement with two stock prosthetic systems. *Br. J. Oral Maxillofac. Surg.* **2020**, *58*, 69–74. [CrossRef] [PubMed]
54. Briceño, F.; Ayala, R.; Delgado, K.; Piñango, S. Evaluation of temporomandibular joint total replacement with alloplastic prosthesis: Observational study of 27 patients. *Craniomaxillofac. Trauma Reconstr.* **2013**, *6*, 171–178. [CrossRef]
55. Alakailly, A.; Schwartz, D.; Alwanni, N.; Demko, C.; Altay, M.A.; Kilinc, Y.; Da Quereshy, B. Patient-centered quality of life (QOL) measures after temporomandibular total joint replacement surgery. *J. Oral Maxillofac. Surg.* **2013**, *71*, e28. [CrossRef]
56. Schuurhuis, J.M.; Dijkstra, P.; de Bont, L.; Spijkervet, K.L.; Dijkstra, P.U.; Stegenga, B. Groningen temporomandibular total joint prosthesis: An 8-year longitudinal follow-up on function and pain. *J. Cranio-Maxillofac. Surg.* **2012**, *40*, 815–820. [CrossRef]
57. List, T.; Jensen, R.H. Temporomandibular disorders: Old ideas and new concepts. *Cephalalgia* **2017**, *37*, 692–704. [CrossRef]

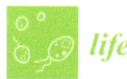

Article

Professional Factors Associated with Case Resolution without Referrals of Orofacial Pain Cases to Secondary Dental Care by Telehealth in Brazil: A Cross-Sectional Study in 2019 and 2020

Ricardo Luiz de Barreto Aranha [1], Renata de Castro Martins [2], Ligia Cristelli Paixão [1] and Mauro Henrique Nogueira Guimarães de Abreu [2,*]

[1] School of Dentistry, Universidade Federal de Minas Gerais, Belo Horizonte 31270-901, Brazil
[2] Department of Community and Preventive Dentistry, School of Dentistry, Universidade Federal de Minas Gerais, Belo Horizonte 31270-901, Brazil
* Correspondence: maurohenriqueabreu@gmail.com

Abstract: This study aimed to identify professional factors associated with case resolution without a referral of orofacial pain to secondary health care by Brazilian Primary Health Care (PHC) practitioners who demanded asynchronous teleconsulting, stratified by year, in 2019 and 2020 (the COVID-19 Pandemic burst). A cross-sectional study employed secondary databases from asynchronous teleconsulting Telehealth Brazil Networks from January 2019 to December 2020. The outcome was the dichotomous variable "If referral to secondary care was avoided." As covariates: sex, healthcare professions, and category of orofacial pain doubts. A negative binomial regression model estimated each covariate's unadjusted and adjusted PR (95%CI) and p values, stratified for 2019 and 2020. There was a difference in descriptive factors associated with case resolution without a referral from 2019 to 2020. Females prevailed in both years, and the total demand decreased to a third from 2019 to 2020. The rate of resoluteness decreased by 19.1%. In 2019, nurses (PR = 0.69 CI 95% 0.57–0.83) and other professionals (PR = 0.84 CI 95% 0.73–0.97) showed less frequency of case resolution without a referral than did general dentists. In 2020, oral-cavity-related doubts (PR = 1.18 CI 95% 1.06–1.32) and temporomandibular disorders (PR = 1.33 95% 1.15–1.54) surpassed other causes of orofacial pain in case resolution without a referral, and female professionals avoided referrals more frequently than men (PR = 1.24 CI 95% 1.21–1.38). In conclusion, in 2019, oral cavity doubts and the PHC profession influenced the case resolution. Female professionals and oral cavity doubts scored the higher case resolution without a referral for the service in 2020.

Keywords: facial pain; telemedicine; community dentistry; public health dentistry; COVID-19

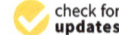

Citation: de Barreto Aranha, R.L.; de Castro Martins, R.; Paixão, L.C.; de Abreu, M.H.N.G. Professional Factors Associated with Case Resolution without Referrals of Orofacial Pain Cases to Secondary Dental Care by Telehealth in Brazil: A Cross-Sectional Study in 2019 and 2020. *Life* **2023**, *13*, 29. https://doi.org/10.3390/life13010029

Academic Editors: Zuzanna Nowak and Aleksandra Nitecka-Buchta

Received: 23 November 2022
Revised: 8 December 2022
Accepted: 20 December 2022
Published: 22 December 2022

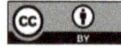

Copyright: © 2022 by the authors. Licensee MDPI, Basel, Switzerland. This article is an open access article distributed under the terms and conditions of the Creative Commons Attribution (CC BY) license (https:// creativecommons.org/licenses/by/ 4.0/).

1. Introduction

The Brazilian National Health System (SUS) is a universal-equity-based public system. The system provides satisfactory health services and privileges primary care in an unequal and complex society [1]. In primary health care (PHC) units, the main objective is the service resolution without an unnecessary referral, in compliance with international statements that underlie the relevant role of primary health care in pursuing integration, comprehensiveness, and social justice in health [2]. This is also the primary resoluteness followed by the Brazilian telehealth program [1]. In addition, telehealth resources can be essential for disseminating knowledge on and elucidating orofacial pain issues in PHC settings. However, little is known about what determines the resolutive capacity of PHC concerning orofacial pain and TMD issues.

Telehealth uses information technology to enhance health care in distant locations. Due to its low cost and functional characteristics, telehealth can lower the inequalities in health services, reaching poorer groups within an adequate time [3]. Telehealth technology, a term that expands the scope beyond the medical area, represents an important tool available to primary care professionals, solving their doubts and increasing the service's resoluteness. This resource is paramount, especially in a country with a continental dimension and a heterogeneous health infrastructure distribution, as is the case in Brazil [1]. Expanded to the entire Brazilian territory, covering all five great Brazilian regions (North, Northeast, Midwest, South, and Southeast), the telehealth initiative of the Brazilian Ministry of Health had its activity guidelines defined in 2015 [4]. One of the Program's strategies is teleconsulting, which consists of bidirectional communication between PHC professionals and teleconsultants (experts in a specific area) for assistance or advanced information on clinical care, health promotion actions, or work process. Teleconsulting is offered by telehealth centers and takes place via synchronous messaging, videoconferences, or asynchronous messages that must be answered within 72 h [5,6]. The primary program goal is to support PHC professionals by offering relevant second opinions. It delivers quick and valuable answers to their questions. This feature enabled a 45% reduction in referrals in some country regions through teleconsulting actions [7].

By contrast, orofacial pain, a broad term encompassing symptoms in the head and neck region, is a frequent form of pain perceived in the face and oral cavity. It may be caused by diseases or disorders of regional structures, nervous system dysfunction, or pain stemming from distant sources [8]. The temporomandibular disorder (TMD), in which painful presentation is a subgroup of orofacial pain, is recognized as a condition of pain or musculoskeletal dysfunction that affects the face in its masticatory structures and encompasses a group of changes involving the temporomandibular joints (TMJ) [9]. It is registered as the primary cause of non-dental pain in the orofacial region and is its most prevalent chronic pain [10]. TMD is defined worldwide as a public health problem [11] in a matrix of multiple possible etiologic factors and interdisciplinary demands [12]. Given its prevalence and relevance in dental practice, knowledge concerning current orofacial pain and temporomandibular disorders in public health services and undergraduate or graduate programs is being debated worldwide [13].

Furthermore, previous evaluation studies with different outcomes have shown that well-structured human resources and management factors have been associated with better performance in Brazilian PHC [14,15]. These topics underline the importance of good health policy initiatives to improve human resources and management in qualified primary care. Hence, spreading and implementing the orofacial pain service in private or public health systems can improve dental practice, providing relief for a series of conditions and avoiding iatrogenic actions or incorrect references.

Therefore, assessing variables of telehealth demands and resolution figures available from the year before the outbreak of the COVID-19 Pandemic and the dissemination of the disease in 2020 is one way to measure and analyze its advantages, shortcomings, and trends over a critical public health period. Accordingly, this study investigated professional factors associated with case resolution without a referral of orofacial pain to secondary health care by Brazilian Primary Health Care (PHC) practitioners who demanded asynchronous teleconsulting, the service dedicated to solving PHC professionals' doubts about diagnoses issues or work processes, stratified by year, in 2019 and 2020 (the COVID-19 Pandemic burst).

2. Materials and Methods

The study used secondary databases from the asynchronous teleconsulting Telehealth Brazil Networks Program from January 2019 to December 2020. The data source was the national database of the Telehealth Results Monitoring and Evaluation System (SMART, the acronym in Portuguese), developed in 2014, provided by the Telehealth Centers that are part of the Telehealth Brazil Networks Program [16]. The telehealth centers were implemented in public universities in 25 out of 26 states in the five Brazilian regions [17]. Duplicate data, incomplete information, or data covering issues other than orofacial pain were excluded. The appropriate University Research Ethics Committee provided ethics approval.

The dichotomous variable "If referral to secondary care was avoided" was the outcome, representing the resolvability of the teleconsulting program. Sex, PHC professional category, and doubts related to orofacial pain were the covariates. Sex was dichotomized in males and females. The categories of PHC practitioners were divided into six groups, according to their relationship with orofacial pain treatment [18] and frequency of appearance in the database, as follows: General Dentists, Specialized Dentists, General Physicians, Specialized Physicians, Nurses, and Others. The "others" embraces administrative staff, auditor-dentists, dental assistants, community health agents, radiology technicians, biomedical, resident physicians, speech therapists, clinical psychologists, physical therapists, pharmacists, occupational therapists, or uninformed.

SMART registered teleconsulting data according to the International Classification of Diseases 10 Version: 2019 (ICD-10) [19] and the International Classification of Primary Care, second edition (ICPC-2) [20]. The last one deals with the reasons for demands beyond the apparent diseases, allowing a better understanding of PHC user problems and perceptions. It is a complementary tool to the traditional ICD and has been gradually recognized as an appropriate classification for family medicine and primary care [21].

The screening of orofacial pain/TMD doubts was based on the American Academy of Orofacial Pain criteria for this study's purposes [22]. After that, the category of doubts gave rise to three groups based on the proximity to the traditional clinical dental practice, coherent with a current orofacial pain international classification (ICOP) [23] highlighting oral cavity-related pain conditions and temporomandibular disorders. Apart from then, a group for "other conditions in the head and neck" represented the demands that, although referring to the structure of the head/neck, are generally related to other distinct medical specialties, such as headaches and sinusitis, and may hinder or overlap in the oral cavity-related pain or TMD diagnosis.

The three demand groups are described in Figure 1.

Group 1 – Oral cavity-related pain conditions
• DS19 Teeth, gum symptom or complaint (ICPC-2)
• DS20 Mouth, tongue, lip symptom or complaint (ICPC-2)
• K03.0 Excessive attrition of teeth (ICD-10)
• K04.0 Pulpitis (ICD-10)
• K05.0 Acute gingivitis (ICD-10)
• K05.2 Acute periodontitis (ICD-10)
• K14.6 Glossodynia (ICD-10)
• S02.5 Fracture of tooth (ICD-10)
Group 2 Temporomandibular Disorder
• K07.6 Temporomandibular joint disorders (ICD-10)
• L07 Jaw symptom/complaint (ICPC-2)
Group 3 - Other pain/condition in head or neck
• H01 Ear pain/earache (ICPC-2)
• N01 Headache (ICPC-2)
• N03 Pain face (ICPC-2)
• N89 Migraine (ICPC-2)
• N91 Facial paralysis/bell's palsy (ICPC-2)
• N92 Trigeminal neuralgia (ICPC-2)
• N95 Tension headache (ICPC-2)
• R09 Sinus symptom/complaint (ICPC-2)
• R75 Sinusitis acute/chronic (ICPC-2)

Figure 1. Description of groups of demands/doubts for orofacial pain.

A descriptive analysis of the data was carried out, using frequency, with data stratification by year of demand (2019 or 2020), for sex and category of the primary care professional, and demands/doubts for orofacial pain. The regression models estimated the prevalence ratios (PR) and the corresponding 95% confidence interval. Initially, it uses unadjusted and adjusted negative binomial regression models to estimate PR (95%CI) and p values for each of the three covariates. Any covariate with a p-value less than 0.25 was a candidate to be tested in the final negative binomial regression model. Only covariates with a p-value less than 0.05 were maintained in the final model [24]. The final model fit was evaluated using a ratio between the residual deviation and the degree of freedom and the chi-square test of the results of the residual deviation. All analyzes were performed in SPSS version 22.0 (SPSS, Chicago, IL, USA).

3. Results

From 10,340 orofacial pain teleconsulting stemming from the original 2019/2020 bank data, 7042 were duplicated or incomplete and excluded. The remaining 3298 were reassessed for compliance with the eligibility criteria, and 669 were discarded. Finally, 2629 integrated the analysis: 1982 referring to 2019 (75.4%) and 647 to 2020 (24.6%) (Figure 2).

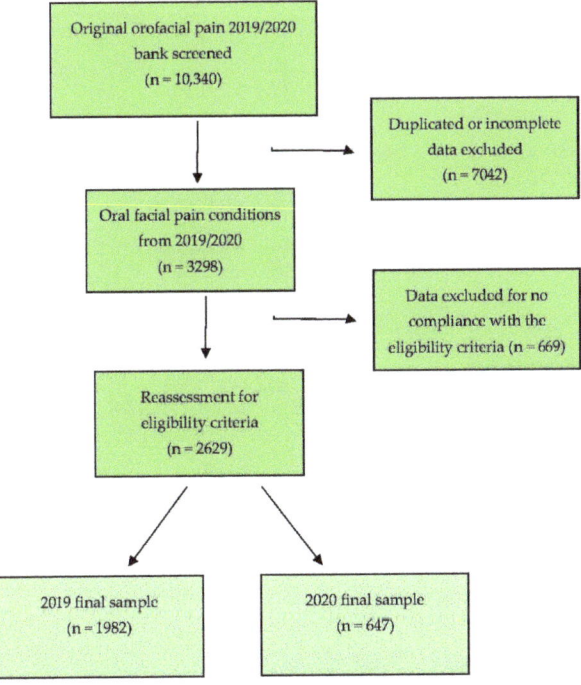

Figure 2. Flow chart showing the criteria of PHC doubts' search and selection.

From these last, in 2019, 1522 (76.8%) avoided referral to secondary care, and in 2020, 373 (57.7%) did so, representing a reduction of 19.1%. For 2020, 403 (62.3%) PHC professionals were females, increasing the prior frequency of 55.3% for women. Physicians were the most frequent professional category in 2019, and dentists in 2020. Regarding doubts recorded in teleconsulting (ICD/ICPC), the "other" group was the most frequent in 2019 (67.1%), and the oral cavity-related pain conditions group in 2020 (65.5%). Despite the relative growth, general physicians, nurses, "others," and the G2 (TMD) diagnostic category still represented a minor fraction in 2020 (Table 1).

Table 1. Description of the characteristics of telehealth for orofacial pain in the Unified Health System, Brazil, 2019 and 2020.

Variable	2019 (N = 1982) Frequency N (%)	2020 (N = 647) Frequency N (%)
If avoided the referral to secondary care		
No	460 (23.2)	274 (42.3)
Yes	1522 (76.8)	373 (57.7)
Sex of PHC * professional		
Female	1096 (55.3)	403 (62.3)
Male	886 (44.7)	244 (37.7)
PHC * profession		
General dentist	171 (8.6)	149 (23.0)
Specialized dentist	332 (16.8)	220 (34.0)
General physician	16 (0.8)	14 (2.2)
Specialized physician	1284 (64.8)	135 (20.9)
Nurse	91 (4.6)	46 (7.1)
Others	88 (4.4)	83 (12.8)
Demands/Doubts		
Group 1	619 (31.2)	424 (65.5)
Group 2	33 (1.7)	27 (4.2)
Group 3	1330 (67.1)	196 (30.3)

* Primary Health Care.

In 2019, nurses (PR = 0.69 CI 95% 0.57–0.83) and "other professionals" (PR = 0.84 CI 95% 0.73–0.97) showed less frequency of avoiding referral of orofacial pain cases to secondary healthcare than general dentists. When the doubts were related to oral cavity pain conditions (G1), there was a lower frequency of avoiding referral (PR = 0.85 CI 95% 0.77–0.94) than other causes of orofacial pain (G3). In 2020, female professionals avoided referrals more frequently than men (PR = 1.24 CI 95% 1.12–1.38). Oral cavity-related pain conditions (G1) doubts (PR = 1.18 CI 95% 1.06–1.32) and temporomandibular disorders (G2) (PR = 1.33 CI 95% 1.15–1.54) surpassed referral avoidance to secondary care than other cases of orofacial pain (G3) (Table 2).

Table 2. Factors associated with avoiding orofacial pain referral to secondary healthcare in the Unified Health System, Brazil, 2019 and 2020 telehealth.

Variables	2019				2020			
	Unadjusted PR (CI 95%)	p-Value	Adjusted PR (CI 95%)	p-value	Unadjusted PR (CI 95%)	p-Value	Adjusted PR (CI 95%)	p-Value
Sex of PHC *								
Female	0.97 (0.94–0.99)	0.015			1.27 (1.14–1.41)	<0.001	1.24 (1.12–1.38)	<0.001
Male	1				1		1	
PHC * profession								
Others	0.88 (0.76–1.01)	0.065	0.84 (0.73–0.97)	0.019	0.90 (0.78–1.04)	0.168		
Nurse	0.75 (0.63–0.89)	0.001	0.69 (0.57–0.83)	<0.001	0.89 (0.74–1.08)	0.232		
Specialized Physician	1.15 (1.08–1.22)	<0.001	0.99 (0.88–1.11)	0.828	0.82 (0.72–0.95)	0.006		
General Physician	0.96 (0.75–1.22)	0.719	0.82 (0.64–1.07)	0.129	0.99 (0.77–1.27)	0.952		
Specialized Dentist	0.96 (0.89–1.04)	0.330	0.96 (0.89–1.04)	0.354	0.95 (0.86–1.05)	0.275		
General Dentist	1		1		1			
Doubts								
Group 1	0.82 (0.79–0.86)	<0.001	0.85 (0.77–0.94)	0.001	1.21 (1.08–1.36)	0.001	1.18 (1.06–1.32)	0.040
Group 2	0.92 (0.81–1.04)	0.175	0.96 (0.82–1.11)	0.551	1.39 (1.19–1.62)	<0.001	1.33 (1.15–1.54)	0.001
Group 3	1		1		1		1	

* Primary Health Care.

4. Discussion

A change was observed in both the descriptive characteristics of asynchronous teleconsulting on orofacial pain and the factors associated with avoiding referrals to secondary health care from 2019 to 2020. In 2019 (before the COVID-19 Pandemic), physicians were the most frequent professionals demanding teleconsulting for orofacial pain. The majority of the demands were related to non-tooth conditions. In 2020, the first year of the COVID-19 Pandemic, dentists were the most frequent professionals, and oral-cavity-related pain conditions doubts were the most frequent. Noteworthy, Teleconsulting's ability to avoid referral to secondary health care and the number of demands decreased from 2019 to 2020. In 2019, professional groups and doubts were associated with avoiding referrals. In 2020, the sex of professionals and doubts were associated with this outcome.

The drop in the total teleconsulting over the assessed period stands out. It may represent a consequence of the general global disarray or disruption in the health system caused by the Pandemic, which forced organizations to focus on COVID-19 issues rather than regular services. Services were suddenly rearranged to deal mainly with pandemic issues or urgencies, leaving behind some previously structured programs and other essential health needs. In Brazil, mobility and non-essential services suffered severe restrictions in 2020, particularly from the second trimester, following the worldwide spread of cases and deaths [25]. Similarly, the apparent drop in physicians' demands in 2020 coincides with the burden of the COVID-19 Pandemic. The mobility restrictions prevented in-person health facility visits and face-to-face patient–doctor interaction, and the shift from traditional care to telehealth occurred for a limited period, demanding rapid training and personnel allocation [26]. In this scenario, the physicians may have initially interrupted regular and elective procedures in favor of medical urgencies, not to mention the staff directly involved with COVID-19 patient management. This fast and somewhat chaotic change may explain the withdrawal of physicians in teleconsulting devoted to orofacial pain issues in the stressful pandemic context of 2020 [27]. Concerning types of doubts, the preeminence of the G3 group over G1 and G2 in 2019 and the reverse in 2020 follows this same scenario, as "other conditions in the head and neck" represented the demands in general related to medical specialties, such as headaches and sinusitis.

The dentists themselves and the doubt categories related to oral cavity conditions (G1) were the most frequent in the 2020 sample. It matches the reallocation of dental professionals in the Public Health System during the Pandemic, leaving their previous routine in favor of managing face-to-face dental urgencies, potentially leading several dental branches to search for information on acute dental conditions in teleconsulting. It is important to note that dental pain is reported as a relevant fraction of dental urgencies [28] and represents the most frequent category of orofacial pain [29]. The general 2020 increase in females in the sample matches the increase in dentists. Women also represent a relevant fraction of Brazilian dental schools in the national dental public health system [30]. In contrast, the G2 (TMD) diagnostic category represented a minor fraction in both years assessed. This situation may reflect the mechanical and technical classical tendencies of dental formation, contrasting with the complexity of chronic conditions such as TMD, which tend to be overlooked in favor of the relative simplicity of acute urgent pathologies. The novelty of the TMD/orofacial pain field in dental schools may also contribute [31].

In 2019 (the pre-pandemic year), nurses and other professionals showed a lower resolution without a referral performance than general dentists. Despite the notorious wide range of diagnostic conditions involved and interdisciplinarity, orofacial pain is traditionally a dental branch that was gradually recognized as a dental specialty. In Brazil, the area has been considered a separate dental specialty from the Federal Council of Dentistry rule since 2002 [31]. This specific dental background in orofacial issues would give dentists a higher capacity for resoluteness in this field than nurses and other professionals. By contrast, in 2019, the lower frequency of case resolution without a referral from oral cavity issues could be partly explained by the full availability of the secondary service chain. In an average period, without pandemic restrictions, the steady health system flow to secondary aid permits PHC professionals to refer a higher number of mild or moderate cases. This standard would change during the Pandemic.

The upsurge in the Pandemic in 2020 marks the preeminence of dentists in the sample. Nurses and "other professionals" in 2020 did not show the same negative association as in 2019. This situation may well reflect the staff reallocation and training in a disruptive period to deal with acute dental concerns, granting fewer referrals (some "other professionals" were already dental practice-related, such as dental assistants). The increase in the proportion of dentists in the sample could result in more resolution capacity of G1 and G2 doubts [31]. Women's higher performance may also be associated with their higher commitment to health care during a pandemic, requiring more in-depth investigation [32,33].

The severe acute respiratory syndrome caused by Coronavirus 2 (SARS-COVID 2), or COVID-19, with the surge in 2020, still represents a massive problem to healthcare systems worldwide, with millions of dead by that year. A "Post-Covid Syndrome" can last beyond the acute 4-week period and affects multiple organs and systems, also related to widespread pain (myalgia) and headaches [34]. Although still under debate and extensive investigation, it will inevitably require interdisciplinary health teams for its study, control, and surveillance, most likely for extended periods. In this regard, telehealth (encompassing teleconsulting) for managing chronic conditions must also find a fertile field of application and expansion ahead [35,36]. Notwithstanding the eventual distortions, challenges in implementation, and lack of randomized controlled assessments of its clinical outcomes and long-term economic analyses [37] these technological advantages are paramount to reducing inequities in periods of high health challenging demands, much like the outbreak of the COVID-19 Pandemic in 2019–2020 [38].

PHC is structured to offer solutions for the basic needs of health, reducing the number of demands for secondary services, mitigating costs, and making the whole system more efficient. The drop in resoluteness recorded in the period of this research following the Pandemic challenges may also reflect a repressed demand for health, making simpler pathologies develop and escalate to a matrix of more complex conditions over the same period [25,27]. It would naturally deflagrate secondary actions, with the potential to decrease the total resoluteness aspect.

This study presents some limitations. First, the short period covering data investigation (2019 and 2020) may not reflect the impact of previous or posterior tendencies upon the Telehealth usage characteristics; therefore, comprehensive time-covering data analysis still needs to be conducted. Second, the cross-sectional study design does not enable inferences regarding causality. Third, the effect of other covariates, such as professional age and patient characteristics on demographic (i.e., age, gender) and clinical status (i.e., the severity of pain and its length and quality, systemic background of the patients) were not available in this dataset, so the study considered only some PHC personnel's dataset. It is important to suggest to the Brazilian Ministry of Health the inclusion of both age of the patient and the professional, a truly confounding variable in quantitative studies [39]. Moreover, more details in the clinical diagnosis of the patient may be also very useful to understand factors associated with our outcome. The access to these variables could impact the quality of the associations identified. Despite these limitations, the study contributes to future analyses regarding the Brazilian orofacial pain teleconsulting program and to elaborate a historical time series research.

5. Conclusions

In 2019, oral cavity doubts scored the lower-case resolution without a referral and PHC profession also influenced this outcome. Female professionals and oral cavity doubts scored the higher case resolution without a referral for the service in 2020.

Author Contributions: Conceptualization, R.L.d.B.A., R.d.C.M. and M.H.N.G.d.A.; data curation, R.L.d.B.A., R.d.C.M., L.C.P. and M.H.N.G.d.A.; formal analysis, R.L.d.B.A., R.d.C.M., L.C.P. and M.H.N.G.d.A.; investigation, R.L.d.B.A., R.d.C.M., L.C.P. and M.H.N.G.d.A.; methodology, R.L.d.B.A., R.d.C.M., L.C.P. and M.H.N.G.d.A.; project administration, R.L.d.B.A., R.d.C.M., L.C.P. and M.H.N.G.d.A.; software, R.L.d.B.A., R.d.C.M., L.C.P. and M.H.N.G.d.A.; writing–original draft, R.L.d.B.A., R.d.C.M. and M.H.N.G.d.A.; writing–review and editing, R.L.d.B.A., R.d.C.M., L.C.P. and M.H.N.G.d.A. All authors have read and agreed to the published version of the manuscript.

Funding: This research received no external funding.

Institutional Review Board Statement: Ethics approval was provided by the Research Ethics Committee of the Federal University of Minas Gerais (UFMG) (CAAE 17400319.9.0000.5149).

Informed Consent Statement: Patient consent was waived due to this study was based on public, secondary and de-identified dataset.

Data Availability Statement: The data presented in this study are available on request from the corresponding author.

Acknowledgments: The authors gratefully acknowledge the Brazilian Ministry of Health by use of data collected from the national database of the Telehealth Results Monitoring and Evaluation System (SMART, by the acronym in Portuguese) and the CAPES (process 001). MHNG Abreu is a research fellow of CNPq (303772/2019-0).

Conflicts of Interest: The authors declare no conflict of interest.

References

1. Castro, M.; Massuda, A.; Almeida, G.; Menezes-Filho, N.; Andrade, M.; Noronha, K.; Rocha, R.; Macinko, J.; Hone, T.; Tasca, R.; et al. Brazil's unified health system: The first 30 years and prospects for the future. *Lancet* **2019**, *394*, 345–356. [CrossRef] [PubMed]
2. World Health Organization. WHO Called to Return to the Declaration of Alma-Ata. *International conference on primary health care*. Available online: https://www.who.int/teams/social-determinants-of-health/declaration-of-alma-ata#:~{}:text=The%20Alma%2DAta%20Declaration%20of,goal%20of%20Health%20for%20Allpdf (accessed on 25 February 2022).
3. Ryu, S. Telemedicine: Opportunities and developments in member states: Report on the second global survey on eHealth 2009 (Global Observatory for eHealth Series, Volume 2). *Healthc Inf. Res.* **2012**, *18*, 153–155. [CrossRef]
4. Diretrizes para oferta de atividades do Programa Nacional Telessaúde Brasil Redes [Guidelines for Offering Activities of the National Telehealth Brasil Redes Program]. Nota Técnica n° 50/2015. Brasília DF. Brazilian. Available online: http://189.28.128.100/dab/docs/portaldab/notas_tecnicas/Nota_Tecnica_Diretrizes_Telessaude.pdf (accessed on 25 February 2022).
5. Ministério da Saúde. Portaria n°. 2.546, de Outubro de 2011. Redefine e Amplia o Programa Telessaúde Brasil, Que Passa a se Chamar Programa Nacional Telessaúde Brasil Redes [Ministry of Health. Ordinance no. 2,546, of October 2011. Redefines and Expands the Telehealth Brazil Program, which Is Now Called National Telehealth Brazil Networks Program]. Available online: https://bvsms.saude.gov.br/bvs/saudelegis/gm/2011/prt2546_27_10_2011.html (accessed on 21 November 2022).
6. Costa, C.B.; Peralta, F.S.; Mello, A.L.S.F. How has teledentistry been applied in public dental health services? An integrative review. *Telemed. J. E-Health* **2020**, *7*, 945–954. [CrossRef] [PubMed]
7. Bavaresco, C.; Hauser, L.; Haddad, A.; Harzheim, E. Impact of teleconsultations on the conduct of oral health teams in the Telehealth Brazil Networks Programme. *Braz. Oral Res.* **2020**, *34*, e011. [CrossRef]
8. International Association for the Study of Pain. Orofacial Pain. International Association for the Study of Pain, 2013–2014. Available online: https://www.iasp-pain.org/advocacy/global-year/orofacial-pain (accessed on 15 May 2022).
9. Ohrbach, R.; Dworkin, S.F. The Evolution of TMD Diagnosis: Past, Present, Future. *J. Dent. Res.* **2016**, *95*, 1093–1101. [CrossRef]
10. Progiante, P.S.; Pattussi, M.P.; Lawrence, H.P.; Goya, S.; Grossi, P.K.; Grossi, M.L. Prevalence of temporomandibular disorders in an adult Brazilian community population using the research diagnostic criteria (Axes I and II) for temporomandibular disorders (The Maringá Study). *Int. J. Prosthodont.* **2015**, *28*, 600–609. [CrossRef]
11. Croft, P.; Blyth, F.M.; van der Windt, D. *Chronic Pain Epidemiology: From Aetiology to Public Health*; Oxford University Press: Oxford, UK; New York, NY, USA, 2010; ISBN 9780191594816.
12. Greene, C.S.; Kusiak, J.W.; Cowley, T.; Cowley, A.W., Jr. Recently released report by major scientific academy proposes significant changes in understanding and managing temporomandibular disorders. *J. Oral Maxillofac. Surg.* **2022**, *80*, 8–9. [CrossRef]
13. Romero-Reyes, M.; Uyanik, J.M. Orofacial pain management: Current perspectives. *J. Pain Res.* **2014**, *7*, 99–115. [CrossRef]
14. Cunha, M.A.; Vettore, M.V.; Santos, T.R.D.; Matta-Machado, A.T.; Lucas, S.D.; Abreu, M.H.N.G. The role of organizational factors and human resources in the provision of dental prosthesis in primary dental care in Brazil. *Int. J. Environ. Res. Public Health* **2020**, *17*, 1646. [CrossRef]
15. da Rocha Mendes, S.; de Castro Martins, R.; de Melo Mambrini, J.V.; Matta-Machado, A.T.G.; Mattos-Savage, G.C.; Gallagher, J.E.; Abreu, M.H.N.G. The Influence of dentists' profile and health work management in the performance of Brazilian dental teams. *Biomed. Res. Int.* **2021**, *2021*, 8843928. [CrossRef]
16. Paiva, J.; Carvalho, T.; Vilela, A.; Nóbrega, G.; Souza, B.; Valentim, R. SMART: A service-oriented architecture for monitoring and assessing Brazil's Telehealth outcomes. *Res. Biomed. Eng.* **2018**, *34*, 317–328. [CrossRef]
17. Ministério da Saúde. Núcleos de Telessaúde no Brasil [Ministry of Health. State Telehealth Centers]. Available online: https://www.gov.br/saude/pt-br/acesso-a-informacao/acoes-e-programas/programa-telessaude/nucleos-de-telessaude-no-brasil (accessed on 20 April 2021).
18. Lobbezoo, F.; Aarab, G.; Kapos, F.; Dayo, A.; Koutris, M.; Thymi; Häggman-Henrikson, B. Leave no one behind: Easy and valid assessment of orofacial pain. *Lancet Glob. Health* **2022**, *10*, e184. [CrossRef] [PubMed]
19. World Health Organization. International Statistical Classification of Diseases and Related Health Problems, 10th revision, 5th ed. 2016. Available online: https://apps.who.int/iris/handle/10665/246208 (accessed on 17 May 2021).
20. World Health Organization. International Classification of Primary Care (ICPC-2), 2nd ed. Available online: https://www.who.int/standards/classifications/other-classifications/international-classification-of-primary-care (accessed on 17 May 2021).
21. Basílio, N.; Ramos, C.; Figueira, S.; Pinto, D. Worldwide Usage of International Classification of Primary Care. *Rev. Bras. Med. Fam. Comunidade* **2016**, *11*, 1–9. [CrossRef]
22. De Leeuw, R.; Klasser, G. *Orofacial Pain: Guidelines for Assessment, Diagnosis, and Management*, 5th ed.; Quintessence Publishing: Chicago, IL, USA, 2018; ISBN 978-0-86715-610-2.
23. International Headache Society (IHS). International Classification of Orofacial Pain, 1st edition (ICOP). *Cephalalgia* **2020**, *40*, 129–221. [CrossRef]
24. Hosmer, D.W.; Lemeshow, S.; Sturdivant, R.X. *Applied Logistic Regression*, 3rd ed.; Wiley: Hoboken, NJ, USA, 2013.
25. World Health Organization. Modelling the Health Impacts of Disruptions to Essential Health Services during COVID-19. UNICEF. Available online: https://data.unicef.org/resources/modelling-the-health-impacts-of-disruptions-to-essential-health-services-during-covid-19 (accessed on 12 February 2022).

26. Garfan, S.; Alamoodi, A.H.; Zaidan, B.B.; Al-Zobbi, M.; Hamid, R.A.; Alwan, J.K.; Ahmaro, I.Y.Y.; Khalid, E.T.; Jumaah, F.M.; Albahri, O.S.; et al. Telehealth utilization during the COVID-19 Pandemic: A systematic review. *Comput. Biol. Med.* **2021**, *138*, 104878. [CrossRef]
27. Verhoeven, V.; Tsakitzidis, G.; Philips, H.; Van Royen, P. Impact of the COVID-19 Pandemic on the core functions of primary care: Will the cure be worse than the disease? A qualitative interview study in Flemish GPs. *BMJ Open* **2020**, *10*, e039674. [CrossRef]
28. Mikkola, M.K.; Gästgifvars, J.J.; Helenius-Hietala, J.S.; Uittamo, J.T.; Furuholm, J.O.; Välimaa, H.; Ruokonen, H.M.A.; Nylund, K.M. Triage and urgent dental care for COVID-19 patients in the Hospital District of Helsinki and Uusimaa. *Acta Odontol. Scand.* **2022**, *80*, 433–440. [CrossRef]
29. Horst, O.V.; Cunha-Cruz, J.; Zhou, L.; Manning, W.; Mancl, L.; DeRouen, T.A. Prevalence of pain in the orofacial regions in patients visiting general dentists in the Northwest Practice-based REsearch Collaborative in Evidence-based DENTistry research network. *J. Am. Dent. Assoc.* **2015**, *146*, 721–728.e3. [CrossRef]
30. Kfouri, M.; Moysés, S.; Gabardo, M.; Nascimento, A.; da Rosa, S.; Moysés, S. The feminization of dentistry and the perceptions of public service users about gender issues in oral health. *Cien Saude Colet.* **2019**, *24*, 4285–4296. [CrossRef]
31. Conselho Federal de Odontologia [Federal Council of Dentistry]. Resolução CFO-25, de 16 de maio de 2002 (16 May 2002). Brazilian. Available online: https://sistemas.cfo.org.br/visualizar/atos/RESOLU%c3%87%c3%83O/SEC/2002/25 (accessed on 12 February 2022).
32. Tay, P.K.C.; Ting, Y.Y.; Tan, K.Y. Sex and Care: The evolutionary psychological explanations for sex differences in formal care occupations. *Front. Psychol.* **2019**, *10*, 867. [CrossRef]
33. Mandil, A.M.; Alhayyan, R.M.; Alshalawi, A.A.; Alemran, A.S.; Alayed, M.M. Preference of physicians' gender among male and female primary health care clinic attendees in a university hospital in Saudi Arabia. *Saudi Med. J.* **2015**, *36*, 1011. [CrossRef]
34. Nalbandian, A.; Sehgal, K.; Gupta, A.; Madhavan, M.V.; McGroder, C.; Stevens, J.S.; Cook, J.R.; Nordvig, A.S.; Shalev, D.; Sehrawat, T.S.; et al. Post-acute COVID-19 syndrome. *Nat. Med.* **2021**, *27*, 601–615. [CrossRef] [PubMed]
35. Achmad, H.; Tanumihardja, M.; Ramadhany, Y.F. Teledentistry as a solution in dentistry during the COVID-19 pandemic period: A systematic review. *Int. J. Pharm. Res.* **2020**, *12*, 272–278.
36. Almeida-Leite, C.M.; Stuginski-Barbosa, J.; Conti, P.C.R. How psychosocial and economic impacts of COVID-19 pandemic can interfere on bruxism and temporomandibular disorders? *J. Appl. Oral Sci.* **2020**, *28*, e20200263. [CrossRef]
37. Flumignan, C.; Rocha, A.; Pinto, A.C.; Milby, K.; Batista, M.; Atallah, Á.; Saconato, H. What do Cochrane systematic reviews say about telemedicine for healthcare? *Sao Paulo Med. J.* **2019**, *137*, 184–192. [CrossRef]
38. Lattimore, C.M.; Kane, W.J.; Fleming, M.A.I.; Martin, A.N.; Mehaffey, J.H.; Smolkin, M.E.; Ratcliffe, S.J.; Zaydfudim, V.M.; Showalter, S.L.; Hedrick, T.L. Disparities in telemedicine utilization among surgical patients during COVID-19. *PLoS ONE* **2021**, *16*, e0258452. [CrossRef]
39. Philipps, L.R. Age: A truly confounding variable. *West J. Nurs. Res.* **1989**, *11*, 181–195. [CrossRef]

Disclaimer/Publisher's Note: The statements, opinions and data contained in all publications are solely those of the individual author(s) and contributor(s) and not of MDPI and/or the editor(s). MDPI and/or the editor(s) disclaim responsibility for any injury to people or property resulting from any ideas, methods, instructions or products referred to in the content.

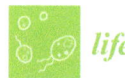

Article

Complicated Relationships between Anterior and Condylar Guidance and Their Clinical Implications—Comparison by Cone Beam Computed Tomography and Electronic Axiography—An Observational Cohort Cross-Sectional Study

Łukasz Lassmann [1,*], Zuzanna Nowak [2], Jean-Daniel Orthlieb [3] and Agata Żółtowska [4]

1 Dental Sense Medicover, ul. Myśliwska 33a, 80-283 Gdańsk, Poland
2 Department of Temporomandibular Disorders, Medical University of Silesia in Katowice, Traugutta sq. 2, 41-800 Zabrze, Poland
3 Faculty of Odontology, Aix-Marseille University, 58 Boulevard Charles Livon, 13007 Marseille, France
4 Department of Conservative Dentistry, Faculty of Medicine, Medical University of Gdańsk, 80-210 Gdańsk, Poland
* Correspondence: lassmann.lukas@gmail.com

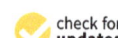

Citation: Lassmann, Ł.; Nowak, Z.; Orthlieb, J.-D.; Żółtowska, A. Complicated Relationships between Anterior and Condylar Guidance and Their Clinical Implications—Comparison by Cone Beam Computed Tomography and Electronic Axiography—An Observational Cohort Cross-Sectional Study. *Life* **2023**, *13*, 335. https://doi.org/10.3390/life13020335

Academic Editor: Marcin Balcerzyk

Received: 21 December 2022
Revised: 18 January 2023
Accepted: 23 January 2023
Published: 26 January 2023

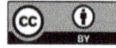

Copyright: © 2023 by the authors. Licensee MDPI, Basel, Switzerland. This article is an open access article distributed under the terms and conditions of the Creative Commons Attribution (CC BY) license (https:// creativecommons.org/licenses/by/ 4.0/).

Abstract: A complex prosthodontic treatment is believed to be more successful when the condylar path is replicated using the articulator. However, there is an ongoing major disagreement between the researchers as the exact relationship between the posterior and anterior determinants has not been clear. The purpose of this study was to investigate whether the protrusive movement of the mandible does correlate with the temporomandibular joint (TMJ) anatomy or with incised features. Subjects (15 males and 15 females) were qualified for this study based on an initial interview including the following criteria: age 21–23 (+/−1), no history of trauma, orthodontic treatment, or temporomandibular disorders (TMD). For each patient, the angle of the condylar path, incisal guidance angle (IGA), interincisal angle, as well as overbite and overjet were measured on cone beam computed tomography (CBCT). This was followed by the examination with the Modjaw® electronic axiograph recording and calculating the functional sagittal condylar guidance angle (SCGA) for the right and left TMJ during the protrusion. The results show that the mean functional axiographic measurement of SCGA in protrusion significantly correlates with the TMJ anatomy presented on CBCT. Moreover, a significant correlation was found between the values of SCGA in the functional and anatomical measurements in all its variants. It turned out that, statistically, the AB measurement was the most accurate. Finally, results showed that incisal relationships of permanent teeth such as overbite, overjet, incisal guidance angle and interincisal angle do not correlate with TMJ anatomy, and therefore, regarding an analyzed study group, do not affect the TMJ formation in young adults.

Keywords: temporomandibular joint; temporomandibular disorders; dental occlusion; dental prosthesis

1. Introduction

The temporomandibular joint (TMJ) is a part of the stomatognathic system that allows the mandible to move. In adults, those movements are dictated by the shape of the articular tubercle, articular disk, the limitation of the associated ligaments, the neuromuscular system, and the guiding planes of the teeth [1]. A sagittal trajectory of the condyle traversing the articular tubercle with any chosen horizontal plane (e.g., Frankfort) creates the sagittal condylar guidance angle (SCGA). The SCGA can be measured radiographically, using a jaw movement recording device, or with a protrusive interocclusal bite registration method [2,3]. In previous decades, pantomograms have sometimes been recommended for measuring SCG [4]. However, they have many disadvantages, including the orientation of the reference plane and the head, and parallax distortions due to the difficulty of distinguishing the outline of the articular elevation from the lower border of the zygomatic arch [5]. Moreover, panoramic images are often not precise for SCGA measurement due to the overlapping of many structures. In contrast, CBCT scans provide a 3D image for both sides without overlapping, so that articular sublimation and acetabular fossa can be clearly distinguished from adjacent structures, and the CBCT SCGA measurement alone gives much more reliable results. With the advent of CBCT, CT scans were associated with less radiation exposure and greater accuracy, which resulted in their widespread use in dentistry [6].

The registered values of SCGA allow for an accurate articulator setting [3,7,8]. A complex prosthodontic treatment is believed to be more successful when the condylar path is replicated using the articulator, since condylar inclination adjustment affects the cusp height and, to a lesser extent, the occlusal ridge and groove positions [9,10]. Studies have shown that it allows the restoration of the effective shape of the occlusal surface without interferences [2,8]. The steep angles of the articular tubercle allow longer cusps and deeper fossae of the posterior teeth, and shallower concavity of the palatal surfaces of the anterior teeth, thanks to a rapid discussion in the molar area during mandibular movements. A flat articular tubercle requires shorter cusps and shallower grooves of the posterior teeth. The incisal overlap is equally important. The greater the amount of vertical overlap and the smaller the horizontal overlap, the longer the cusps and the deeper the fissures may be [11].

However, there is an ongoing major disagreement between the researchers as the exact relationship between the posterior and anterior determinants has not been clear. Different authors have attempted to confirm or deny the relationship between the posterior determinant—corresponding to the condylar guidance path within the TMJ and the anterior determinant—the incisal, and canine guidance, and their findings vary [12]. The first group claims that there is no correlation between the path of the condyle and the anterior incisal slope [13–15]. According to that approach, the anterior guidance must be reconstructed in line with aesthetics, anatomical, and phonetic criteria and provide a posterior disclusion during movements [13]. Dawson emphasizes the importance of adequate concavity or occlusal clearance for anterior guidance to prevent restriction of the mandibular movements and its reduction to simple rotational movement [16].

The opposing group advocates the existence of a connection between the anterior slope and the path of the condyle [12]. As the gnathological approach matured, an anterior guidance steeper than the condylar guidance became a mandatory rule as it provided the elimination of all horizontal forces from the posterior teeth [17]. Brose et al. claim that the incisal guidance angle should always be steeper than the condylar guidance, whereas the height and slope angles of the cusps of the posterior teeth should be harmonious with the condylar and anterior guidance, and where such harmony does not exist, the teeth can be reshaped to a more desirable contour by adjusting or restoring them to eliminate trauma and lessen the harmful effects of parafunction [11]. There are reports suggesting that the steep incisal guidance (IG) may cause the temporomandibular joint to malfunction [18]. It has been hypothesized that IG influences the movements of the condyles, which in turn modifies the growth and morphology of TMJ [19]. However, so far, no one has proven this causation in a meaningful way. Han et al. showed weak but statistically significant correlations between the incisal angle (IGA) and the size of the condyle and fossa centroid [19].

On the other hand, Luca et al. in their study found that there are no differences in the relation between the mandibular fossa features and the inclination of the upper incisors in people with different types of faces, and there is no clinically significant relationship between the shape of the joint and the inclination of the incisors [20]. However, the age of the population in this study ranged from 18 to 40. It is an important factor as TMJ develops between 21 and 23 y.o., and after its peak in growth and development after 17 years of age, TMJ gradually exhibits various modes of adaptation that may be associated with IGA [21]. It is not likely that the morphology and position of incisors have a significant impact on shaping a developing TMJ since incisal guidance seems to be of recent origin.

This hypothesis is supported by a study of plague victims in the south of France from 1720 in which a vertical overbite was not present. Some authors argue that incisal guidance did not appear until the Middle Ages, when the use of a fork became common [22–24].

1.1. Objectives

In view of the controversy raised by the literature, the aim of this study was to investigate the existence of a statistically significant correlation between the incisal features (IGA, interincisal angle, overbite, and overjet), TMJ morphology, and its function.

Therefore, the following null hypotheses were set:

I. The protrusive movement of the mandible does correlate with the TMJ anatomy.
II. The protrusive movement of the mandible does not correlate with the incisal features.
III. The position and relationship of upper and lower permanent incisors do not have a direct and significant effect on the TMJ morphology in young adults.

1.2. Clinical Implications

Incisal relationships of permanent dentition should not be considered as impacting TMJ morphology and function at an early age. Therefore, the orthodontist should not overestimate the role of overbite and overjet in the aspect of preventing TMJ disorders, and should focus their attention on more important issues, such as the angle of inclination of the occlusal plane.

If the CBCT scans are available, the AB measurement method allows one to accurately determine the condylar guidance angle and aids in the programming of virtual or analog articulators. Otherwise, electronic axiography is a reliable tool for transferring these data to virtual articulators as a part of prosthetic rehabilitation.

2. Materials and Methods

2.1. Study Participants

This study was approved by the Independent Bioethics Committee for Scientific Research at Medical University of Gdańsk (number NKBBN/1043/2021-2022) and is retrospectively registered at ClinicalTrials.gov (NCT05637372). Patients received verbal and written information describing the trial and gave their consent to participate in this study.

Subjects were qualified for this study based on an initial interview including the following criteria: age 21–23 (+/−1), no history of trauma, orthodontic treatment, or TMD. Previous studies by Sulün et al. confirmed that the articular eminence reaches its full size between 21 and 30 years of age in healthy patients and decreases after the age of 31 [25]. Similarly, the articular condyle is fully developed between the ages of 21 and 22 [26]. For this reason, we decided to construct the study group including subjects exactly in 21–23 (+/−1) age range, so the correlation between occlusal and joint features is not falsified by any form of adaptation within the TMJ. The interview was followed by an examination performed in accordance with the Polish version of the RDC/TMD criteria, which disqualified one patient diagnosed with myofascial pain [27]. Eventually, 30 patients qualified for this study.

2.2. Study Protocol

For each patient, the angle of the condylar path, incisal guidance angle, the interincisal angle, as well as overbite and overjet were measured on CBCT, followed by the examination with the Modjaw® (MODJAW, Lyon, France) electronic axiograph recording and calculating the functional SCGA for right and left TMJ during the protrusion.

Each CBCT examination was conducted by an experienced radiologist technician with the use of Carestream 9300 device (Carestream Dental, Altanta, GA, USA), set to following parameters: 120 kV, 3.20 mA, 40 s with 1698.19 mGy/cm^2 delivered. The patient was in standing position with the mandible in the maximum intercuspation position (MIP). Obtained images were analyzed in CS Imaging 8.0.5 program. To measure the SCGA on the obtained imaging examination, the Frankfort horizontal plane (FHP) was marked as a horizontal reference plane. It was constructed by connecting the left Orbitale and Porion points on both sides (Figure 1A) [28]. Next, in the sagittal view, a layer perpendicular to one running through the innermost and outermost point of the condyle in transverse cross-section was selected for each joint separately (Figure 1B).

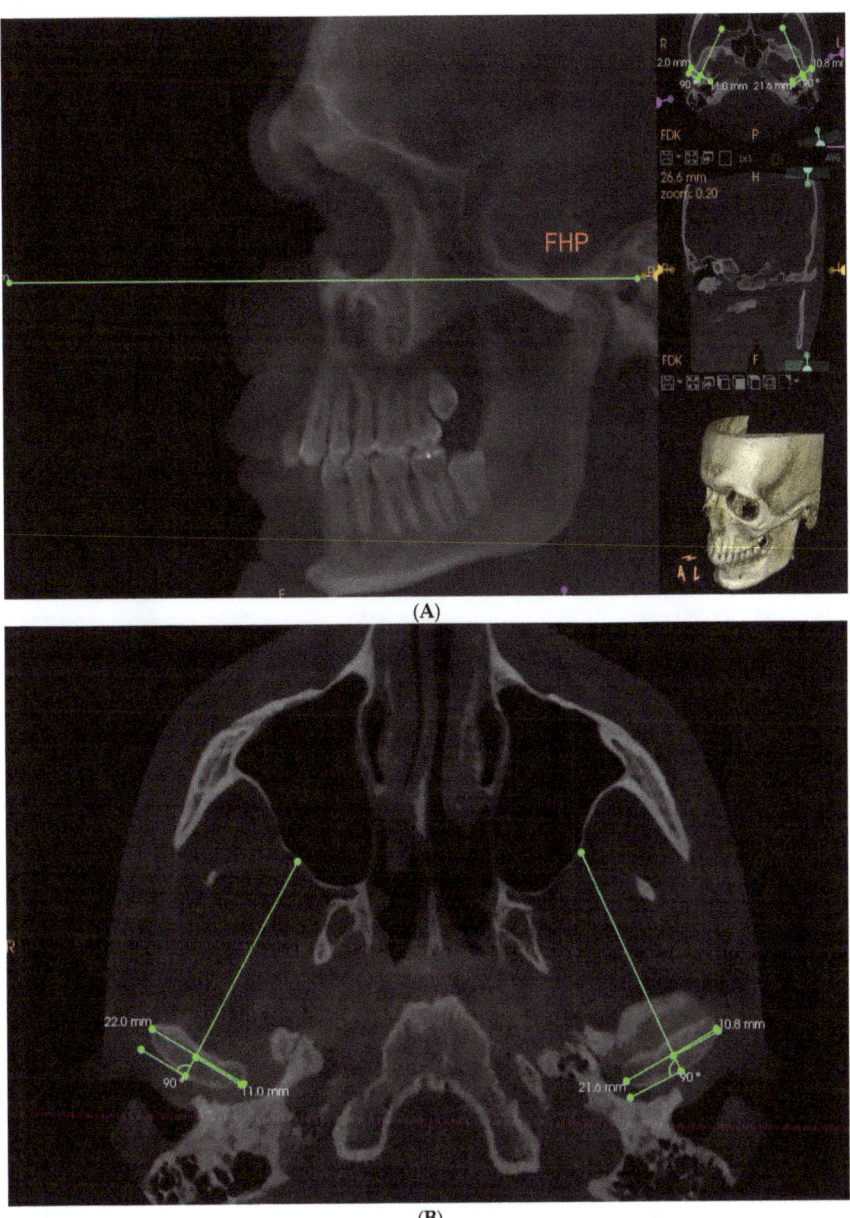

Figure 1. (**A**,**B**) Establishing a Frankfort reference plane and a proper CBCT layer to obtain reproducible measurements for all the patients according to anatomical landmarks (FHP—Frankfort horizontal plane).

The temporomandibular joint space was described by marking the antero-superior space (ASS) and superior space (SS). ASS indicates the thickness of the intermediate band of the disc, while SS indicates the thickness of the posterior band of the disc. Additionally, the vertical height of the fossa (H) was marked (Figure 2A). Then, to achieve the most objective data, three different methods of measuring the SCGA were proposed. First—the AB measurement, which indicates the angle between FHP and the line connecting point A at the deepest point of the articular fossa to point B at the highest point of the articular eminence (Figure 2B). Second—the AT measurement, which indicates the angle between FHP and the line connecting point A at the deepest point of the articular fossa with the tangent point T adjacent to the articular eminence (Figure 2C). Additionally, third—the CD measurement, which indicates angle between Frankfurt plane and a line connecting the highest point C of the condyle to point D, which is below the highest point of the articular tubercle (B), considering the change in the thickness of the disc above the condyle during protrusive movement (Figure 2D). The distance BD reflects intermediate discal space that in vertical dimension is equal to ASS. The numerical data were collected for both joints of each patient and tabulated for further analyses.

Likewise, the data concerning the incisors were collected. The cross-section view of left and right incisors was examined, and, for each patient, the pair of central incisors presenting the higher value of IGA was selected for further measurements of the incisal features [19,29]. We measured the incisal guidance angle—the angle between the line connecting the incisal margin of the maxillary and mandibular incisors with the FHP (Figure 3A); the interincisal angle—between long axis of upper and lower incisors (Figure 3B); overbite—vertical and perpendicular to FHP distance between incisal margins; and overjet—horizontal and parallel to FHP distance between incisal margin of upper incisor and transverse to the FHP projection of the lower incisal edge (Figure 3C).

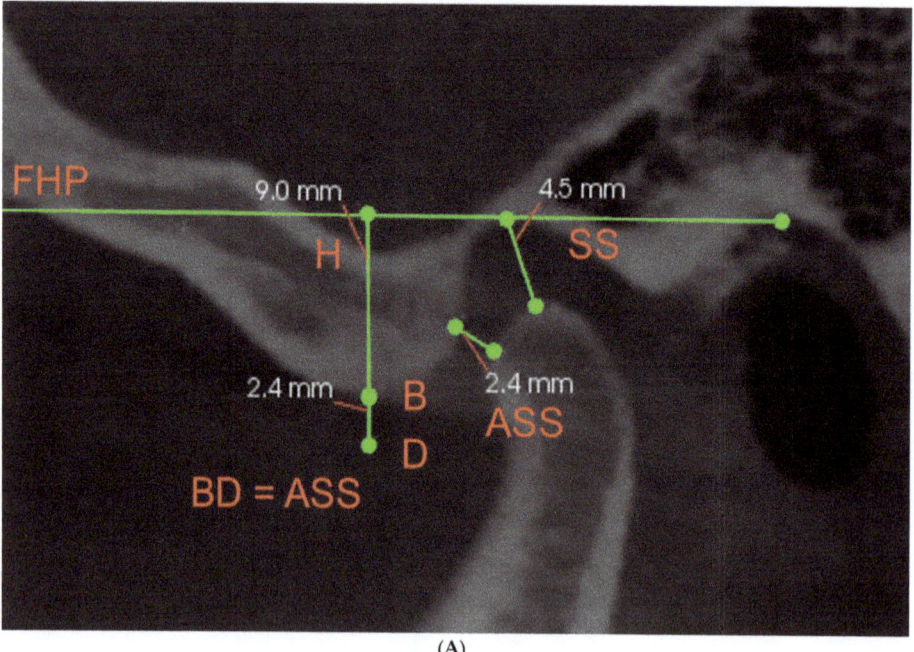

(A)

Figure 2. *Cont.*

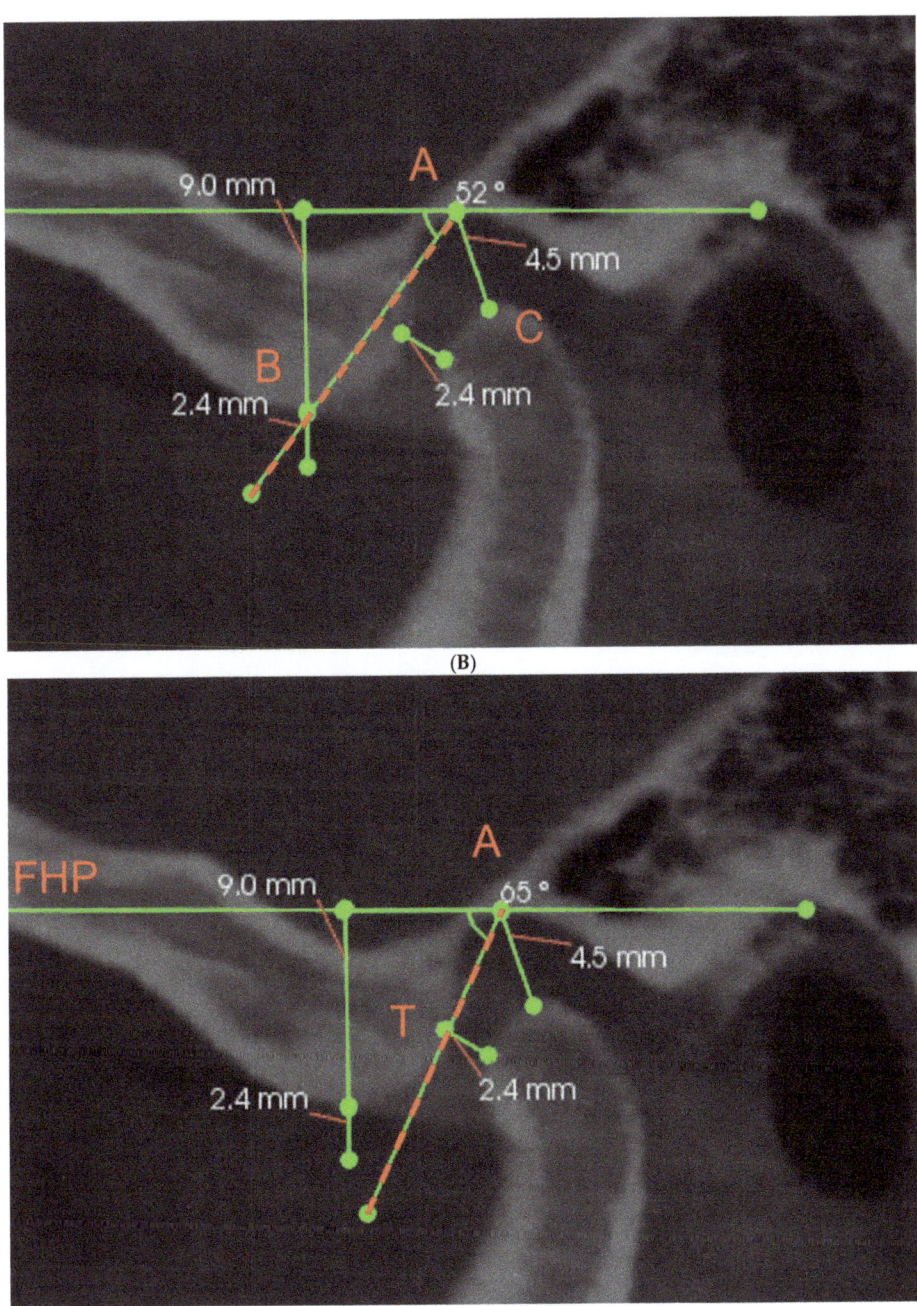

Figure 2. *Cont.*

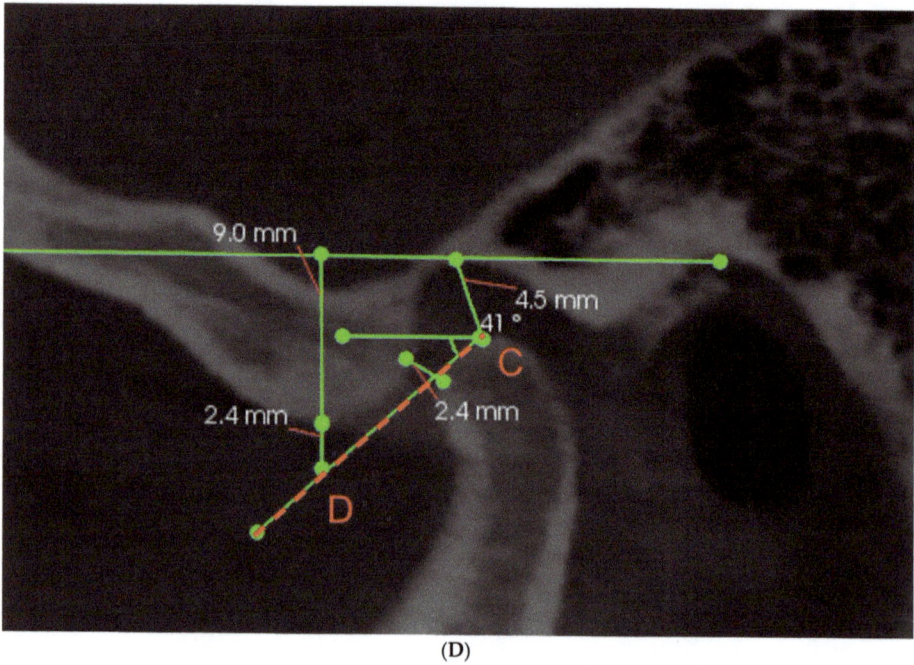

(D)

Figure 2. (A–D) The sagittal view of the TMJ with marked landmarks and illustration of three different methods of measuring the SCGA (ASS—antero-superior space; SS—superior space; H—vertical height of the fossa; FHP—Frankfort horizontal plane; A—deepest point of the articular fossa; B—highest point of the articular eminence; T—tangent point adjacent to the articular eminence; C—highest point of the condyle; D—point below the highest point of the articular tubercle).

Afterward, intraoral scans of qualified patients were conducted with the use of the Carestream 3600 scanner. The obtained STL files were transferred to the Modjaw® measuring device to record the mandible movements in real time (Figure 4). The Modjaw® was designed as a substitute for the facebow, axiograph, and mechanical articulator at the same time, with the possibility to transfer obtained data along with the patient's individual reference plane to CAD/CAM software (Exocad GmbH, Darmstadt, Germany) [30]. To obtain an individual value of the SCGA, the following actions were performed: fixing the hinge axis by means of repetitive opening and closing movements with the tongue positioned on the palate, and protrusive movement from MIP to edge-to-edge position. The SCGA during function for each patient was computed in the Modjaw® software between the path of the moving condyle and the individual reference plane set by the line connecting the hinge axis to the line created between the Nasion and Subnasale point.

2.3. Statistical Analysis

All calculations have been carried out by means of Microsoft Excel 2019 spreadsheet and STATISTICA (TIBCO Software Inc., Palo Alto, CA, USA; 2020) Data Science Workbench, version 14. In the statistical description of quantitative data, classical measures of location, such as arithmetic means and median, and measures of variation, such as standard deviation and range, were used. The normality of distribution of the variables was tested using Shapiro–Wilk's test. To assess the linear correlation between two variables, Pearson's correlation and Spearman's correlation were used with respect to the type of distribution of the variables tested. To estimate best predictors for a particular dependent variable, multiple regression models were created. In all the calculations, the statistical significance level was set to $p < 0.05$.

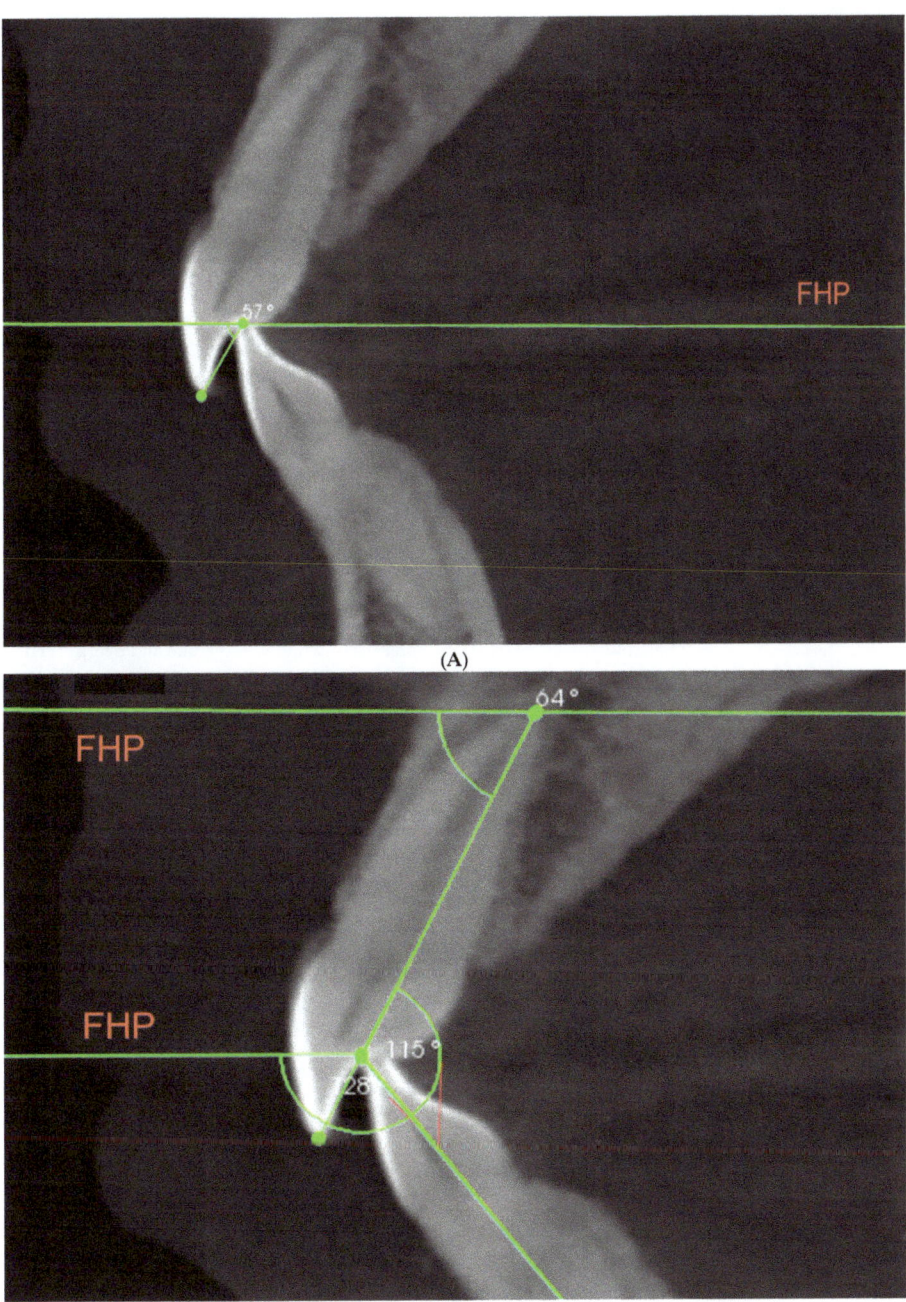

Figure 3. *Cont.*

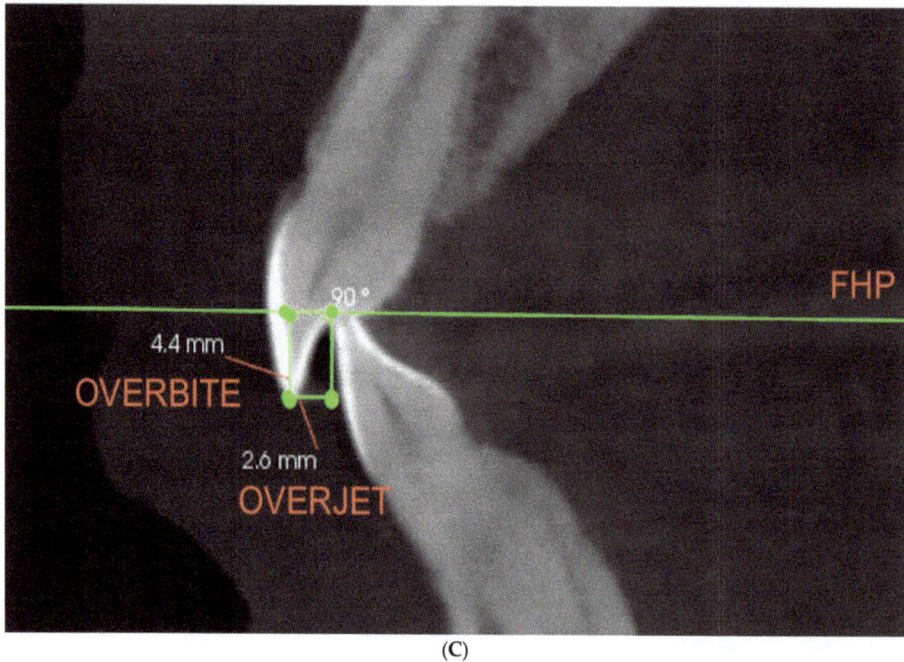

(**C**)

Figure 3. (**A**–**C**) Illustration of measurements concerning the anterior determinant—the incisors: A—incisal guidance angle (IGA), B—interincisal angle, C—overbite and overjet (FHP—Frankfort horizontal plane).

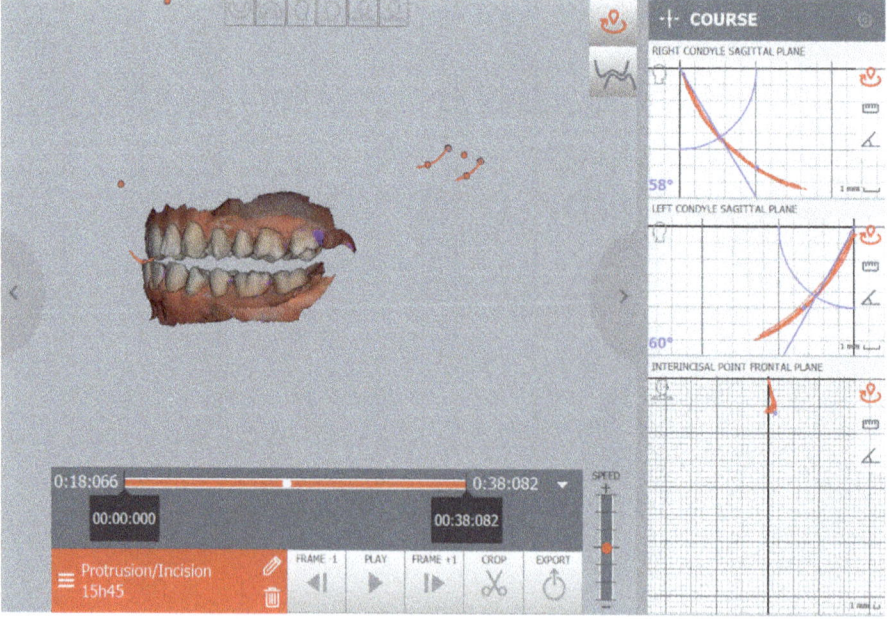

Figure 4. An example of SCGA measured by Modjaw axiography.

2.4. Limitations

We are aware of some limitations of this work, which is mostly a small study group, and the fact that the Modjaw® axiograph uses an individual reference pane for each patient. However, due to the heterogeneity of the reference plane and its individual character for each patient, it was not possible to directly compare the angles obtained on Modjaw® and on CBCT; the statistical analysis was applied to check the correlations.

3. Results

The measurements of the parameters for all 30 patients (60 TMJ) were collated and subjected to statistical analysis. The aim was to test the correlation between the values of axiographic SCGA during protrusion with SCGA on CBCT (Table 1), the axiographic SCGA during protrusion with the incisal parameters on CBCT (Table 2), and the SCGA with the incisal parameters both measured on CBCT (Table 3), which are presented in the tables below accordingly.

Table 1. Correlation between mean SCGA during protrusion and mean SCGA in CBCT measurements.

Variables	n	Mean	SD	r (X, Y)	r^2	p
Mean SCGA during protrusion Mean vertical height of the TMJ fossa	30	56.6000 8.2467	6.6299 0.8467	0.496253	0.246267	0.005285
Mean SCGA during protrusion Mean SCGA in AB measurement	30	56.6000 41.1167	6.6299 6.2694	0.551815	0.304500	0.001571
Mean SCGA during protrusion Mean SCGA in AT measurement	30	56.6000 52.4167	6.6299 7.9525	0.532373	0.283421	0.002459
Mean SCGA during protrusion Mean SCGA in CD measurement	30	56.6000 36.4833	6.6299 5.8509	0.449854	0.202368	0.012623

Table 2. Correlation between mean SCGA during protrusion and the incisal parameters measured on CBCT.

Variables	n	Mean	SD	r (X, Y)	r^2	p
Mean SCGA during protrusion Overbite	30	56.6000 3.5400	6.6299 1.2544	−0.173606	0.030139	0.358898
Mean SCGA during protrusion Overjet	30	56.6000 2.4067	6.6299 0.7701	0.022152	0.000491	0.907500
Mean SCGA during protrusion Interincisal angle	30	56.6000 134.6000	6.6299 11.7403	−0.183319	0.033606	0.332212
Mean SCGA during protrusion Incisal guidance angle	30	56.6000 53.1333	6.6299 12.1789	−0.173343	0.030048	0.359636

Table 3. The correlation between the incisal guidance angle and mean SCGA in AB measurements.

Variables	n	Mean	SD	r (X, Y)	r^2	p
Incisal guidance angle Mean SCGA in AB measurement	30	53.13333 41.11667	12.17893 6.26936	−0.069985	0.004898	0.713254
Incisal guidance angle Mean SCGA in AT measurement	30	53.13333 52.41667	12.17893 7.95254	−0.062899	0.003956	0.741250
Incisal guidance angle Mean SCGA in CD measurement	30	53.13333 36.48333	12.17893 5.85085	−0.129900	0.016874	0.493869

The results show that the mean functional axiographic measurement of SCGA in protrusion significantly correlates with the TMJ anatomy described by the mean vertical height of the fossa (Figure 5) and the angle of the articular tubercle corresponding to SCGA on CBCT (Figure 6). Moreover, a significant correlation was found between the values of SCGA in the functional and anatomical measurements in all its variants. It turned out that statistically, the AB measurement was the most accurate; however, the AT measurement and the CD method show the least correlation (Table 1). Therefore, this leads to proving the first null hypothesis.

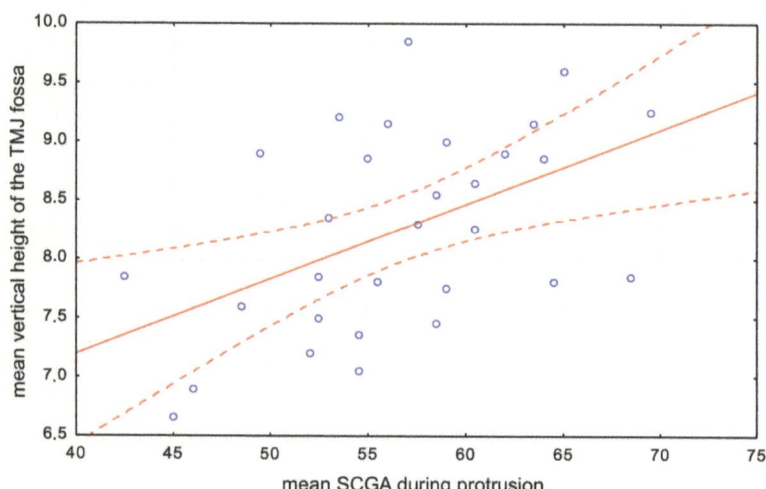

Figure 5. Correlation between mean SCGA during protrusion and mean vertical height of the TMJ fossa.

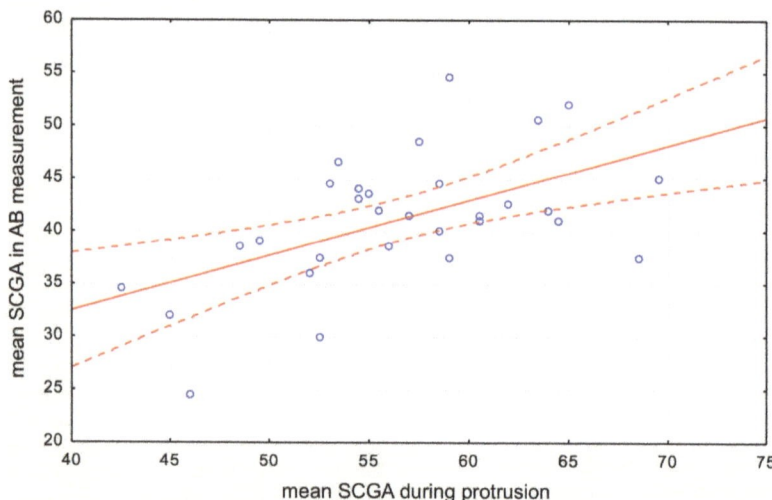

Figure 6. Correlation between mean SCGA during protrusion and mean SCGA in AB measurement.

Subsequent analysis of the mean functional axiographic measurement of SCGA in protrusion collated with the incisal features allowed the confirmation of the second null hypothesis. According to the resolution, the values describing the function of the TMJ did not correlate with any of the incisal parameters: IGA, interincisal angle, overjet, or overbite (Table 2, Figure 7).

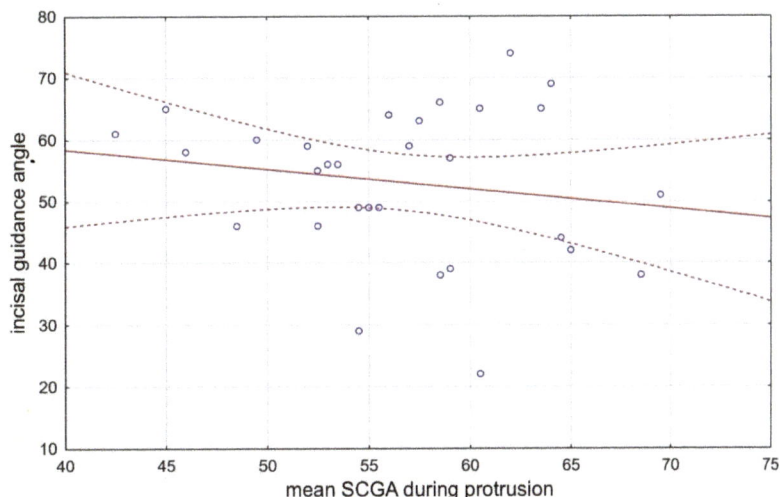

Figure 7. Correlation between mean SCGA during protrusion and the incisal guidance angle.

Similarly, the third null hypothesis was successfully proved as the incisal parameters did not show a correlation with any of the anatomical CBCT measurements within the TMJ. Regardless of a reference line and slight differences in measurements, no correlation was found between the SCGA on CBCT and front teeth relationships (Table 3, Figure 8).

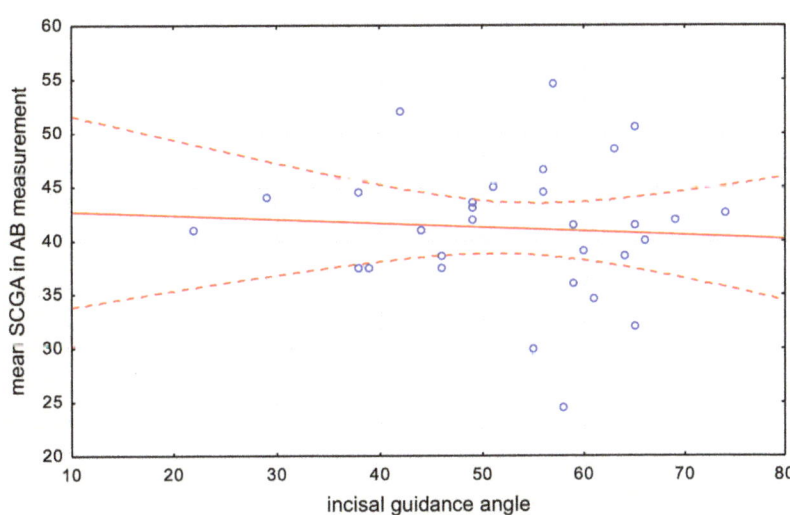

Figure 8. The correlation between the incisal guidance angle and mean SCGA in AB measurement.

4. Discussion

Many researchers support the assumption that the shape of the temporomandibular joint is related to its function and that specific functional patterns will provide correlating changes in both dentition and TMJ [31–34]. The lack of a relationship between the position of the incisors and the morphology of the joint, however, is a much more debatable subject. Our results suggest that while the protrusive movement recorded with the axiograph is correlated with the height and inclination angle of the articular tubercle, the position and mutual relations of the front teeth do not show any correlation to the structure of the temporomandibular joint, regardless of which reference points in the joint are used for measurements.

The evident lack of influence of the anterior guidance and overlapping of the anterior permanent teeth on the formation of the temporomandibular joint early in life is not surprising, considering the age range during which the eminence develops and the hypothesis that the overbite appeared only in the Middle Ages. Articular tuberosity develops in more than 50% of people by the age of five, and almost 90% by the age of eight. The remaining 10% of the eminence angle forms during the teenage years [35]. Therefore, it would be surprising if permanent incisors significantly influenced the structure of the TMJ. An interesting example of a relatively recent change was found in the study of the Maïdu Indians from California. This population showed a straight edge-to-edge bite up to colonization. Later studies showed that the occlusion changed to include the incisal bite, "locking" canine occlusion, and these changes happened probably due to the introduction of a soft diet. The study by Laplanche et al., 2010 also showed more than a doubled incidence of class 3 in 1870 and almost doubled incidence of class 2 in 1970 [22].

Another interesting piece of evidence for modern changes in the relationship of the anterior teeth was provided by the linguist Charles Hockett [33]. He suggested that the use of teeth as tools in hunter–gatherer populations used to wear them down; thus, the production of "f" and "v" consonants between the lower lip and upper teeth was much more difficult. Therefore, there was a hypothesis that these sounds were a recent innovation in human language. Blasi et al. confirmed this hypothesis using paleoanthropology, speech sciences, historical linguistics, and methods from evolutionary biology in their research and provided evidence that labiodental sounds (such as "f" and "v") were introduced after the Neolithic period [36]. It has also been confirmed that the current front teeth overlap is a relatively new phenomenon caused by recent centuries' dietary modifications. It can therefore be concluded that the soft diet has made a significant contribution to changing the human bite from edge-to-edge configuration to what we now consider to be the norm, including incisal guidance, which some consider mandatory and necessary [37].

Additional evidence of lack of influence of both the bite type and the diet on the TMJ anatomy emerged from a study carried out on 120 human dry skulls divided into four groups: Forest Period Illinois population (900 to 1500 CE); Archaic Period Kentucky population (500 BC to AD 500), African Americans (20th century), and Caucasian Americans (20th century). Both the height and angle of the articular tubercle did not differ significantly between all studied populations. Thus, results do not support the hypothesis of microevolutionary changes in the temporomandibular joint caused by changes in the types of food or the way of food preparation over 2500 years [37].

In describing the complicated relationship between the teeth and the temporomandibular joint, one cannot omit the most controversial aspect, which is the impact of occlusion on TMD. Many recent studies report that occlusion is not a significant factor in disorders of masticatory muscles and the TMJ, as it has been repeated many times over the years. Authors in their current research more often highlight the need to evaluate the patients holistically and focus on various factors beyond the head and neck area [38–40]. On the other hand, multiple studies present the correlation between occlusion and the prevalence of TMD. A broad view of the etiology and diagnostics of TMD ensures the further development of more effective and modern treatment methods, which underlines a persistent need to reevaluate our knowledge all over in light of more current research [41–45]. Celebic et al. report that different indicators of condylar and incisal guidance affect the activity of anterior and posterior temporal muscles [30]. Tinastepe et al. found that patients with increased vertical overlapping occlusions and minimal horizontal overlap had more clinical symptoms associated with TMD than patients with physiological mandibular morphology [46]. In a study by Williamson et al., it was reported that masseter and temporalis muscle activity could only be reduced when anterior guidance causes disclusion in the molar region [47]. In the same study, authors stated that muscle activity is not eliminated by the specific relationships of the anterior teeth but by the elimination of contacts on the molars, which is also true for the therapy with the use of anterior jigs [48,49]. Obtaining an immediate disclusion in the posterior region with a protrusive movement may also protect the structure of the posterior teeth by the elimination of the balancing contacts; thus, incisal guidance is still considered to be an important factor in prosthetic rehabilitation and reconstruction. However, it still is a controversial subject whether the existence of balancing contacts can be a cause of TMD. Interestingly, a study by Kahn et al. proves that the balancing occlusal contacts were present much more often in patients without TMD, whereas the patients presenting the symptoms associated with TMD would mostly show an uninterrupted canine guidance [50]. A possible explanation of such an outcome could be the fact that people with TMD tend to clench more, whereas healthy, asymptomatic people grind more often, so they are more likely to show signs of interferences and group contacts during eccentric movements [51]. Moreover, it was proven in a 30 years long cohort study including 1037 patients that abnormal occlusal features such as posterior crossbite and high and low overbite in adolescence are not associated with a higher incidence of TMD later in life [52].

Additionally, according to the results of previous longitudinal studies, high overbite (≥ 4 mm) at the age of 15 was negatively associated with TMJ abnormalities at the age of 45 [53]. It is also worth answering the question of whether deep bite really protects the TMJ. It turns out that a high overbite is a feature common among people with hypodivergent facial patterns, who generally have larger temporomandibular joint condyles than hyperdivergent individuals [54]. There is a hypothesis that large condyles, due to the larger force distribution area, are less susceptible to mechanical stress than small ones, thus protecting against subsequent disc disturbances [55]. This hypothesis seems to be consistent with the results of a systematic review by Manfredini et al., indicating that facial hyperdivergence is a risk factor for degenerative disorders and temporomandibular disc dysfunction [56]. The following points toward the conclusion that the relationship of the incisors in terms of TMD might be significantly less important than the initial cause of their disrupted relationship, which is the vertical growth pattern. This pathology is also associated with a less favorable composition of the muscle fibers. The fibrous composition of the masseter muscle was studied based on a biopsy performed during the surgical correction of malocclusion. It turned out that the occupancy of type I fibers and areas of hybrid I/II fibers increased in open bites, and vice versa; the occupancy of type II fibers increased in deep bites [57]. This means that the masseter muscles of people presenting with an open bite are not predisposed to long and firm contractions characteristic of clenching activity. Further confirmation that skeletal abnormalities, rather than anterior tooth relationships, may contribute to TMD emerged in a study by Cifter et al. in 2022 [58]. It was found that clockwise jaw rotation, a frequent consequence of disrupted vertical facial growth, causes increased compression within the TMJ. Focusing on the occlusion, it could be once again considered that an impaired anterior teeth relationship is the cause of the muscular disorders, while it appears to be only secondary to skeletal disorders caused by abnormal facial growth.

5. Conclusions

1. The SCGA, during the protrusive movement recorded by the axiograph, is correlated with the features of the articular fossa, such as the height and inclination angle of the articular tubercle, suggesting that the TMJ anatomy dictates its function.

2. The SCGA, during the protrusive movement, is not correlated with the relations between the incisors, pointing towards the conclusion that the TMJ function does not depend on the incisal features (IGA, interincisal angle, overbite, and overjet).
3. Incisal relationships of permanent teeth such as overbite, overjet, IGA, and interincisal angle do not correlate with TMJ anatomy; therefore, they do not affect TMJ formation in young adults in regard to analyzed study group.
4. The AB line is the most reliable reference for measuring the SCGA on CBCT.
5. While processed foods contributed significantly to the change in the bite, neither a soft diet nor a change in the bite modified the structure of the temporomandibular joint, either now or in antiquity.

Author Contributions: Ł.L.: conceptualization, methodology, validation, investigation, resources, data curation, and writing—original draft; Z.N.: conceptualization, methodology, investigation, data curation, and writing—original draft; J.-D.O.: methodology, writing—review and editing, supervision; A.Ż. methodology, and supervision. All authors have read and agreed to the published version of the manuscript.

Funding: This research received no external funding.

Institutional Review Board Statement: The study was conducted in accordance with the Declaration of Helsinki, and approved by the Independent Bioethics Committee for Scientific Research at Medical University of Gdańsk (number NKBBN/1043/2021-2022).

Informed Consent Statement: Informed consent was obtained from all subjects involved in this study.

Data Availability Statement: Not applicable.

Conflicts of Interest: The authors declare no conflict of interest.

Abbreviations

Abbreviation	Meaning
TMJ	Temporomandibular joint
TMD	Temporomandibular disorders
IGA	Incisal guidance angle
CBCT	Cone beam computed tomography
SCGA	Sagittal condylar guidance angle
SCG	Sagittal condylar guidance
IG	Incisal guidance
MIP	Maximum intercuspation position
FHP	Frankfort horizontal plane
ASS	Antero-superior space
SS	Superior space

References

1. Kubein-Meesenburg, D.; Fanghänel, J.; Ihlow, D.; Lotzmann, U.; Hahn, W.; Thieme, K.M.; Proff, P.; Gedrange, T.; Nägerl, H. Functional state of the mandible and rolling–gliding characteristics in the TMJ. *Ann. Anat. Anat. Anz.* **2007**, *189*, 393–396. [CrossRef] [PubMed]
2. Gilboa, I.; Cardash, H.S.; Kaffe, I.; Gross, M.D. Condylar guidance: Correlation between articular morphology and panoramic radiographic images in dry human skulls. *J. Prosthet. Dent.* **2008**, *99*, 477–482. [CrossRef]
3. Shreshta, P.; Jain, V.; Bhalla, A.; Pruthi, G. A comparative study to measure the condylar guidance by the radiographic and clinical methods. *J. Adv. Prosthodont.* **2012**, *4*, 153–157. [CrossRef] [PubMed]
4. Tannamala, P.K.; Pulagam, M.; Pottem, S.R.; Swapna, B. Condylar Guidance: Correlation between Protrusive Interocclusal Record and Panoramic Radiographic Image: A Pilot Study. *J. Prosthodont.* **2012**, *21*, 181–184. [CrossRef] [PubMed]
5. Muddugangadhar, B.C.; Mawani, D.; Das, A.; Mukhopadhyay, A. Comparative evaluation of condylar inclination in dentulous subjects as determined by two radiographic methods: Orthopantomograph and cone-beam computed tomography—An in vivo study. *J. Indian Prosthodont. Soc.* **2019**, *19*, 113–119. [CrossRef]
6. Seth, V.; Kamath, P.; Vaidya, N. Cone beam computed tomography: Third eye in diagnosis and treatment planning. *Int. J. Orthod.* **2012**, *23*, 17–22.

7. Utz, K.-H.; Muller, F.; Luckerath, W.; Fuss, E.; Koeck, B. Accuracy of check-bite registration and centric condylar position. *J. Oral Rehabil.* **2002**, *29*, 458–466. [CrossRef]
8. Shah, N.; Hegde, C.; Prasad, K.D. A clinico-radiographic analysis of sagittal condylar guidance determined by protrusive interocclusal registration and panoramic radiographic images in humans. *Contemp. Clin. Dent.* **2012**, *3*, 383–387. [CrossRef]
9. Price, R.B.; Kolling, J.N.; Clayton, J.A. Effects of changes in articulator settings on generated occlusal tracings. Part I: Condylar inclination and progressive side shift settings. *J. Prosthet. Dent.* **1991**, *65*, 237–243. [CrossRef]
10. Lundeen, H.C.; Shryock, E.F.; Gibbs, C.H. An evaluation of mandibular border movements: Their character and significance. *J. Prosthet. Dent.* **1978**, *40*, 442–452. [CrossRef]
11. Brose, M.O.; Tanquist, R.A. The influence of anterior coupling on mandibular movement. *J. Prosthet. Dent.* **1987**, *57*, 345–353. [CrossRef] [PubMed]
12. Zoghby, A.E.; Ré, J.-P.; Perez, C. Functional harmony between the sagittal condylar path inclination and the anterior guidance inclination. *Int. J. Stomatol. Occlusion Med.* **2009**, *2*, 131–136. [CrossRef]
13. Broderson, S.P. Anterior guidance—The key to successful occlusal treatment. *J. Prosthet. Dent.* **1978**, *39*, 396–400. [CrossRef] [PubMed]
14. Pelletier, L.B.; Campbell, S.D. Evaluation of the relationship between anterior and posterior functionally disclusive angles. Part I: Literature review, instrumentation, and reproducibility. *J. Prosthet. Dent.* **1990**, *63*, 395–403. [CrossRef]
15. Pelletier, L.B.; Campbell, S.D. Evaluation of the relationship between anterior and posterior functionally disclusive angles. Part II: Study of a population. *J. Prosthet. Dent.* **1990**, *63*, 536–540. [CrossRef]
16. E Dawson, P. Determining the determinants of occlusion. *Int. J. Periodontics Restor. Dent.* **1983**, *3*, 8–21.
17. Kepron, D. Experiences with Modern Occlusal Concepts. *Dent. Clin. North Am.* **1971**, *15*, 595–610. [CrossRef]
18. Thompson, J.R. Abnormal function of the temporomandibular joints and related musculature. Orthodontic implications. Part II. *Angle Orthod.* **1986**, *56*, 181–195.
19. Han, S.; Shin, S.M.; Choi, Y.-S.; Kim, S.Y.; Ko, C.-C.; Kim, Y.-I. Morphometric analysis for evaluating the relation between incisal guidance angle, occlusal plane angle, and functional temporomandibular joint shape variation. *Acta Odontol. Scand.* **2018**, *76*, 287–293. [CrossRef]
20. Luca, L.; Manfredini, D.; Arveda, N.; Rossi, L.; Siciliani, G. A cone-beam computerized tomography assessment of the relationship between upper incisors inclination and articular eminence features in orthodontically untreated patients with different facial type. *J. World Fed. Orthod.* **2016**, *5*, 56–63. [CrossRef]
21. Li, Y.; Zhou, W.; Wu, Y.; Dai, H.; Zhou, J. The relation between incisal guidance angle and the growth and development of tem-poromandibular joint: A multi-cross-sectional retrospective study. *BMC Oral Health* **2021**, *21*, 380. [CrossRef]
22. Laplanche, O.; Orthlieb, J.D.; Laurent, M.; Vyslozil, O.; Dutour, O. Evolution of the incisal relationship in a Central European population (1870/1970). *Int. J. Stomatol. Occlusion Med.* **2010**, *3*, 2–9. [CrossRef]
23. Kaifu, Y.; Kasai, K.; Townsend, G.C.; Richards, L.C. Tooth wear and the design of the human dentition: A perspective from evolutionary medicine. *Am. J. Phys. Anthr.* **2003**, *122*, 47–61. [CrossRef] [PubMed]
24. Brace, C.L. Egg on the Face, f in the Mouth, and the Overbite. *Am. Anthropol.* **1986**, *88*, 695–697. [CrossRef]
25. Sülün, T.; Cemgil, T.; Duc, J.-M.P.; Rammelsberg, P.; Jäger, L.; Gernet, W. Morphology of the mandibular fossa and inclination of the articular eminence in patients with internal derangement and in symptom-free volunteers. *Oral Surg. Oral Med. Oral Pathol. Oral Radiol. Endodontol.* **2001**, *92*, 98–107. [CrossRef]
26. Lei, J.; Liu, M.-Q.; Yap, A.U.J.; Fu, K.-Y. Condylar subchondral formation of cortical bone in adolescents and young adults. *Br. J. Oral Maxillofac. Surg.* **2013**, *51*, 63–68. [CrossRef]
27. Osiewicz, M.A.; Lobbezoo, F.; Loster, B.W.; Wilkosz, M.; Naeije, M.; Ohrbach, R. Research Diagnostic Criteria for Temporomandibular Disorders (RDC/TMD)—The Polish version of a dual-axis system for the diagnosis of TMD. RDC/TMD Form. *J. Stomatol.* **2013**, *66*, 576–649. [CrossRef]
28. Chae, J.-M.; Park, J.H.; Tai, K.; Mizutani, K.; Uzuka, S.; Miyashita, W.; Seo, H.Y. Evaluation of condyle-fossa relationships in adolescents with various skeletal patterns using cone-beam computed tomography. *Angle Orthod.* **2020**, *90*, 224–232. [CrossRef]
29. Celebic, A.; Alajbeg, Z.I.; Kraljevic-Simunkovic, S.; Valentic-Peruzovic, M. Influence of different condylar and incisal guidance ratios to the activity of anterior and posterior temporal muscle. *Arch. Oral Biol.* **2007**, *52*, 142–148. [CrossRef]
30. Bapelle, M.; Dubromez, J.; Savoldelli, C.; Tillier, Y.; Ehrmann, E. Modjaw® device: Analysis of mandibular kinematics recorded for a group of asymptomatic subjects. *Cranio®* **2021**, 1–7. [CrossRef]
31. Mongini, F. Remodelling of the mandibular condyle in the adult and its relationship to the condition of the dental arches. *Cells Tissues Organs* **1972**, *82*, 437–453. [CrossRef] [PubMed]
32. Mongini, F. Dental abrasion as a factor in remodeling of the mandibular condyle. *Cells Tissues Organs* **1975**, *92*, 292–300. [CrossRef]
33. Katsavrias, E.G.; Halazonetis, D. Condyle and fossa shape in Class II and Class III skeletal patterns: A morphometric tomographic study. *Am. J. Orthod. Dentofac. Orthop.* **2005**, *128*, 337–346. [CrossRef] [PubMed]
34. Tanne, K.; Tanaka, E.; Sakuda, M. Stress distributions in the TMJ during clenching in patients with vertical discrepancies of the craniofacial complex. *J. Orofac. Pain* **1995**, *9*, 153–160. [PubMed]
35. Nickel, J.C.; McLachlan, K.R.; Smith, D.M. Eminence Development of the Postnatal Human Temporomandibular Joint. *J. Dent. Res.* **1988**, *67*, 896–902. [CrossRef] [PubMed]
36. Blasi, D.E.; Moran, S.; Moisik, S.R.; Widmer, P.; Dediu, D.; Bickel, B. Human sound systems are shaped by post-Neolithic changes in bite configuration. *Science* **2019**, *363*, 6432. [CrossRef]

37. Kranjčić, J.; Hunt, D.; Peršić Kiršić, S.; Kovačić, I.; Vukšić, J.; Vojvodić, D. Articular Eminence Morphology of American Historic and Contemporary Populations. *Acta Stomatol. Croat.* **2021**, *55*, 397–405. [CrossRef] [PubMed]
38. Hirsch, C.; John, M.T.; Drangsholt, M.T.; A Mancl, L. Relationship between overbite/overjet and clicking or crepitus of the temporomandibular joint. *J. Orofac. Pain* **2005**, *19*, 218–225.
39. Manfredini, D.; Lombardo, L.; Siciliani, G. Temporomandibular disorders and dental occlusion. A systematic review of association studies: End of an era? *J. Oral Rehabil.* **2017**, *44*, 908–923. [CrossRef] [PubMed]
40. Lassmann, Ł.; Pollis, M.; Żółtowska, A.; Manfredini, D. Gut Bless Your Pain—Roles of the Gut Microbiota, Sleep, and Melatonin in Chronic Orofacial Pain and Depression. *Biomedicines* **2022**, *10*, 1528. [CrossRef] [PubMed]
41. Nowak, Z.; Chęciński, M.; Nitecka-Buchta, A.; Bulanda, S.; Ilczuk-Rypuła, D.; Postek-Stefańska, L.; Baron, S. Intramuscular Injections and Dry Needling within Masticatory Muscles in Management of Myofascial Pain. Systematic Review of Clinical Trials. *Int. J. Environ. Res. Public Health* **2021**, *18*, 9552. [CrossRef] [PubMed]
42. Chęciński, M.; Chęcińska, K.; Turosz, N.; Kamińska, M.; Nowak, Z.; Sikora, M.; Chlubek, D. Autologous Stem Cells Transplants in the Treatment of Temporomandibular Joints Disorders: A Systematic Review and Meta-Analysis of Clinical Trials. *Cells* **2022**, *11*, 2709. [CrossRef]
43. Turosz, N.; Chęcińska, K.; Chęciński, M.; Kamińska, M.; Nowak, Z.; Sikora, M.; Chlubek, D. A Scoping Review of the Use of Pioglitazone in the Treatment of Temporo-Mandibular Joint Arthritis. *Int. J. Environ. Res. Public Health* **2022**, *19*, 16518. [CrossRef] [PubMed]
44. Minervini, G.D.; Del Mondo, D.D.; Russo, D.D.; Cervino, G.D.; D'Amico, C.D.; Fiorillo, L.D. Stem Cells in Temporomandibular Joint Engineering: State of Art and Future Perspectives. *J. Craniofacial Surg.* **2022**, *33*, 2181–2187. [CrossRef] [PubMed]
45. Ferrillo, M.; Nucci, L.; Giudice, A.; Calafiore, D.; Marotta, N.; Minervini, G.; D'Apuzzo, F.; Ammendolia, A.; Perillo, L.; de Sire, A. Efficacy of conservative approaches on pain relief in patients with temporomandibular joint disorders: A systematic review with network meta-analysis. *Cranio®* **2022**, 1–17. [CrossRef] [PubMed]
46. Tinastepe, N.; Oral, K. Investigation of the Relationship between Increased Vertical Overlap with Minimum Horizontal Overlap and the Signs of Temporomandibular Disorders. *J. Prosthodont.* **2015**, *24*, 463–468. [CrossRef]
47. Williamson, E.; Lundquist, D. Anterior guidance: Its effect on electromyographic activity of the temporal and masseter muscles. *J. Prosthet. Dent.* **1983**, *49*, 816–823. [CrossRef]
48. Lukic, N.; Saxer, T.; Hou, M.; Wojczyńska, A.Z.; Gallo, L.M.; Colombo, V. Short-term effects of NTI-tss and Michigan splint on nocturnal jaw muscle activity: A pilot study. *Clin. Exp. Dent. Res.* **2021**, *7*, 323–330. [CrossRef]
49. MacDonald, J.W.C.; Hannam, A.G. Relationship between occlusal contacts and jaw-closing muscle activity during tooth clenching: Part I. *J. Prosthet. Dent.* **1984**, *52*, 718–729. [CrossRef]
50. Kahn, J.; Tallents, R.H.; Katzberg, R.W.; Ross, M.E.; Murphy, W.C. Prevalence of dental occlusal variables and intraarticular temporomandibular disorders: Molar relationship, lateral guidance, and nonworking side contacts. *J. Prosthet. Dent.* **1999**, *82*, 410–415. [CrossRef]
51. Rompré, P.; Daigle-Landry, D.; Guitard, F.; Montplaisir, J.; Lavigne, G. Identification of a Sleep Bruxism Subgroup with a Higher Risk of Pain. *J. Dent. Res.* **2007**, *86*, 837–842. [CrossRef] [PubMed]
52. Olliver, S.; Broadbent, J.; Thomson, W.; Farella, M. Occlusal Features and TMJ Clicking: A 30-Year Evaluation from a Cohort Study. *J. Dent. Res.* **2020**, *99*, 1245–1251. [CrossRef]
53. Mohlin, B.O.; Derweduwen, K.; Pilley, R.; Kingdon, A.; Shaw, W.C.; Kenealy, P. Malocclusion and temporomandibular disorder: A comparison of adolescents with moderate to severe dysfunction with those without signs and symptoms of temporoman-dibular disorder and their further development to 30 years of age. *Angle Orthod.* **2004**, *74*, 319–327. [PubMed]
54. Ma, Q.; Bimal, P.; Mei, L.; Olliver, S.; Farella, M.; Li, H. Temporomandibular condylar morphology in diverse maxillary-mandibular skeletal patterns: A 3-dimensional cone-beam computed tomography study. *J. Am. Dent. Assoc.* **2018**, *149*, 589–598. [CrossRef]
55. Nickel, J.; Iwasaki, L.; Gonzalez, Y.; Gallo, L.; Yao, H. Mechanobehavior and Ontogenesis of the Temporomandibular Joint. *J. Dent. Res.* **2018**, *97*, 1185–1192. [CrossRef] [PubMed]
56. Manfredini, D.; Segù, M.; Arveda, N.; Lombardo, L.; Siciliani, G.; Rossi, A.; Guarda-Nardini, L. Temporomandibular Joint Disorders in Patients With Different Facial Morphology. A Systematic Review of the Literature. *J. Oral Maxillofac. Surg.* **2015**, *74*, 29–46. [CrossRef] [PubMed]
57. Rowlerson, A.; Raoul, G.; Daniel, Y.; Close, J.; Maurage, C.-A.; Ferri, J.; Sciote, J.J. Fiber-type differences in masseter muscle associated with different facial morphologies. *Am. J. Orthod. Dentofac. Orthop.* **2005**, *127*, 37–46. [CrossRef] [PubMed]
58. Cifter, E.D. Effects of Occlusal Plane Inclination on the Temporomandibular Joint Stress Distribution: A Three-Dimensional Finite Element Analysis. *Int. J. Clin. Pract.* **2022**, *2022*, 2171049. [CrossRef] [PubMed]

Disclaimer/Publisher's Note: The statements, opinions and data contained in all publications are solely those of the individual author(s) and contributor(s) and not of MDPI and/or the editor(s). MDPI and/or the editor(s) disclaim responsibility for any injury to people or property resulting from any ideas, methods, instructions or products referred to in the content.

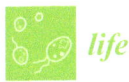

Systematic Review

Comparative Evaluation of Condylar Guidance Angles Measured Using Arcon and Non-Arcon Articulators and Panoramic Radiographs—A Systematic Review and Meta-Analysis

Amjad Obaid Aljohani [1], Mohammed Ghazi Sghaireen [1,*], Muhammad Abbas [1], Bader Kureyem Alzarea [1], Kumar Chandan Srivastava [2,*], Deepti Shrivastava [3,4], Rakhi Issrani [3], Merin Mathew [1], Ahmed Hamoud L Alsharari [5], Mohammed Ali D. Alsharari [5], Naif Abdulrahman Aljunaydi [5], Saif Alanazi [5], Mosheri Muslem S. Alsharari [5] and Mohammad Khursheed Alam [6,7,8]

1. Department of Prosthodontics, College of Dentistry, Jouf University, Sakaka 72345, Saudi Arabia; dr.amjad.johani@jodent.org (A.O.A.); mayali@ju.edu.sa (M.A.); bkzarea@jodent.org (B.K.A.); dr.merin.mathew@jodent.org (M.M.)
2. Division of Oral Medicine & Maxillofacial Radiology, Department of Oral & Maxillofacial Surgery & Diagnostic Sciences, College of Dentistry, Jouf University, Sakaka 72345, Saudi Arabia
3. Preventive Dentistry Department, Division of Periodontics, College of Dentistry, Jouf University, Sakaka 72345, Saudi Arabia; sdeepti20@gmail.com (D.S.); dr.rakhi.issrani@jodent.org (R.I.)
4. Department of Periodontics, Saveetha Dental College and Hospitals, Saveetha Institute of Medical and Technical Sciences, Saveetha University, Chennai 602105, India
5. Dental Intern, College of Dentistry, Jouf University, Sakaka 72345, Saudi Arabia; ahsharari@gmail.com (A.H.L.A.); mohmmad.123678@gmail.com (M.A.D.A.); dr.naifaljunaydi@gmail.com (N.A.A.); saif.alanazi1122@gmail.com (S.A.); mosheri1417@gmail.com (M.M.S.A.)
6. Orthodontic Division, Preventive Dentistry Department, College of Dentistry, Jouf University, Sakaka 72345, Saudi Arabia; mkalam@ju.edu.sa or dralam@gmail.com
7. Department of Dental Research Cell, Saveetha Institute of Medical and Technical Sciences, Saveetha Dental College and Hospitals, Chennai 602105, India
8. Department of Public Health, Faculty of Allied Health Sciences, Daffodil international University, Dhaka 1216, Bangladesh

* Correspondence: dr.mohammed.sghaireen@jodent.org (M.G.S.); drkcs.omr@gmail.com or kchandan@ju.edu.sa (K.C.S.)

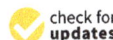

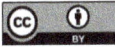

Abstract: The condylar guidance value (CGV) measurement constitutes an important part of a holistic prosthodontic treatment plan, with horizontal CGVs (HCGVs) and lateral CGVs (LCGVs) being two of the most prominently recognized. This systematic review aimed at evaluating the efficacy of two different types of CGV measurement protocols—articulators (both arcon and non-arcon) and panoramic radiographs. Additionally, it attempts to determine which of the mentioned methods performs better across several parameters. Several important web databases were searched using search terms derived from medical subject headings (MeSH), using keywords linked to "Arcon articulator", "Condylar guidance angle", "non-arcon articulator", "Panoramic x-ray" and "Radiographic examination", which constituted the first step in the study selection strategy. After completion, the search strategy which initially turned up to 831 papers, eventually ended up with 13 studies. The review and subsequent meta-analysis revealed that panoramic radiographs had noticeably greater efficacy in terms of the CGVs as compared to the articulators in the majority of the studies. Within the articulators, the arcon types recorded slightly higher CGVs than the non-arcon variety owing to the precision of jaw movement simulation in the former. However, further studies are required to validate these findings and establish more precise guidelines for the use of CGV measurement protocols in prosthodontic practice.

Keywords: temporomandibular joint; arcon articulator; condylar guidance angle; non-arcon articulator; panoramic radiographs; radiographic examination

1. Introduction

One of the most common methods for measuring condylar guidance values (CGVs) is through panoramic radiographs [1–3]. Panoramic radiographs are two-dimensional images of the entire jaw and provide a panoramic view of the maxilla and mandible [4]. They allow for the measurement of the angle between the occlusal plane and the condylar path inclination [5]. The average CGVs range from 30 to 60 degrees, with higher values indicating a steeper condylar path. The CGVs are useful in determining the treatment plan for prosthodontic patients including the use of orthognathic surgery to correct severe jaw discrepancies.

An articulator is a mechanical device that simulates the movement of the jaws and teeth, allowing the prosthodontist to accurately diagnose and plan prosthodontic treatment [6,7]. There are different types of articulators: simple-hinge or plane-line articulators, fixed condylar path (mean-value) articulators, and adjustable articulators. The adjustable articulators can be classified into semi-adjustable and fully adjustable groups. The fully adjustable articulators can be adjusted to simulate a wide range of movements of the jaw, including lateral and protrusive movements. The semi-adjustable articulators are designed to reproduce a fixed relationship between the maxilla and the mandible, and it can be classified into two types: arcon and non-arcon [8].

Arcon articulators have a condylar ball and socket mechanism that mimics the natural movement of the jaw. They are named after the German manufacturer who first developed this type of articulator. In an arcon articulator, the lower member, which represents the patient's mandible, has two metal balls attached to it that fit into the corresponding sockets on the upper member, which represents the maxilla [8]. The arcon articulator allows easy adjustment of the occlusal plane, inclination of the occlusal plane, and lateral and protrusive movements of the mandible. Accuracy and reliability are the main advantages of arcon articulators. They closely mimic the natural movement of the jaw and provide a stable platform for prosthodontic diagnosis and treatment planning [9]. They are also highly durable and long-lasting.

Non-arcon articulators do have a condylar ball and socket mechanism but the condyle is located in the upper member of the articulator. Instead, they use a hinge mechanism to simulate the movement of the jaw. They are less expensive than arcon articulators and are often used in dental schools and clinics that cannot afford expensive arcon articulators [7]. The main disadvantage of non-arcon articulators is their limited accuracy. They do not mimic the natural movement of the jaw as closely as arcon articulators and may not provide as stable a platform for prosthodontic diagnosis and treatment planning. However, they are still useful tools for many prosthodontic procedures, particularly in clinics and dental schools with limited resources [7].

Arcon and non-arcon articulators are important tools in prosthodontics that allow accurate diagnosis and treatment planning. The choice of articulator depends on the needs and resources of the individual prosthodontist or clinic [8].

Condylar guidance values (CGVs) are an essential parameter in the diagnosis and treatment planning of prosthodontic patients. They refer to the angle formed between the horizontal plane and the condylar path inclination during protrusive movement over the posterior slope of the articular eminence. This angle helps in determining the movement of the mandible during various functions such as chewing and speaking. These values can be measured using various methods, including clinical examination, radiographs, and digital imaging techniques.

Panoramic radiographs are commonly used to measure CGVs and help in determining the movement of the mandible during various functions such as chewing and speaking [10]. There are two different CGVs that are used in prosthodontics, including the horizontal condylar guidance value (HCGV), the lateral condylar guidance value (LCGV), protrusive guidance, and immediate lateral translation. The Bennett angle is the angle formed between the sagittal plane and condylar path inclination on the non-working side during lateral movement. It represents the lateral movement of the mandible during chewing and speaking. The average Bennett angle is around 15 degrees, with higher values indicating a more lateral mandibular movement [11]. The Immediate Lateral Translation (ILT) is the amount of lateral movement of the mandible during the initial opening of the mouth. This movement is important in the diagnosis and treatment planning of patients with temporomandibular joint (TMJ) disorders and during the fabrication of prosthesis. The average ILT is around 1.5 to 2.5 mm. The average protrusive guidance angle is around 30 degrees.

Measuring these angles can be conducted through various methods, including clinical and laboratory examination, radiographs, and digital imaging techniques [11]. However, the cone beam-computed tomography is becoming popular, with wider applications such as the identification of osteoporosis [12] and the tracing of inferior alveolar nerve canal [13]; nonetheless, panoramic radiographs still remain the most common method for measuring CGVs [14,15]. The CGVs also play a significant role in the design and construction of occlusal splints, which are used to treat patients with TMJ disorders [16,17]. So, this systematic review and meta-analysis aimed to determine the accuracy of arcon and non-arcon articulators in measuring condylar guidance angles compared to panoramic radiographs. It also attempts to compare the differences in condylar guidance angle measurements between arcon and non-arcon articulators and panoramic radiographs. The secondary objectives include the identification of the factors affecting the accuracy of condylar guidance angle measurements using arcon and non-arcon articulators and panoramic radiographs. Additionally, this review attempts to assess the reliability and reproducibility of condylar guidance angle measurements using arcon and non-arcon articulators and panoramic radiographs.

2. Materials and Methods

2.1. Protocol and Research Framework

The current systematic review was registered on the International Prospective Register of Systematic Reviews (PROSPERO; registration number: CRD42023404427. The PICO (Population, Intervention, Comparison, Outcome) strategy for this study can be summarized as follows: The population of interest included patients or individuals who required evaluation of condylar guidance angles. The intervention under investigation was the measurement of condylar guidance angles using arcon articulators. The comparison involved the measurement of condylar guidance angles using non-arcon articulators. Additionally, the outcome of interest was the comparison of condylar guidance angles obtained from panoramic radiographs in relation to arcon and non-arcon articulators. The research question addressed in this study was whether there is any difference in the measurement of condylar guidance angles when using arcon and non-arcon articulators, as well as panoramic radiographs.

The study followed a well defined framework to ensure a rigorous and comprehensive analysis. Initially, an extensive search was conducted across multiple electronic databases and relevant sources were manually searched to identify eligible studies. During the study selection phase, pre-defined inclusion and exclusion criteria were applied to select studies that directly compared the measurement of condylar guidance angles using both arcon and non-arcon articulators, incorporating panoramic radiographs. Data extraction involved collecting relevant information such as study characteristics, participant demographics, and condylar guidance angle values obtained through different techniques. The quality assessment phase involved evaluating the methodological rigor and risk of bias in the included studies. A meta-analysis was then performed to synthesize the condylar guidance angle measurements from the selected studies, utilizing appropriate statistical methods to calculate pooled effect estimates and associated confidence intervals. Heterogeneity among the studies was assessed, and subgroup and sensitivity analyses were conducted to explore potential sources of heterogeneity.

2.2. Database Search Protocol

Following databases were searched using MeSH keywords for the extraction of relevant papers for this review:

- PubMed: ((systematic review[Title/Abstract] OR meta-analysis[Title/Abstract]) AND ("condylar guidance"[MeSH Terms] OR "condylar guidance"[Title/Abstract]) AND ("arcon articulator"[MeSH Terms] OR "arcon articulator"[Title/Abstract]) AND ("non-arcon articulator"[MeSH Terms] OR "non-arcon articulator"[Title/Abstract]) AND ("panoramic radiography"[MeSH Terms] OR "panoramic radiography"[Title/Abstract]));
- Google Scholar: "systematic review" OR "meta-analysis" AND "condylar guidance" AND ("arcon articulator" OR "non-arcon articulator") AND "panoramic radiography";
- Web of Science: TS = ("systematic review" OR "meta-analysis") AND TS = ("condylar guidance" AND ("arcon articulator" OR "non-arcon articulator")) AND TS = ("panoramic radiography");
- Scopus: TITLE-ABS-KEY ("systematic review" OR "meta-analysis") AND TITLE-ABS-KEY("condylar guidance" AND ("arcon articulator" OR "non-arcon articulator")) AND TITLE-ABS-KEY("panoramic radiography");
- EMBASE: ("condylar guidance angles" OR "condylar inclination" OR "condylar path" OR "mandibular movement") AND ("arcon articulator" OR "arcon condylar guidance" OR "arcon condylar inclination" OR "arcon condylar path") AND ("non-arcon articulator" OR "non-arcon condylar guidance" OR "non-arcon condylar inclination" OR "non-arcon condylar path") AND ("panoramic radiograph" OR "orthopantomogram" OR "OPG");
- LILACS: ("condylar guidance angles" OR "condylar inclination" OR "condylar path" OR "mandibular movement") AND ("arcon articulator" OR "Arcon Condylar Guidance" OR "arcon condylar inclination" OR "arcon condylar path") AND ("non-arcon articulator" OR "non-arcon condylar guidance" OR "non-arcon condylar inclination" OR "non-arcon condylar path") AND ("panoramic radiograph" OR "Orthopantomogram" OR "OPG");
- DOSS: ("condylar guidance angles" OR "condylar inclination" OR "condylar path" OR "mandibular movement") AND ("arcon articulator" OR "arcon condylar guidance" OR "arcon condylar inclination" OR "arcon condylar path") AND ("non-arcon articulator" OR "non-arcon condylar guidance" OR "non-arcon condylar inclination" OR "non-arcon condylar path") AND ("panoramic radiograph" OR "orthopantomogram" OR "OPG");
- Cochrane: ("condylar guidance angles" OR "condylar inclination" OR "condylar path" OR "mandibular movement") AND ("arcon articulator" OR "Arcon Condylar Guidance" OR "Arcon condylar inclination" OR "arcon condylar path") AND ("non-arcon articulator" OR "non-arcon condylar guidance" OR "non-arcon condylar inclination" OR "non-arcon condylar path") AND ("panoramic radiograph" OR "Orthopantomogram" OR "OPG").

2.3. Inclusion Criteria

- Studies that evaluated the efficacy of two different types of CGV measurement protocols—articulators (both arcon and non-arcon) and panoramic radiographs;
- Studies that compared the efficacy of the two CGV measurement protocols across several parameters;
- Studies that were in accordance with the search terms derived from MeSH-linked keywords such as "arcon articulator", "condylar guidance angle", "non-arcon articulator", "panoramic radiographs" and "radiographic examination";
- Studies that provided information on the CGVs measured using both the articulators and panoramic radiographs;
- Studies published from 2011 to date.

2.4. Exclusion Criteria

- Studies that did not evaluate the efficacy of the two different types of CGV measurement protocols;
- Studies that did not compare the efficacy of the two CGV measurement protocols across several parameters;

- Studies that did not provide information on the CGVs measured using both the articulators and panoramic radiographs;
- Studies that did not reveal key information related to measurement of the type of CGV that was being assessed;
- Articles published before 2011;
- Studies that were case reports, seminar articles or thesis articles.

2.5. Reviewer Assessment and Bias Evaluation

Two independent reviewers who had expertise in prosthodontics and experience in conducting systematic reviews and meta-analyses were identified and recruited. Later, they independently evaluated the selected study to determine if it was relevant to the research question and meets the eligibility criteria. The PRISMA tool (Figure 1) was selected for the purpose of analyzing different types of studies and their relevance to this investigation, i.e., whether they were in accordance with the inclusion and exclusion criterion [18]. The reviewers evaluated the study's objectives, methodology, and results. They also assessed its validity and reliability. They were also asked to document their evaluations independently and provide a summary of the reasons for their inclusion or exclusion of a certain study. Subsequently, they compared the evaluations and any discrepancies that arose were discussed and ironed out through discussion and consensus with another reviewer. They extracted the relevant data from the included studies, including the number of participants, type of measurement protocol, type of articulator used, type of panoramic radiograph used, CGV measurements, and any other relevant information. As for the bias assessment, the quality of studies being selected was evaluated using the RoB-2 tool (Figure 2). This tool assesses the risk of bias in studies by evaluating five different domains, the results of which were categorically separated into 'low', 'moderate', and 'high' risk of bias, respectively [19]. A meta-analysis of the assessed data was performed after the completion of the search strategy to evaluate the efficacy of the two different types of CGV measurement protocols, the results of which were interpreted, and conclusions were drawn.

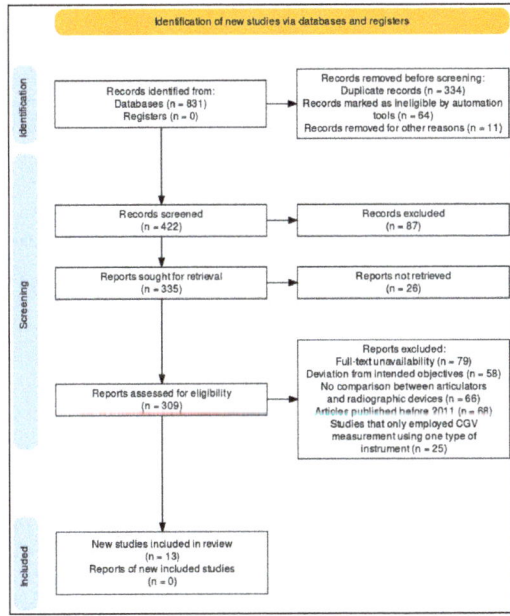

Figure 1. Study selection framework using the PRISMA protocol for this review.

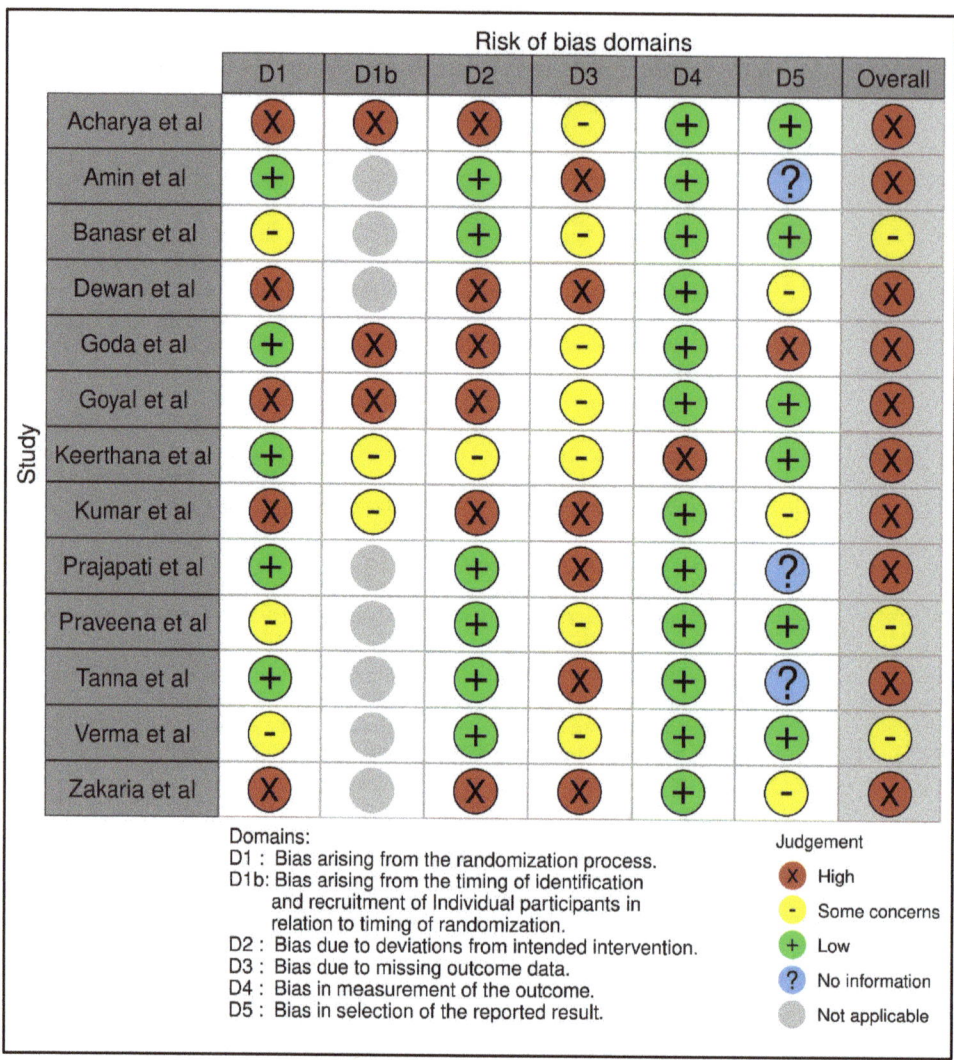

Figure 2. Bias assessment of individual studies using RoB-2 tool across five different domains [20–32].

2.6. Protocol for Meta-Analysis

Using the RevMan 5 software (Version 5.3, The Cochrane Collaboration), a meta-analysis was conducted. The objective was to determine the pooled effect size for the effectiveness of the two different types of articulators in comparison to the panoramic radiograph for measuring CGVs. Data on the type of measurement protocol and CGV type assessed were extracted from each included study, along with information on the mean age, parity, number of participants, type of measurement protocol, type of articulator used, and any other pertinent data (CIs). The risk ratio (RR) and risk differential (RD) were given with their own forest plot. In addition to the overall pooled estimate and its 95% CI, each forest plot also contained the summary estimate and its 95% CI for each research.

3. Results

In order to provide an updated review and assessment of CGVs, a keyword search was first conducted on various databases from the years 2011 to 2022. Following the implementation of the MeSH search strategy, initially a total of 831 papers were surfaced. Based on duplication and ineligibility by automation tools, the studies were filtered, resulting in a total of 422 papers. To make sure that only original papers were included, further screening of articles was conducted, which resulted in a total of 309 papers.

The titles and summaries of these 309 papers were scrutinized, and 296 additional papers that did not meet the inclusion/exclusion standards were ignored. Finally, we selected thirteen articles, which mainly contained in vivo and in vitro experiments, that met the required standards. These made up the final group of articles that were taken into account for the meta-analysis.

Five of the thirteen investigations [20–24] evaluated the measurement of sagittal CGV; the HCGV in was covered in seven [25–31]. (Table 1). The variety of studies that were reviewed leads one to believe that this significant issue may require a multi-disciplinary strategy to be addressed. OPG was used to produce panoramic radiographs in all of the studies that were considered for the evaluation. Individuals ranging in age from 18 to 75 were included in the research. Only three studies [22,29,31] considered CGV values acquired using a non-arcon articulator, while all studies [20–32] used an arcon articulator for CGV analysis. In the majority of studies [21,24,25,30–32], radiographs evaluated significantly higher values compared to the articulator, with panoramic X-rays evaluating higher CGVs compared to their mechanical measurement counterparts. Although in one study [31], males scored higher total mean values than females using both articulators for both HCGV and LCGV, with the arcon articulator obtaining higher overall mean values than the non-arcon articulator, gender correlation was not frequently sought.

Figures 3–5 show, respectively, the forest plots from the 13 studies that were considered for the study. The data were entered into the RevMan 5 software after taking into account all relevant aspects of the papers, and three separate forest plots displaying the odds ratio, risk ratio, and risk difference related to the measurement of the CGV, using either the articulator or the panoramic X-ray that was noted in that study, were generated and evaluated. A random effects model with a 95% confidence interval was used in the meta-analysis. The overall number of events was the sample size for each paper.

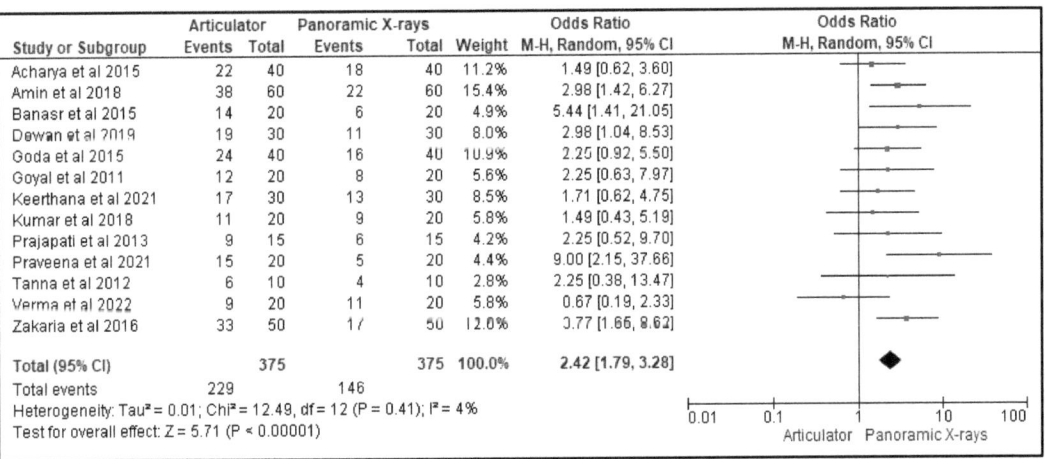

Figure 3. Forest plot representing the odds ratio of the efficacy of an articulator as compared to a panoramic X-ray for measuring CGVs in the 13 studies that were evaluated in this review [20–32].

Table 1. Description of the variables evaluated in the 13 studies selected for review and subsequent meta-analysis.

Paper ID	Year	Region of Investigation	Study Design	Age Range (in Years)	Number of Participants	Type of Articulator Used	Type of CGV Assessed	Clinical Inference
Banasr et al. [20]	2015	Saudi Arabia	In-vitro	21–35	20	Arcon	Sagittal CGV	Similar values obtained from the articulator and radiographic images (little to no difference)
Dewan et al. [21]	2019	Saudi Arabia	In-vivo	20–40	30	Arcon	Sagittal CGV	Radiographs measured noticeably higher values as compared to the articulator
Goyal et al. [22]	2011	India	In-vivo	19–35	20	Arcon and Non-arcon	Sagittal CGV	Similar values obtained from the two types of articulators (little to no difference)
Kumar et al. [23]	2018	India	In-vitro	20–35	20	Arcon	Sagittal CGV	Similar values obtained from the articulator and radiographic images (little to no difference)
Tanna et al. [24]	2012	India	Prospective	-	10	Arcon	Sagittal CGV	Radiographs measured noticeably higher values as compared to the articulator
Acharya et al. [25]	2015	India	In-vivo	18–30, 40–75	40 (20 edentulous, 20 dentulous)	Arcon	HCGV	Radiographs measured noticeably higher values as compared to the articulator
Amin et al. [26]	2018	India	In-vivo	40–60	60	Arcon	HCGV	In dentulous subjects, statistically significant values were found using the articulator and radiographic method.
Goda et al. [27]	2015	India	In-vitro	20–30, 40–65	40 (20 edentulous, 20 dentulous)	Arcon	HCGV	Radiographs measured similar values as the articulator but only in edentulous individuals
Keerthana et al. [28]	2021	India	In-vivo	20–40	30	Arcon	HCGV	Similar values obtained from the articulator and radiographic images (little to no difference)
Prajapati et al. [29]	2013	India	In-vitro	20–30	15	Arcon and Non-arcon	zHCGV	Statistically insignificant values between the arcon-type, Non-arcon type and radiographic images were obtained across all parameters
Verma et al. [30]	2022	India	In-vivo	40–75	20	Arcon	HCGV	Radiographs measured higher values as compared to the articulator
Zakaria et al. [31]	2016	Iraq	In-vivo	30–65	50	Arcon and Non-arcon	HCGV and LCGV	Males scored higher total mean values than females using both articulators for both HCGV and LCGV, with the arcon articulator scoring higher overall mean values than the non-arcon articulator.
Praveena et al. [32]	2021	India	In-vitro	40–60	20	Arcon	LCGV	Radiographs measured noticeably higher values as compared to the articulator

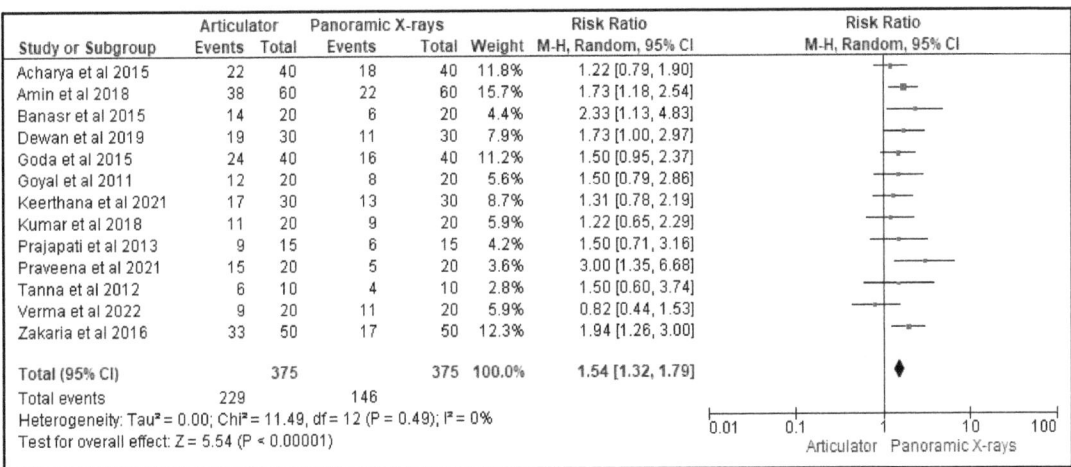

Figure 4. Forest plot representing the risk ratio of the efficacy of an articulator compared to a panoramic X-ray for measuring CGVs in the 13 studies that were evaluated in this review [20–32].

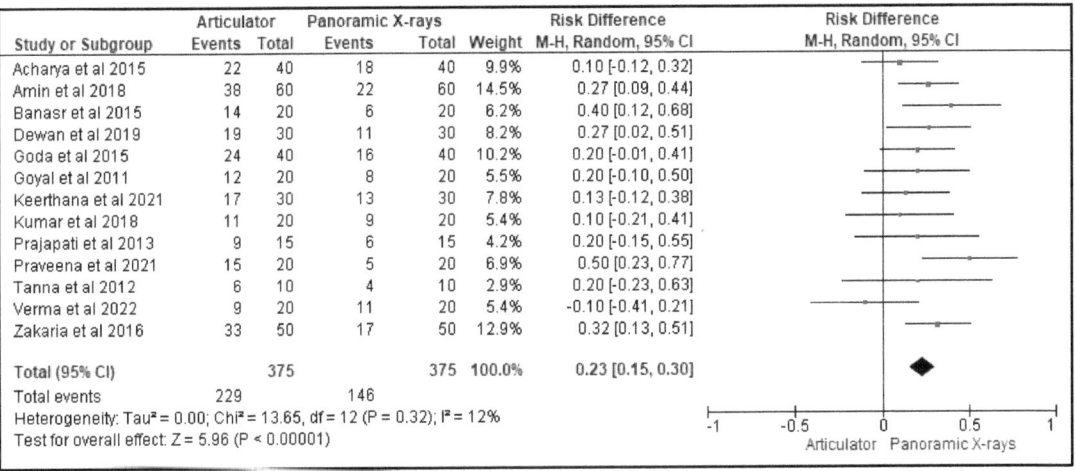

Figure 5. Forest plot representing the risk difference of the efficacy of an articulator compared to a panoramic X-ray for measuring CGVs in the 13 studies that were evaluated in this review [20–32].

Figure 3 is a forest plot that presents the odds ratio of the effectiveness of using an articulator versus a panoramic X-ray for measuring condylar guidance values (CGVs) in 13 studies. The random-effects model was used, and the confidence interval was set at 95%. The individual study results are represented as squares, with their size corresponding to the weight of the study, and the horizontal line across each square indicates the 95% confidence interval. The diamond at the bottom represents the summary effect estimate, with its width showing the confidence interval. The overall odds ratio was in favor of the panoramic X-ray, indicating that it was more effective in measuring CGVs compared to the articulators that were utilized in the studies.

Figure 4 is a forest plot that represents the risk ratio of the effectiveness of using an articulator versus a panoramic X-ray for measuring CGVs in the 13 studies evaluated in this review. The random-effects model was used, and the confidence interval was set at

95%. The individual study results are represented as squares, with their size corresponding to the weight of the study, and the horizontal line across each square indicates the 95% confidence interval. The diamond at the bottom represents the summary effect estimate, with its width showing the confidence interval. The overall odds ratio was also in favor of the panoramic X-ray, indicating that it was more effective in measuring CGVs compared to the articulators that were utilized in the studies.

Figure 5 is a forest plot that represents the risk difference of the effectiveness of using an articulator versus a panoramic X-ray for measuring CGVs in the 13 studies evaluated in this review. The random-effects model was used, and the confidence interval was set at 95%. The individual study results are represented as squares, with their size corresponding to the weight of the study, and the horizontal line across each square indicates the 95% confidence interval. The diamond at the bottom represents the summary effect estimate, with its width showing the confidence interval. The overall odds ratio was, again, in favor of the panoramic X-ray, indicating that it was more effective in measuring CGVs compared to the articulators that were utilized in the studies.

4. Discussion

Prosthodontics is a branch of dentistry which is concerned with the detection, prevention, and treatment of dental and facial abnormalities. Prosthodontic treatment involves fixed prosthesis, removable prosthesis, and maxillofacial prosthesis to improve the esthetics and rehabilitation of the oral cavity [33]. A holistic approach of prosthodontic treatment takes into account various factors including the CGVs. This measurement is an essential part of the prosthodontic treatment plan as it helps determine the ideal position of the mandible in relation to the maxilla during jaw movements. Cases with improper assessment of CGVs eventually lead to prothesis, which brings discomfort to oral functions, including the TMJ. Improper measurement of angle can also worsen the existing TMJ disorders affecting children, adults, and special patients [34,35]. It will eventually affect their quality of life [36]. In the current systematic review, the majority of the studies found that the panoramic radiographs had a noticeably greater efficacy in terms of the CGVs in contrast to the articulators. Within the articulators, the arcon recorded slightly higher CGVs than the non-arcon owing to the precision of jaw movement simulation. These findings provide important guidance for the prosthodontist to select the appropriate CGV measurement protocol. Therefore, the primary significance of the present systematic review lies in its contribution to the field of prosthodontics by evaluating the efficacy of two different CGV measurement protocols and providing important guidance for clinical practice. The findings have important implications in terms of improving the quality of care for patients; at the same time, they highlight the need for further research in this area.

The research methodologies that were observed in this systematic review were unique in a variety of ways. The condylar elements of the articulator are set in the clinical method so that they will replicate the inclinations close to the patient's temporomandibular articulation using protrusive jaw relation. In the included experiments, the condylar guidance in semi-adjustable articulators was set using interocclusal protrusive wax records, Lucia jig, and gothic arch tracers. In studies using protrusive wax records, the amount of protrusion was maintained as constant for all patients at 6 mm, and the same protrusive records were used for programming the articulator. Hence, it is important to maintain protrusion distance as a constant as the HCGV changes with amount of protrusion [26,37]. The majority of studies used a Hanua Wide Vue semi-adjustable articulator after the protrusive jaw relation was determined, while a few studies used a whip mix semi-adjustable articulator to measure horizontal condylar inclination. To determine the horizontal condylar inclination, a reference line is used. The whip mix uses the nasion–porion as a reference plane; whereas Hanua articulators mount the cast in relation to the Frankfort horizontal plane, producing more precise angles [38,39]. Due to the substantial differences in the instruments, a slightly modified method for detecting SCGVs is inconsistent, lacks precision, and has lower levels of reproducibility [40,41]. The reasons for the compressed or deformed records include tipped casts due to incorrect cast adaptation, force exerted by the operator on the record, and records whose values have changed depending on the amount of protrusion, overjet, and overbite [1,41,42]. Additionally, because set inter-condylar distance and straight condylar pathway, the semi-adjustable articulators are unable to properly reconstruct the condylar movements [41].

One of the studies showed that intraoral recording methods produced lower values for condylar angles compared with the radiographic measurements. The man's dynamic mandibular locomotor system appears to be incompatible with the fixed mechanical principles governing the movements of an adjustable articulator [25,43]. Hence, the diagnosis is now frequently made using CBCT, lateral cephalograms and panoramic radiographs. In the current review, significantly higher CGVs were found in panoramic radiographs than in protrusive interocclusal records. The findings of the review can be justified by the following rationales. In research by Gilboa et al. [44], it was shown that the panoramic radiographic method frequently produces a value that is higher than the actual value. In dry skulls, they found that the average sagittal CGV was seven degrees higher than its true anatomic contour. The resilient oral mucosa is depressed, and the inter-ridge distance is shortened when the occlusal rims are kept in a protruded mandibular position. It results in a narrower triangular wedge-shaped space between the posterior part of the occlusal rims. This space is similar to the Christensen's space found in natural dentition and documented by protrusive interocclusal records [26,45,46].

Despite the fact that all of the included studies used the same reference line, there were differences in the results of the included patients. The observed variations can be due to patients' head positioning, which causes parallax errors, the models of the panoramic machine, magnification variations, image distortions, overlapping of the anatomic structures such as mandibular notch, the coronoid process, and the zygomatic arch around TMJ [7,24,27,47–49].

Due to the fact that CBCT provides three-dimensional information for both sides without superimpositions, the glenoid fossa and other landmarks can be readily identified. The mean sagittal CGVs obtained from CBCT are marginally higher than those acquired from other techniques on both sides for dentate and edentulous individuals. Similar outcomes were found in the individual studies that were excluded from the review. For instance, in the study by Kumar et al. [50], condylar guidance values obtained from CBCT measurements were 5°–6° higher than those from protrusive occlusal records, while values obtained from clinical methods were attested in three studies mentioned in the literature [40,41,51]. The major benefit of CBCT over intraoral, panoramic, and cephalometric is the production of distinctive images that show 3D features. Cursor-driven measurement techniques give clinicians the ability to evaluate dimensions interactively and instantly. Additionally, the on-screen measurements are free from amplification and distortion.

Other benefits of CBCT include better image quality, smaller fields, faster scans, compatibility with different radiographic setups for image output, and simplicity of setup for minimal units in a general clinical setting. In edentulous and dentulous patients, these CBCT preferences may be used to identify the condylar position during dynamic registration and accurately locate the condyle [10,51]. The primary reason we did not include studies that used this measurement procedure was the high cost of the equipment, which is the main disadvantage of using CBCT.

Carossa et al. [52] provide another method; they use a jaw movement analyzer in conjunction with a robotic device to correctly record and duplicate mandibular movements. The system employs optoelectronic motion technology with markers attached to the jaw, allowing for quick and exact movement recording. Unlike earlier robotic systems, this one featured fewer mechanical components, which reduced tolerances and production costs. The results showed that the system accurately records and reproduces maxillomandibular relations in both static and dynamic settings. The authors stated that this robotic system represents a major advancement over existing analog and digital alternatives, providing cost savings, precision, and time-saving opportunities, and making it attractive for both clinical and research applications.

The study has a few limitations that need to be addressed. Firstly, the number of studies included in the review was relatively small, which may limit the generalizability of the findings. Secondly, the quality of the studies varied, and some of them had a high risk of bias, which may affect the validity of the results. Thirdly, the search strategy used in the study may have missed some relevant studies that could have contributed to the analysis. Finally, the study only evaluated the efficacy of two CGV measurement protocols and did not consider other potential measurement methods that may be available. Moreover, all the selected studies were from the South Asian region. Therefore, the results should be interpreted with caution, and further research is needed to confirm the findings and explore additional measurement protocols.

5. Conclusions

To conclude, this systematic review and meta-analysis evaluated the efficacy of two different types of CGV measurement protocols—articulators (both arcon and non-arcon) and panoramic radiographs. Moreover, it attempted to determine which performed better across several parameters. Based on the data from majority of the includes studies, the review found that panoramic radiographs had noticeably greater efficacy in terms of the CGVs. Within the articulators themselves, the arcon types recorded slightly higher CGVs than the non-arcon variety owing to the precision of jaw movement simulation in the former. This information can be useful for prosthodontic practitioners to make an informed decision about the type of CGV measurement protocol they choose to use for their patients. However, further studies are required to validate these findings and establish more precise guidelines for the use of CGV measurement protocols in prosthodontic practice.

Author Contributions: Conceptualization, M.G.S. and K.C.S.; methodology, A.O.A., M.G.S., M.A. and B.K.A.; data search, D.S., R.I., M.M., A.H.L.A., M.A.D.A., N.A.A., S.A. and M.M.S.A.; formal analysis, K.C.S. and M.K.A.; resources, M.G.S., A.H.L.A., M.A.D.A., N.A.A. and S.A.; writing—original draft preparation, M.G.S., D.S., K.C.S. and M.K.A.; writing—review and editing, A.O.A., M.A., B.K.A., K.C.S., D.S., R.I., M.M., A.H.L.A., M.A.D.A., N.A.A., S.A., M.M.S.A. and M.K.A.; supervision, M.G.S.; project administration, K.C.S.; funding acquisition, K.C.S., A.H.L.A., M.A.D.A., N.A.A., S.A. and M.M.S.A. All authors have read and agreed to the published version of the manuscript.

Funding: This research received no external funding.

Institutional Review Board Statement: Not applicable.

Informed Consent Statement: Not applicable.

Data Availability Statement: All data are available within the manuscript.

Conflicts of Interest: The authors declare no conflict of interest.

References

1. Borse, S.; Chaware, S. Tooth shade analysis and selection in prosthodontics: A systematic review and meta-analysis. *J. Indian Prosthodont. Soc.* **2020**, *20*, 131. [CrossRef] [PubMed]
2. Sghaireen, M.G.; AlZarea, B.K.; Kundi, I.; Farhat, C.; Alam, M.K.; Alruwaili, H.H.T.; Al-Omiri, M.K. Application of Hanau equation to a Saudi population. *Int. Med. J.* **2020**, *27*, 95–97.
3. Lal, A.; Alam, M.K.; Ahmed, N.; Maqsood, A.; Al-Qaisi, R.K.; Shrivastava, D.; Alkhalaf, Z.A.; Alanazi, A.M.; Alshubrmi, H.R.; Sghaireen, M.G.; et al. Nano Drug Delivery Platforms for Dental Application: Infection Control and TMJ Management—A Review. *Polymers* **2021**, *13*, 4175. [CrossRef] [PubMed]
4. Srivastava, D.; Shrivastava, D.; Austin, D. Journey towards the 3D Dental Imaging—The Milestones in the Advancement of Dental imaging. *Int. J. Adv. Res.* **2016**, *4*, 377–382. [CrossRef]
5. Mishra, A.; Palaskar, J. Effect of direct and indirect face-bow transfer on the horizontal condylar guidance values: A pilot study. *J. Dent. Allied Sci.* **2014**, *3*, 8. [CrossRef]
6. Pelletier, L.B.; Campbell, S.D. Comparison of condylar control settings using three methods: A bench study. *J. Prosthet. Dent.* **1991**, *66*, 193–200. [CrossRef]

7. Galagali, G.; Kalekhan, S.; Nidawani, P.; Naik, J.; Behera, S. Comparative analysis of sagittal condylar guidance by protrusive interocclusal records with panoramic and lateral cephalogram radiographs in dentulous population: A clinico-radiographic study. *J. Indian Prosthodont. Soc.* **2016**, *16*, 148. [CrossRef]
8. Singh, K.; Singh, A.; Jayam, C.; Singh, R.; Huda, I.; Nabi, A.T. Assessment of Sagittal Condylar Guidance with Protrusive Inter-occlusal Method, Panoramic Radiographs, and Lateral Cephalogram: A Comparative Study. *J. Contemp. Dent. Pract.* **2021**, *22*, 47–50. [CrossRef]
9. Gosavi, S.S.; Ghanchi, M.; Patil, S.; Sghaireen, M.G.; Ali, A.H.; Aber, A.M. Original Research The Study of the Effect of Altering the Vertical Dimension of Occlusion on the Magnitude of Biting Force. *J. Int. Oral Health* **2015**, *11*, 110.
10. Loster, J.; Groch, M.; Wieczorek, A.; Muzalewska, M.; Skarka, W. An evaluation of the relationship between the range of mandibular opening and the condyle positions in functional panoramic radiographs. *Dent. Med. Probl.* **2017**, *54*, 347–351. [CrossRef]
11. Amarnath, G.S.; Kumar, U.; Hilal, M.; Muddugangadhar, B.C.; Anshuraj, K.; Shruthi, C.S. Comparison of Cone Beam Computed Tomography, Orthopantomography with Direct Ridge Mapping for Pre-Surgical Planning to Place Implants in Cadaveric Mandibles: An Ex-Vivo Study. *J. Int. Oral Health* **2015**, *7* (Suppl. 1), 38–42. [PubMed]
12. Sghaireen, M.G.; Ganji, K.K.; Alam, M.K.; Srivastava, K.C.; Shrivastava, D.; Ab Rahman, S.; Patil, S.R.; Al Habib, S. Comparing the Diagnostic Accuracy of CBCT Grayscale Values with DXA Values for the Detection of Osteoporosis. *Appl. Sci.* **2020**, *10*, 4584. [CrossRef]
13. Srivastava, K.C. A CBCT aided assessment for the location of mental foramen and the emergence pattern of mental nerve in different dentition status of the Saudi Arabian population. *Braz. Dent. Sci.* **2020**, *24*, 10-P. [CrossRef]
14. Das, A.; Muddugangadhar, B.C.; Mawani, D.P.; Mukhopadhyay, A. Comparative evaluation of sagittal condylar guidance obtained from a clinical method and with cone beam computed tomography in dentate individuals. *J. Prosthet. Dent.* **2021**, *125*, 753–757. [CrossRef] [PubMed]
15. Shreshta, P.; Jain, V.; Bhalla, A.; Pruthi, G. A comparative study to measure the condylar guidance by the radiographic and clinical methods. *J. Adv. Prosthodont.* **2012**, *4*, 153. [CrossRef] [PubMed]
16. Srivastava, K.C.; Shrivastava, D.; Khan, Z.A.; Nagarajappa, A.K.; Mousa, M.A.; Hamza, M.O.; Al-Johani, K.; Alam, M.K. Evaluation of temporomandibular disorders among dental students of Saudi Arabia using Diagnostic Criteria for Temporomandibular Disorders (DC/TMD): A cross-sectional study. *BMC Oral Health* **2021**, *21*, 211. [CrossRef]
17. Pontual, M.D.A.; Freire, J.; Barbosa, J.; Frazão, M.; Pontual, A.D.A.; da Silveira, M.F. Evaluation of bone changes in the temporomandibular joint using cone beam CT. *Dentomaxillofac. Radiol.* **2012**, *41*, 24–29. [CrossRef]
18. Page, M.J.; McKenzie, J.E.; Bossuyt, P.M.; Boutron, I.; Hoffmann, T.C.; Mulrow, C.D.; Shamseer, L.; Tetzlaff, J.M.; Akl, E.A.; Brennan, S.E.; et al. The PRISMA 2020 statement: An updated guideline for reporting systematic reviews. *BMJ* **2021**, *372*, n71. [CrossRef]
19. Haddaway, N.R.; Page, M.J.; Pritchard, C.C.; McGuinness, L.A. *PRISMA2020*: An R package and Shiny app for producing PRISMA 2020-compliant flow diagrams, with interactivity for optimised digital transparency and Open Synthesis. *Campbell Syst. Rev.* **2022**, *18*, e1230. [CrossRef]
20. Banasr, F.H.; Shinawi, L.A.; Soliman, I.S.A. A Comparative Evaluation to Measure the Sagittal Condylar Guidance Values between the Semiadjustable Articulators and Radiographic Images. *Smile Dent. J.* **2015**, *10*, 12–18. [CrossRef]
21. Dewan, H.; Akkam, T.I.; Chohan, H.; Sherwani, A.; Masha, F.; Dhae, M. Comparison of Sagittal Condylar Guidance Determined by Panoramic Radiographs to the One Determined by Conventional Methods Using Lateral Interocclusal Records in the Saudi Arabian Population. *J. Int. Soc. Prev. Community Dent.* **2019**, *9*, 597. [PubMed]
22. Goyal, M.; Goyal, S. A comparative study to evaluate the discrepancy in condylar guidance values between two commercially available arcon and non-arcon articulators: A clinical study. *Indian J. Dent. Res.* **2011**, *22*, 880. [CrossRef] [PubMed]
23. Kumar, N.; Sirana, P.; Malhotra, A.; Singhal, N.; Chaudhary, N. Comparative Analysis of Sagittal Condylar Guidance Recorded by Intraoral Gothic Arch Tracing and Panoramic Radiograph in Completely Edentulous Patients. *J. Contemp. Dent. Pract.* **2018**, *19*, 1301–1305. [CrossRef]
24. Tannamala, P.K.; Pulagam, M.; Pottem, S.R.; Swapna, B. Condylar Guidance: Correlation between Protrusive Interocclusal Record and Panoramic Radiographic Image: A Pilot Study. *J. Prosthodont.* **2012**, *21*, 181–184. [CrossRef]
25. Acharya, S.; Pandey, A.; Sethi, S.; Meena, M. A Comparative Study of Condylar Guidance Setting Obtained From Interocclusal Records and Panoramic Radiographs in Both Dentulous and Edentulous Subjects. *Dent. J. Adv. Stud.* **2015**, *03*, 085–090. [CrossRef]
26. Kumar, G.S.; Shetty, A.; Amin, B.; Raj, B.; Mithra, A. Assessment and Comparison of the Condylar Guidance by Protrusive Interocclusal Records and Panoramic Radiographic Imaging in Edentulous and Dentulous Individuals. *Int. J. Prosthodont. Restor. Dent.* **2018**, *8*, 10–16. [CrossRef]
27. Godavarthi, A.S.; Sajjan, M.C.S.; Raju, A.V.R.; Rajeshkumar, P.; Premalatha, A.; Chava, N. Correlation of Condylar Guidance Determined by Panoramic Radiographs to One Determined by Conventional Methods. *J. Int. Oral Health* **2015**, *7*, 123–128.
28. Keerthana, S.; Mohammed, H.; Hariprasad, A.; Anand, M.; Ayesha, S. Comparative evaluation of condylar guidance obtained by three different interocclusal recording materials in a semi-adjustable articulator and digital panoramic radiographic images in dentate patients: An in vivo study. *J. Indian Prosthodont. Soc.* **2021**, *21*, 397. [CrossRef]

29. Prajapati, P.; Sethuraman, R.; Naveen, Y.; Patel, J. A clinical study of the variation in horizontal condylar guidance obtained by using three anterior points of reference and two different articulator systems. *Contemp. Clin. Dent.* **2013**, *4*, 162. [CrossRef] [PubMed]
30. Verma, S.; Kalra, T.; Kumar, M.; Bansal, A. Comparative Analysis of Condylar Guidance Angle Obtained by Protrusive Interocclusal Records and Radiographic Methods in Edentulous Patients: An In Vivo Study. *Dent. J. Adv. Stud.* **2022**, *10*, 87–94. [CrossRef]
31. Ma'an Rasheed Zakaria, B.D.S. A Comparison between the Horizontal Condylar and Bennett Angles of Iraqi Full Mouth Rehabilitation Patients by Using Two Different Articulator Systems (An In-Vivo Study). *J. Bagh Coll. Dent.* **2016**, *28*, 26–35. [CrossRef]
32. Praveena, K.; Ajay, R.; Devaki, V.; Balu, K.; Preethisuganya, S.; Menaga, V. A comparative evaluation of lateral condylar guidance by clinical and radiographic methods—Hanau's formula revisited. *J. Pharm. Bioallied Sci.* **2021**, *13*, 537. [CrossRef]
33. Ahmad, P.; Alam, M.K.; Aldajani, A.; Alahmari, A.; Alanazi, A.; Stoddart, M.; Sghaireen, M.G. Dental Robotics: A Disruptive Technology. *Sensors* **2021**, *21*, 3308. [CrossRef] [PubMed]
34. Minervini, G.; Franco, R.; Marrapodi, M.M.; Fiorillo, L.; Cervino, G.; Cicciù, M. Prevalence of temporomandibular disorders in children and adolescents evaluated with Diagnostic Criteria for Temporomandibular Disorders: A systematic review with meta-analysis. *J. Oral Rehabil.* **2023**, *50*, 522–530. [CrossRef] [PubMed]
35. Minervini, G.; Franco, R.; Marrapodi, M.M.; Fiorillo, L.; Cervino, G.; Cicciù, M. Prevalence of temporomandibular disorders (TMD) in pregnancy: A systematic review with meta-analysis. *J. Oral Rehabil.* **2023**. [CrossRef]
36. Qamar, Z.; Alghamdi, A.M.S.; Haydarah, N.K.B.; Balateef, A.A.; Alamoudi, A.A.; Abumismar, M.A.; Shivakumar, S.; Cicciù, M.; Minervini, G. Impact of temporomandibular disorders on oral health-related quality of life: A systematic review and meta-analysis. *J. Oral Rehabil.* **2023**. [CrossRef]
37. Posselt, U.; Skytting, B. Registration of the condyle path inclination: Variations using the Gysi technique. *J. Prosthet. Dent.* **1960**, *10*, 243–247. [CrossRef]
38. Prakash, S. A Study to Evaluate the Horizontal Condylar Inclination in Dentulous Patients Using Clinical and Two Radiographic Techniques. Master's Thesis, Raja's Dental College and Hospital, Tirunelveli, India, 2019.
39. Santos, J.D.; Nelson, S.J.; Nummikoski, P. Geometric Analysis of Occlusal Plane Orientation Using Simulated Ear-Rod Facebow Transfer. *J. Prosthodont.* **1996**, *5*, 172–181. [CrossRef]
40. Kwon, O.-K.; Yang, S.-W.; Kim, J.-H. Correlation between sagittal condylar guidance angles obtained using radiographic and protrusive occlusal record methods. *J. Adv. Prosthodont.* **2017**, *9*, 302. [CrossRef]
41. Naqash, T.A.; Chaturvedi, S.; Yaqoob, A.; Saquib, S.; Addas, M.K.; Alfarsi, M. Evaluation of sagittal condylar guidance angles using computerized pantographic tracings, protrusive interocclusal records, and 3D-CBCT imaging techniques for oral rehabilitation. *Niger. J. Clin. Pract.* **2020**, *23*, 550–554.
42. Patel, P.S.; Shah, J.S.; Dudhia, B.B.; Butala, P.B.; Jani, Y.V.; Macwan, R.S. Comparison of panoramic radiograph and cone beam computed tomography findings for impacted mandibular third molar root and inferior alveolar nerve canal relation. *Indian J. Dent. Res.* **2020**, *31*, 91–102. [CrossRef] [PubMed]
43. LChristensen, V.; Slabbert, J.C.G. The concept of the sagittal condylar guidance: Biological fact or fallacy? *J. Oral Rehabil.* **1978**, *5*, 1–7. [CrossRef] [PubMed]
44. Gilboa, I.; Cardash, H.S.; Kaffe, I.; Gross, M.D. Condylar guidance: Correlation between articular morphology and panoramic radiographic images in dry human skulls. *J. Prosthet. Dent.* **2008**, *99*, 477–482. [CrossRef] [PubMed]
45. Alkhalaf, Z.A.; Sghaireen, M.G.; Issrani, R.; Ganji, K.K.; Alruwaili, N.N.; Alsaleh, R.M.; Alruwaili, M.R.S.; Alabdali, M.F.; Alsirhani, M.A.R.; Alam, M.K. The Effect of Accentuation of Curve of Spee on Masticatory Efficiency—A Systematic Review and Meta-Analysis. *Children* **2023**, *10*, 511. [CrossRef]
46. AL-Omiri, M.K.; Sghaireen, M.G.; Alhijawi, M.M.; Alzoubi, I.A.; Lynch, C.D.; Lynch, E. Maximum bite force following unilateral implant-supported prosthetic treatment: Within-subject comparison to opposite dentate side. *J. Oral Rehabil.* **2014**, *41*, 624–629. [CrossRef]
47. Bhandari, A.; Manandhar, A.; Singh, R.K.; Suwal, P.; Parajuli, P.K. A Comparative study to measure the horizontal condylar guidance obtained by protrusive interocclusal records and panoramic radiographic images in completely edentulous patients. *J. Coll. Med. Sci.-Nepal* **2018**, *14*, 21–27. [CrossRef]
48. Kumari, V.V.; Anehosur, G.; Meshramkar, R.; Nadiger, R.; Lekha, K. An in vivo study to compare and correlate sagittal condylar guidance obtained by radiographic and extraoral gothic arch tracing method in edentulous patients. *Eur. J. Prosthodont.* **2016**, *4*, 12. [CrossRef]
49. Shetty, S.; Kunta, M.; Shenoy, K. A clinico-radiographic study to compare and co-relate sagittal condylar guidance determined by intraoral gothic arch tracing method and panoramic radiograph in completely edentulous patients. *J. Indian Prosthodont. Soc.* **2018**, *18*, 19. [CrossRef]
50. Kumar, R.V.; Gowda, M.; Shashidhar, M. Clinicoradiographic comparison of sagittal condylar guidance angle determined by dynamic and radiographic methods. *J. Dent. Def. Sect.* **2022**, *16*, 123. [CrossRef]

51. Jerath, S.; Rani, S.; Kumar, M.; Agarwal, C.D.; Kumar, S.; Rathore, A. Clinico-radiographic comparative evaluation of horizontal condylar guidance angle by interocclusal wax record, cbct and gothic arch tracing method-an in vivo study. *Int. J. Recent Sci. Res.* **2019**, *10*, 33715–33720.
52. Carossa, M.; Cavagnetto, D.; Ceruti, P.; Mussano, F.; Carossa, S. Individual mandibular movement registration and reproduction using an optoeletronic jaw movement analyzer and a dedicated robot: A dental technique. *BMC Oral Health* **2020**, *20*, 271. [CrossRef] [PubMed]

Disclaimer/Publisher's Note: The statements, opinions and data contained in all publications are solely those of the individual author(s) and contributor(s) and not of MDPI and/or the editor(s). MDPI and/or the editor(s) disclaim responsibility for any injury to people or property resulting from any ideas, methods, instructions or products referred to in the content.

Article

Operative Findings of over 5000 Microvascular Decompression Surgeries for Hemifacial Spasm: Our Perspective and Current Updates

Jae Sung Park [1] and Kwan Park [2,3,*]

1 Department of Neurosurgery, Konyang University Hospital, 158, Gwanjeodong-ro, Seo-gu, Daejeon 35365, Republic of Korea; nsjasonpark@hotmail.com
2 Department of Neurosurgery, Konkuk University Medical Center, 120-1, Neungdong-ro, Gwangjin-gu, Seoul 05030, Republic of Korea
3 Department of Neurosurgery, Sungkyunkwan University School of Medicine, Seoul 06351, Republic of Korea
* Correspondence: kwanpark@skku.edu

Abstract: Hemifacial spasm (HFS) is a hyperactive cranial neuropathy, and it has been well established that the cause of primary HFS is compression on the root exit zone (REZ) of the facial–vestibulocochlear nerve complex (CN VII-VIII) by a vessel or vessels. MVD is the only curative treatment option for HFS with a high success rate and low incidence of recurrence and complications. We categorize six classical compressive patterns on the REZ as well as five challenging types. Knowledge of these patterns may help in achieving a better surgical outcome.

Keywords: hemifacial spasm; microvascular decompression; compressive patterns

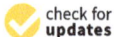

Citation: Park, J.S.; Park, K. Operative Findings of over 5000 Microvascular Decompression Surgeries for Hemifacial Spasm: Our Perspective and Current Updates. Life 2023, 13, 1904. https://doi.org/10.3390/life13091904

Academic Editor: Katalin Prokai-Tatrai

Received: 6 July 2023
Revised: 7 August 2023
Accepted: 11 September 2023
Published: 13 September 2023

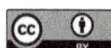

Copyright: © 2023 by the authors. Licensee MDPI, Basel, Switzerland. This article is an open access article distributed under the terms and conditions of the Creative Commons Attribution (CC BY) license (https://creativecommons.org/licenses/by/4.0/).

1. Introduction

Hemifacial spasm (HFS) is a hyperactive cranial neuropathy, and it has been well established that the cause of primary HFS is compression on the root exit zone (REZ) of the facial–vestibulocochlear nerve complex (CN VII-VIII) by a vessel or vessels [1,2]. The modern understanding of its etiology has contributed to the development of microvascular decompression (MVD) which can offer a cure in a non-destructive way [3,4]. Accordingly, MVD has been accepted as the treatment of choice for medically intractable primary HFS [5]. An uncountable number of HFS patients have been benefited by MVD around the globe, but there still remains much to discover. We believe this report stands out in that it is used to describe detailed operative findings of more than 5000 MVD procedures performed by a single surgeon in a single institution. A brief overview and current updates of HFS from our experience and perspective are to be presented.

2. Materials and Methods

From January 2004 to March 2020, 5026 MVDs were performed for HFS by a single surgeon in a single institution. All patients had been diagnosed with medically intractable primary HFS and underwent an MVD via a lateral retrosigmoid suboccipital approach. Preoperative evaluation included computed tomography (CT), magnetic resonance imaging (MRI) along with T2 weighted sequences, and three-dimensional time of flight MR angiography (3D TOF MRA). Neurovascular conflict is better visualized by high resolution T2 weighted images than 3D TOF MRA, especially in cases of venous compression. Pure tone audiometry along with speech audiometry were carried out before and after the MVD.

Under general anesthesia, a lateral retrosigmoid suboccipital craniotomy was performed, followed by incision of the dura, careful dissection of the arachnoid layer, and gentle retraction of the flocculus. Upon exposure of the REZ of CN VII-VIII complex, the compressing vessel, or offending vessel, was identified. A Teflon sponge was inserted between the REZ and the offending vessel, which completed the decompression process. Throughout the surgery, electrophysiological evaluation was used to monitor the facial nerve, i.e., the disappearance of the lateral spread response (LSR), free running electromyography (EMG) and direct nerve stimulation, as well as brainstem auditory evoked potentials (BAEP), in all patients. The compression patterns were described and categorized by the surgeon (K.P.), and, according to the categorization, they were illustrated by the first author (J.P.).

Preoperative and postoperative evaluation for symptoms were described and collected by a single nurse practitioner to minimize response bias. The data processing was carried out using commercially available software (IBM SPSS Statistics, version 24). The Chi-square test and Fisher's exact test were employed when analyzing cross tables between compression patterns and clinical outcomes. Patient consent was not necessary because of the retrospective nature of the study, and the validity of the findings would not be affected by the absence of patient consent. Moreover, no additional risk to patient safety was expected from this study without patient consent. The first author, J.P, owns all copyright privileges regarding all illustrations.

3. Results

Over the past 16 years, operative findings were described and recorded by the surgeon (K.P.). When the REZ was inspected through a microscope, how it was compressed by a vessel or vessels was not uniform. After around 5–7 years in his career as a neurosurgeon specialized in MVD, the surgeon noticed that in the vast majority of cases, there was a contributing factor that made compression somewhat inevitable. A thickened arachnoid membrane was the first thing that inspired him to pursue this categorization process according to the contributing factors, which eventually led to the creation of the "compression patterns". When the thickened arachnoid membrane was found around the compressing vessels, dissection of the arachnoid membrane often led to the disappearance of the LSR, which could indicate that the thickened arachnoid membrane was the cause of the compression. The surgeon hypothesized that the vessel was "forced" to compress the REZ by the thickened arachnoid membrane pushing it to the REZ (Figure 1B). Indeed, the arachnoid type, the most frequently observed one, accounts for 27.9% of all cases [6]. Under the same hypothesis, other forms of compression were described. When short and tight perforating arteries from the offending vessel were tethering the vessel to the REZ, we named it the "perforator" type (Figure 1C). This perforator type was also grouped in the challenging ones because the short and tight perforating arteries limited the working space for decompression, and they must not be injured to avoid any irreversible sequelae such as brain stem infarction or intracranial hemorrhage (Figure 2A). The compressing vessels of overall HFS, in order of frequency, consisted of the anterior inferior cerebellar artery (AICA, 51.7%), the posterior inferior cerebellar artery (PICA, 21.6%), and the vertebral artery (VA) [6]. AICA was involved in the perforating type in 84.5% of instances, which was disproportionately higher than in other type ($p < 0.005$) [6]. The branch type (Figure 1D) referred to a compression where the REZ was caught between branches of the offending artery, while the sandwich type (Figure 1E) illustrated a compression of the REZ by two independent arteries on each side. The two arteries in the sandwich type were either AICA + PICA or AICA + another branch of AICA; the VA was not involved in any sandwich types. In the tandem type, on the contrary, the VA was one of the two arteries in 61.5% of instances [6]. Figure 1F depicts the tandem type where a larger artery, most commonly the vertebral artery, compresses a smaller one that is in contact with the REZ. The tandem type was also categorized as a challenging one (Figure 2B), since Teflon pieces inserted between the REZ and the smaller offending artery might not be sufficient for a complete decompression; the smaller artery must be released from the pressure by the larger one as well. When there was no contributing factor other than the vascular loop itself, they were categorized as the "loop type" (Figure 1A). PICA was responsible for 72.7% of the loop types.

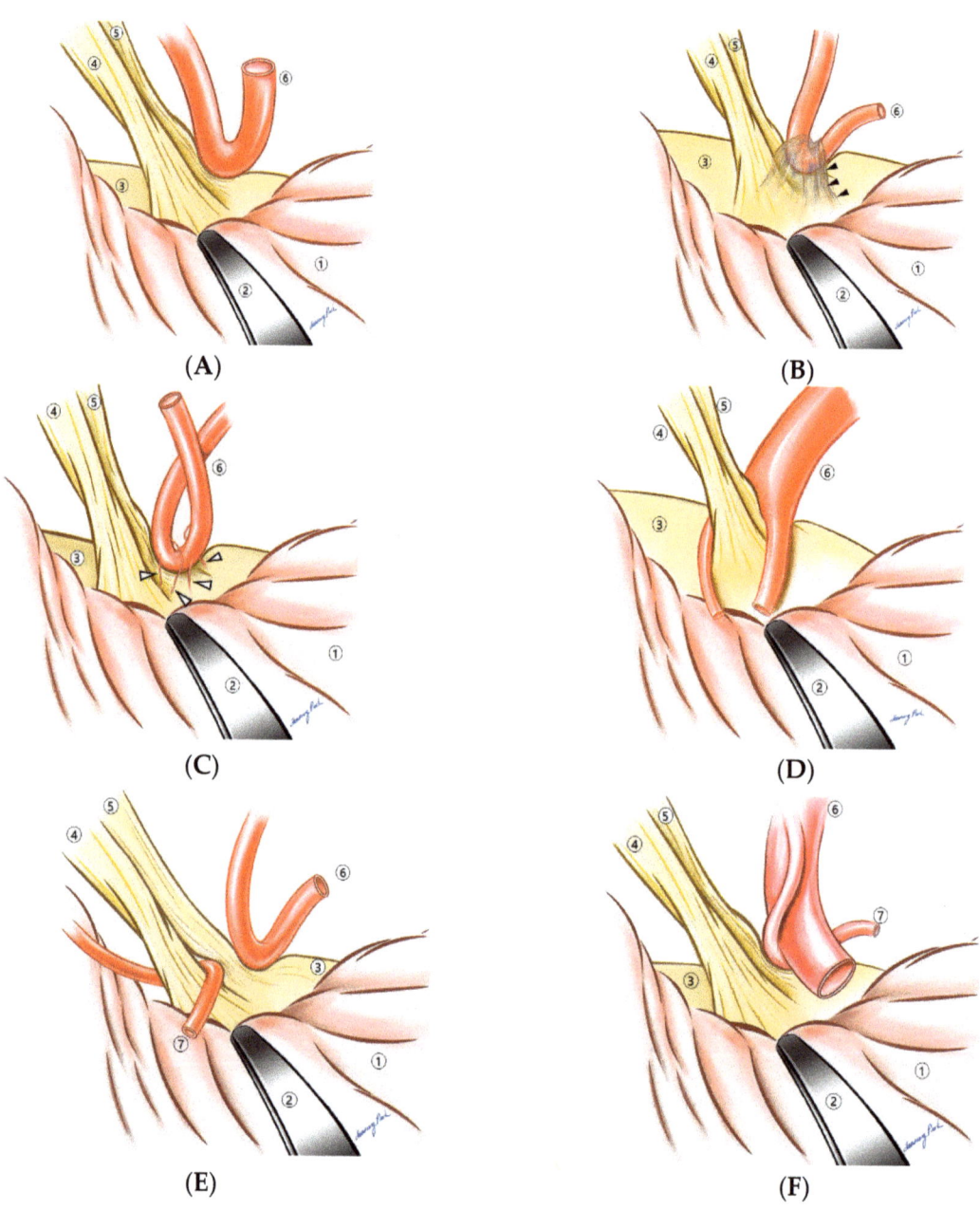

Figure 1. Classic compression patterns. (**A**) Loop type, (**B**) arachnoid type, black arrow heads: thickened arachnoid membrane, (**C**) perforator type, hollow arrow heads: perforating arteries, (**D**) branch type, (**E**) sandwich type, and (**F**) tandem type. ① Cerebellum, ② brain retractor, ③ brain stem, ④ vestibulocochlear nerve, ⑤ facial nerve, ⑥ primary offending vessel, and ⑦ secondary offending vessel.

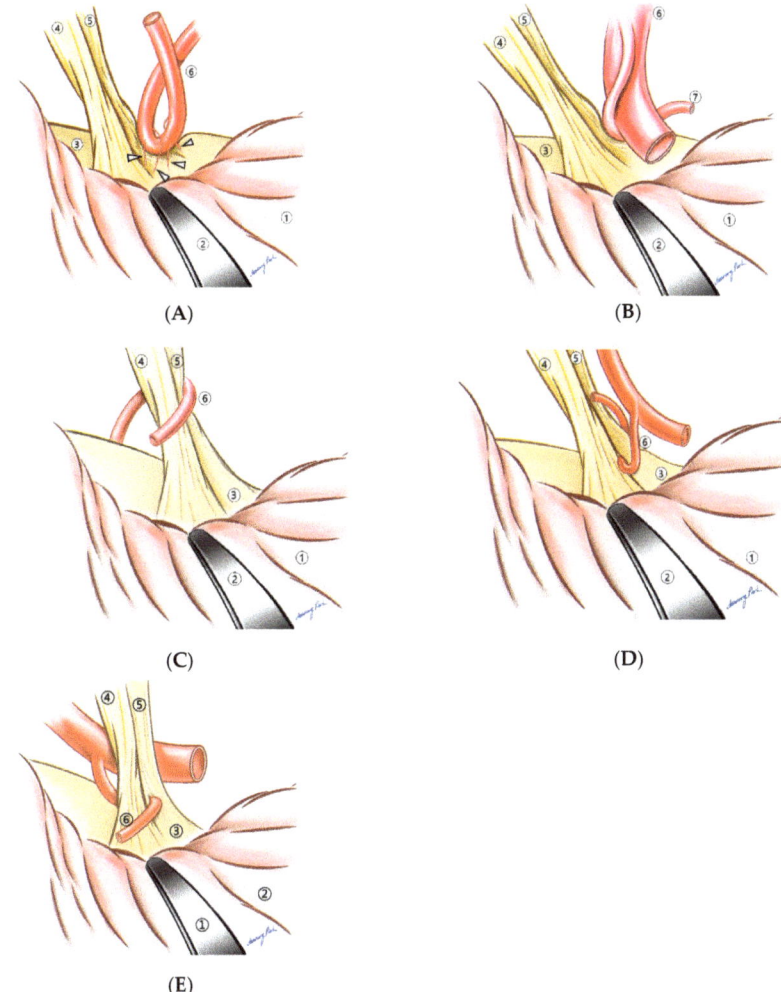

Figure 2. Challenging patterns. (**A**) Perforator type, hollow arrow heads: perforating arteries, (**B**) tandem type, (**C**) cisternal type, (**D**) encircling type, and (**E**) penetrating type. ① Cerebellum, ② brain retractor, ③ brain stem, ④ vestibulocochlear nerve, ⑤ facial nerve, ⑥ primary offending vessel, and ⑦ secondary offending vessel.

As an addendum to the original "compression patterns", we selected five types as "challenging patterns", for they were found to pose an additional challenge during the process of decompression. Besides the two aforementioned types, i.e., the perforator and tandem, three unusual ones were added: cisternal, encircling, and penetrating (Figure 2). The combined number of these five types accounted for 50.4% of instances (1527 of 3028) [7]. Although these five types were named "challenging", the clinical outcome, in terms of improvement of symptoms and postoperative complications, did not differ from that of the overall cases. The success rate of the challenging group was 88.6% whereas that of total cases was 90.1%. Likewise, the complication rate of the former was 0.71 while that of the latter was 0.89% [7]. Re-do surgeries (13 out of 1527), however, yielded a lower spasm-free rate (10 of 13, 76.9%) along with a substantially higher incidence of intraoperative BAEP change (7 of 13, 53.8%), postoperative facial palsy (6, 46.2%), and deafness (1, 7.7%) [7].

4. Discussion

A bibliometric analysis of hemifacial spasm (HFS) in 2022 reported that the second largest number (3.26%) of all HFS-related articles in the world were published from Sungkyunkwan university in South Korea where Prof. Kwan Park initiated the hemifacial clinic and personally performed over 5000 microvascular decompressions (MVD) for HFS [8]. We hereby present a concise overview with current updates of HFS.

4.1. Overview of HFS

HFS is defined as contractions on one side of the face. The clinical term, HFS, refers to involuntary facial contractions that are irregular, unilateral, and tonic or clonic. Those twitches usually start with the periorbital muscles and then they can spread to the perinasal, perioral, zygomaticus, and platysma muscles [9]. The diagnosis of HFS is primarily based on clinical history in accordance with the definition of HFS: involuntary facial contractions that are unilateral, irregular, and tonic or clonic. As an adjunctive maneuver, the "other Babinski sign", also known as the Babinski-2 sign, may be useful. It refers to a synchronized contraction of the frontalis muscle or orbicularis oculi muscle, induced by an attempt to lift up one's eyebrow while the eye is being closed [10]. This maneuver assists in the diagnosis of HFS with a sensitivity of 86% and a specificity of 100% [10]. Electromyography (EMG), computed tomography (CT), or magnetic resonance imaging (MRI) also can be adopted to confirm the diagnosis. Time of flight (TOF) of an MR angiography may delineate the proximity or contact of an offending vessel with the REZ. According to more recent studies where 3D MRI volumetric analysis was applied to evaluate the size of the CSF space in the posterior fossa, it appeared to be smaller in HFS patients compared to that of the control group [11]. The characteristic feature of EMG in HFS can be described as spontaneous and high-frequency synchronized firing, which may be helpful to differentiate HFS from other movement disorders, such as myokymia, blepharospasm, craniocervical dystonia (Meige syndrome), post-facial palsy synkinesia, tic disorders, myokymia, neuromyotonia, and tardive dyskinesias (TD) as well as phychogenic HFS [9]. According to an epidemiological study based on a Norwegian population, the prevalence of HFS was about 9.8 per 100,000 persons [12]. Another study from the USA reported the prevalence rate of HFS as 7.4 per 100,000 men and 14.5 per 100,000 women [13]. Data from our own institute revealed the male-to-female ratio to be 1:2.28 with an average age of 52.2 years [14].

The pathophysiology of HFS, as widely accepted, is explained by vascular compression on the root entry zone (REZ) of the facial nerve. When the compression of the REZ is the sole cause of HFS, it is defined as primary HFS, whereas any impairment of the facial nerve due to a pre-existing condition can constitute a secondary HFS. A modern-day concept of vascular compression syndrome that included trigeminal neuralgia, HFS, and glossopharyngeal neuralgia was introduced by McKenzie in 1936 [9]. Based on its pathophysiological background, vascular decompression for HFS was first introduced by Gardner in 1962, following which, a more modern technique with a minimal approach, i.e., MVD via retrosigmoid craniotomy, was first performed by Bremond in 1974 [9,15,16]. The current concept of the pathophysiology and surgical treatment of HFS was established and popularized by Jannetta, and it started with his article in 1975, titled *"Neurovascular cross-compression in patients with hyperactive dysfunction symptoms of the eighth cranial nerve"* [9,17]. When a vascular curvature causes the compression on the REZ, the anterior inferior cerebellar artery (AICA) is most commonly involved, followed by posterior inferior cerebellar artery (PICA), and the vertebral artery (VA). A single artery could be the sole cause of the neurovascular compression, but it is rather infrequent (4.7%) according to our previous report [9,18]. In consideration of other additional factors, a total of six compressive patterns in HFS were proposed: loop, arachnoid, perforator, branch, sandwich, and tandem types [9,18]. Regarding a more detailed mechanism of HFS in addition to the microscopic disruption of myelin in the REZ, there are two major hypotheses: the central (hyperexcitability of the facial motor nucleus) vs the peripheral (ephaptic transmission between the facial nerve bundles) hypothesis [9,19]. An increasing amount of micro-anatomical and neurophysiological research is dedicated to elucidating the precise pathway of HFS; but one hypothesis cannot explain all the phenomena without the other.

Pharmaceutical medicine in general has failed to provide long-term improvement for HFS. Anticonvulsants or GABAergic medicines may lessen symptoms partially and temporarily, but the effectiveness of those medicines cannot be comparable to botulinum neurotoxin (BTX) injection, not to mention microvascular decompression. BTX injection is the most preferred non-surgical treatment for HFS, yielding up to 85% of symptomatic relief, and among the seven serotypes of BTX, serotypes A and B are currently commercialized [9]. Following injections, symptomatic improvement occurs in 1–3 days, and it usually reaches its peak effect in 5 days [9,20]. The duration of clinical benefit varies center to center by 3–6 months [9,21,22]. Repeated injections of BTX are unavoidable, and tolerance can naturally develop in some subjects, although a 10-year multicenter study reported that the average duration of improvement did not change from the first year of injection to the 10th year of treatment with a similar dose of BTX [9,23]. Additionally, they insisted that the adverse responses derived from BTX injections decreased throughout the 10-year course. Local complications of BTX injection include ptosis, blurred vision, and diplopia, but they are rarely permanent [9,24]. Incidence of overall adverse effects was estimated as ranging from 20 to 53%, and the most frequent one was ptosis [21,22,25]. Despite its relatively high success rate of symptomatic improvement, one cannot ignore the fact that BTX injection fundamentally requires repeated sessions, which leads to emotionally and financially non-negligible burdens on the patients [9].

MVD is the only curative treatment option for HFS with a high success rate and low incidence of recurrence and complications. According to a systemic review on 22 studies with 5700 patients who underwent MVD, a complete resolution was achieved in 91.1% (95% CI: 90.3–91.8%) of patients [9,26]. Recurrence occurred in 2.4% (95% CI: 1.9–2.9%) of patients, and postoperative complications included transient complications including facial palsy (9.5% [95% CI:8.8–10.3%]), hearing deficit (3.2% [95% CI: 2.7–3.7%]), and cerebrospinal fluid leak (1.4% [95% CI: 1.1–1.7%]) [9,26]. Permanent complications included hearing deficit in 2.3% (95% CI: 1.9–2.7%) and facial palsy in 0.9% (95% CI: 0.7–1.2%) of patients, the risk of stroke was 1 in 1800, and risk of death was 1 in 5500 [9,26].

The basic concept of MVD is well described in the literature, but the detailed techniques vary depending on institutions and surgeons. Once a lateral retro-sigmoid sub-occipital craniectomy or craniotomy is performed under a general anesthesia, the dura is incised to reveal the cerebellar cortex. With or without traction of the flocculus, the root entry zone (REZ) of the facial nerve is to be observed. Upon the identification of the compressing vessels, or the offending arteries, they are separated from the seventh nerve, which then can be perpetuated by insertion of Teflon pieces. A few more additional techniques, including transposition of the vessels, snare technique, vascular sling, etc., have been proposed [9,27–29]. Intraoperative EMG monitoring can be beneficial for improvement of surgical outcomes. Lateral spread response (LSR) is one of the most commonly employed neurophysiologic tests for HFS since Moller and Jannetta suggested that properly performed decompression would be accompanied with the disappearance of the LSR [9,30]. However, persistence of the LSR did not necessarily indicate a poor outcome, which precludes the LSR from being a reliable predictor for the long-term prognosis of HFS after MVD [9,31]. Furthermore, to properly monitor the integrity of the eighth nerve (CN VIII) during MVD, intraoperative brain stem auditory evoked potential (BAEP) can be employed, which has been accepted by numerous institutions in decreasing the risk of hearing impairment during MVD [9].

Clinical courses following MVD are not identical. According to our own report, 737 (92.8%) of 807 patients who had undergone MVD for HFS became absolutely or nearly spasm free by the 2-year postoperative follow-up [9,18]. However, not everyone became asymptomatic immediately after the surgery; 140 (19.0%) of 737 patients still experienced residual spasms for more than a month, and some of them lasted more than a year [9,18]. These inhomogeneous courses of MVD for HFS may indicate that microscopic changes in the REZ, facial nerve, or facial nucleus in each patient can be diverse; some may have reversible compression without any structural changes, whereas others may have gone through microscopic changes in their facial nerve or nucleus. We believe that one cannot easily conclude the two aforementioned hypotheses of pathophysiology, i.e., hyperexcitability of the facial nucleus vs. ephaptic transmission of the facial nerve, are mutually exclusive.

4.2. Compressive Patterns

Since we introduced six compression patterns of HFS which included the loop, arachnoid, perforator, branch, sandwich, and tandem in 2008, we have received many questions concerning the significance of this categorization. As reported, one type was not necessarily associated with a better outcome compared to another, which indicated that a specific compression pattern could not determine indications for MVD. In 2020, we selected five types that can be technically challenging during MVD, but these also did not necessarily contribute to poorer results [7]. The only cases that significantly resulted in unfavorable outcomes are re-do surgeries, which underscores the importance of an accurate diagnosis, proper determination of surgical indication, thorough exploration around the REZ during MVD, and avoidance of iatrogenic compression on the REZ [7]. The significance of our categorization system can be rephrased as knowledge on these patterns may help in achieving a better surgical outcome. By being aware that there could be more than one artery causing the compression, as in the sandwich or tandem type, an incomplete decompression can be avoided. Additionally, when the vessel on the REZ is not easily movable, one must consider the possibility of the perforator type to prevent a devastating complication such as brain stem infarction or hemorrhage. Although each type did not directly impact the postoperative results, the understanding of these patterns seemed to improve the overall outcome in our institution.

A brief summary of the features and some useful tips for surgery are presented in Table 1. In the arachnoid type, the offending vessel may no longer be located on the REZ after the arachnoid dissection, which can coincide with the disappearance of the LSR. When the preoperative MRI delineates the VA near the REZ, the tandem type should be the first one to rule out. If the tandem type is confirmed during the surgery, one should be reminded of the fact that the simple insertion of Teflon pieces between the REZ and the smaller artery may not guarantee a satisfactory outcome, because the larger artery, most likely the VA, would probably continue to derive throbbing forces to the smaller one. The larger artery must be detached from the smaller one, and furthermore, it would be ideal if the larger one could be transposed so that the trajectory of the throbbing force can be re-directed. The loop type is the least challenging since the approach to the REZ is not hindered by any obstacles and there is enough working space for decompression. The involvement of PICA is most frequent in this type. The perforator type is one of the challenging ones. Owing to the tight perforators, manipulation of the compressing artery can be highly difficult and sometimes potentially dangerous. Any disruption to one or more of the perforators can result in permanent impairment to the brain stem. When the REZ is caught between the branches, the main trunk must be moved off the REZ, so that the inserted Teflon does not cause an iatrogenic compression. The sandwich type can be overlooked if the medial side of the REZ is not thoroughly inspected. After one compression on the dorsal side of the REZ is successfully decompressed, the medial side also should be carefully observed.

The arachnoid type was most frequently observed (27.9%), followed by the tandem (24.6%) and the perforator (22.0%) types based on our own research in 2008 [6]. The addendum classification was published in 2021, where 1527 (50.4%) of 3027 MVD for HFS cases were selected as such [7]. Among the challenging types, the tandem (40.2%) and the perforator (31.1%) accounted for the majority, and the remaining three types included cisternal, encircling, and penetrating ones in order of frequency; the penetrating type was the most extreme one (4 out of 3027, 0.13%). In the cisternal type, it is sometimes difficult to find the compression, because the usual compression site, i.e., the REZ, appears to be compression-free. Exploration towards the cisternal portion of the facial nerve often demands further retraction of the cerebellum, but special attention must be paid not to retract it excessively. BAEP monitoring is mandatory. When the encircling artery is found around the REZ, the decompression process should be carried out from the medial to the lateral side of the REZ, because the insertion of Teflon pieces on the lateral side may hinder the medial side from being properly maneuvered. The penetrating type is the most rare and probably the most challenging of all. These challenging types did not necessarily lead to poorer outcomes, whereas revision cases resulted in a significantly lower spasm-free rate (10 of 13, 76.9%) along with a substantially higher incidence of intraoperative BAEP change (7 of 13, 53.8%), postoperative facial palsy (6, 46.2%), and deafness (1, 7.7%) [7].

Table 1. Features and surgical tips for each type.

	Distinctive Feature	Tips for Operation
Classic compression patterns		
Loop type	Compression most commonly by PICA ¶	Technically least challenging
Arachnoid type	Thickened arachnoid membrane	1. Careful and thorough dissection of the arachnoid membrane is the key ¶ 2. LSR * may disappear upon the release of the arachnoid membrane
Perforator type	Tight perforators	Do not attempt to move the vessel off the REZ forcefully or excessively
Branch type	Caught between branches	Make sure the main trunk is moved off the REZ
Sandwich type	Two independent arteries from each side	After a successful decompression, always consider another possible source of compression
Tandem type	Larger vessel (most commonly VA $^\beta$) compressing a smaller one	Trajectory of the larger vessel must be altered to accomplish a full decompression
Challenging patterns		
Perforator type	Written above	Written above
Tandem type	Written above	Written above
Cisternal type	Compression on a cisternal portion of the facial nerve, instead of the REZ $^\delta$	Be careful not to excessively retract the cerebellum
Encircling type	More than 270° contact with the nerve	Decompression process should be carried out from medial to lateral side of the REZ
Penetrating type	Most rare (0.13%)	Extra care must be taken not to injure the facial nerve

¶: Posterior inferior cerebellar artery, $^\beta$: vertebral artery, $^\delta$: root exit zone, *: lateral spread response.

Veins were found to be responsible for HFS in 6 (1.1%) out of 528 HFS patients, according to our previous study; 2 of them were solely caused by venous compression, whereas the remaining 4 cases were due to a combination of arterial and venous compression [32]. We did not cauterize the vein as it may result in venous infarction or brain stem injury. After careful manipulation of the vein, the REZ was decompressed using a small piece of Teflon. Although we do not have statistically significant data, HFS due to venous compression appeared to be associated with rather unfavorable outcomes because it was not always possible to detach the vein from the REZ and manipulation of the facial nerve was sometimes inevitable.

The importance of a thorough 360° inspection around the REZ cannot be overemphasized. Even after one offending artery is successfully detached and insulated, the medial and cisternal sides of the REZ should also be free from any compression. The LSR tends to disappear when the REZ is no longer compressed, but it is questionable if the disappearance of the LSR can be a predictor of the long-term prognosis [18,24]. If the LSR still exists after a decompression process, it could indicate either incomplete decompression with a secondary cause of compression untreated, or complete decompression with lingering hyperexcitability of the facial nucleus or ephaptic transmission between nerve fibers [2,14,33]. Since it is not possible to discriminate the latter from the former during a surgery, a hypothetical secondary cause should always be ruled out to achieve a long-term cure.

4.3. Brief Summary of Current Updates

A recent randomized clinical trial (RCT) on BTX injections for HFS revealed that bilateral injection of BTX decreased facial asymmetry more than ipsilateral injection did [34]. In a related study, MR tractography findings were evaluated in HFS patients following injection of BTX, where apparent diffusion coefficient (ADC) and fractional anisotropy (FA) values in the contralateral motor cortex were found to be close to those of the pathological side [35]. The authors suggested that this result might indicate an impact of peripherally injected BTX on the central nervous system [35]. Another double blinded, RCT demonstrated that pretarsal injection of BTX was more efficient than preseptal injection in terms of better symptom control and longer duration of efficacy [36].

Surgical techniques have evolved over time as well. Since the concept of MVD initiated by Jannetta et al. has been employed for HFS, trigeminal neuralgia, and glossopharyngeal neuralgia, newer techniques have emerged. The "transposition technique" differs from the simple insertion of Teflon pieces as it aims to alter the location and trajectory of the offending vessel so that the vessel can no longer convey the pulsating force to the REZ [37]. This technique can be roughly rephrased as "off the REZ", since the REZ is free not only from the offending vessel but also from any iatrogenic Teflon pieces [37]. MVD using this transposition technique, with or without the help of a fibrin coated sling, demonstrated a higher success and lower recurrence rate [37]. As we emphasized, the re-do surgeries resulted in significantly poorer outcomes [7]. During a revision MVD, previously inserted Teflon pieces were often found near the REZ, and they were thought to have accounted for the residual or recurrent symptoms. Iatrogenic compression must be avoided at all costs, and we believe that this "off the REZ" policy may be the key to prevent a recurrence, and accordingly, a re-do intervention.

Endoscope-assisted MVD and fully endoscopic surgery have gained increasing popularity. A meta-analysis comparing the traditional and endoscopic MVD, with a total of 12 studies and 1122 patients, reported that the endoscopic MVD yielded a higher success rate (97% vs. 89%), lower recurrence rate (5.7% vs. 0.3%), as well as a lower complication rate (12% vs. 27%) than the microscopic MVD did [38]. Another study in 2019 also insisted that a fully endoscopic MVD is both safe and feasible in the treatment of HFS since it can provide a better visualization of the neurovascular conflict, despite its original shortcomings, e.g., being prone to blood soiling, lacking 3D information, or having a longer learning curve [39].

The disappearance of the LSR is still a useful parameter during MVD, either traditional or endoscopic, as the majority of researchers concur. A meta-analysis on intraoperative monitoring of the LSR reported that an intraoperative disappearance of the LSR could predict a favorable clinical outcome with a high specificity of 90% at discharge and after 1 year, whereas the sensitivity was only 40% at discharge and after 1 year [40]. We believe this lower sensitivity of the LSR might be derived from the hyperexcitability of the facial motor nucleus in HFS, which could be sustained even after a successful decompression. A neurophysiological study using a novel parameter in the future may distinguish the hyperexcitability of the facial motor nucleus from the ephaptic transmission.

5. Conclusions

We believe the categorization of compressing patterns on the REZ of HFS patients as well as insightful technical tips in accordance with each individual pattern, may contribute to a safer and more efficient MVD for HFS. The golden rules of successful MVD for HFS are accurate diagnosis, proper indication for surgery, thorough and careful exploration around the REZ, and avoidance of iatrogenic compression on the REZ.

Author Contributions: Conceptualization, K.P.; Methodology, J.S.P.; Resources, J.S.P.; Data curation, J.S.P.; Writing—original draft, J.S.P.; Writing—review & editing, K.P.; Visualization, J.S.P.; Supervision, K.P. All authors have read and agreed to the published version of the manuscript.

Funding: This research received no external funding.

Institutional Review Board Statement: Institutional review board of Samsung medical center: SMC (2020-04-008).

Informed Consent Statement: Patient consent was not necessary because of the retrospective nature of the study, and the validity of the findings would not be affected by the absence of patient consent. Moreover, no additional risk to patient safety was expected from this study without patient consent.

Data Availability Statement: Data available on request due to restrictions eg privacy or ethical.

Conflicts of Interest: The authors declare no conflict of interest.

References

1. Møller, A.R. The cranial nerve vascular compression syndrome: II. A review of pathophysiology. *Acta Neurochir.* **1991**, *113*, 24–30. [CrossRef] [PubMed]
2. Møller, A.R.; Jannetta, P.J. On the origin of synkinesis in hemifacial spasm: Results of intracranial recordings. *J. Neurosurg.* **1984**, *61*, 569–576. [CrossRef] [PubMed]
3. Barker, F.G.; Jannetta, P.J.; Bissonette, D.J.; Shields, P.T.; Larkins, M.V.; Jho, H.D. Microvascular decompression for hemifacial spasm. *J. Neurosurg.* **1995**, *82*, 201–210. [CrossRef] [PubMed]
4. Møller, A.R.; Jannetta, P.J. Microvascular decompression in hemifacial spasm: Intraoperative electrophysiological observations. *Neurosurgery* **1985**, *16*, 612–618. [CrossRef] [PubMed]
5. Jo, K.W.; Kong, D.-S.; Park, K. Microvascular decompression for hemifacial spasm: Long-term outcome and prognostic factors, with emphasis on delayed cure. *Neurosurg. Rev.* **2013**, *36*, 297–302. [CrossRef]
6. Park, J.S.; Kong, D.-S.; Lee, J.-A.; Park, K. Hemifacial spasm: Neurovascular compressive patterns and surgical significance. *Acta Neurochir.* **2008**, *150*, 235–241. [CrossRef]
7. Lee, S.; Joo, K.M.; Park, K. Challenging microvascular decompression surgery for hemifacial spasm. *World Neurosurg.* **2021**, *151*, e94–e99. [CrossRef]
8. Fang, L.-J.; Wang, C.-Y. Bibliometric analysis of studies on the treatment of hemifacial spasm. *Front. Neurol.* **2022**, *13*, 931551. [CrossRef]
9. Park, K.; Park, J.S. *Hemifacial Spasm: A Comprehensive Guide*; Springer Nature: London, UK, 2020.
10. Pawlowski, M.; Gess, B.; Evers, S. The Babinski-2 sign in hemifacial spasm. *Mov. Disord.* **2013**, *28*, 1298–1300. [CrossRef]
11. Chan, L.-L.; Ng, K.-M.; Fook-Chong, S.; Lo, Y.-L.; Tan, E.-K.J.N. Three-dimensional MR volumetric analysis of the posterior fossa CSF space in hemifacial spasm. *Neurology* **2009**, *73*, 1054–1057. [CrossRef]
12. Nilsen, B.; Le, K.-D.; Dietrichs, E. Prevalence of hemifacial spasm in Oslo, Norway. *Neurology* **2004**, *63*, 1532–1533. [CrossRef] [PubMed]
13. Auger, R.G.; Whisnant, J.P. Hemifacial spasm in Rochester and Olmsted county, Minnesota, 1960 to 1984. *Arch. Neurol.* **1990**, *47*, 1233–1234. [CrossRef] [PubMed]
14. Park, J.S.; Lee, S.; Park, S.-K.; Lee, J.-A.; Park, K. Facial motor evoked potential with paired transcranial magnetic stimulation: Prognostic value following microvascular decompression for hemifacial spasm. *J. Neurosurg.* **2018**, *131*, 1780–1787. [CrossRef] [PubMed]
15. Rand, R.W. Gardner's neurovascular decompression for hemifacial spasm. *Arch. Neurol.* **1982**, *39*, 510–511. [CrossRef]
16. Bremond, G.; Garcin, M.; Magnan, J.; Bonnaud, G. L'abord a minima de l'espace pontocerebelleux. *Cah ORL* **1974**, *19*, 443–460.
17. Jannetta, P. Neurovascular cross-compression in patients with hyperactive dysfunction symptoms of the eighth cranial nerve. *Surge Forum* **1975**, *26*, 467–469.
18. Park, J.S.; Kong, D.-S.; Lee, J.-A.; Park, K. Chronologic analysis of symptomatic change following microvascular decompression for hemifacial spasm: Value for predicting midterm outcome. *Neurosurg. Rev.* **2008**, *31*, 413–419. [CrossRef]
19. Campos-Benitez, M.; Kaufmann, A.M. Neurovascular compression findings in hemifacial spasm. *J. Neurosurg.* **2008**, *109*, 416–420. [CrossRef]
20. Dutton, J.J.; Buckley, E.G. Long-term Results and Complications of Botulinum A Toxin in the Treatment of Blepharospasm. *Ophthalmology* **1988**, *95*, 1529–1534. [CrossRef]
21. Dutton, J.J.; Fowler, A.M. Botulinum toxin in ophthalmology. *Surv. Ophthalmol.* **2007**, *52*, 13–31. [CrossRef]
22. Ababneh, O.H.; Cetinkaya, A.; Kulwin, D.R. Long-term efficacy and safety of botulinum toxin A injections to treat blepharospasm and hemifacial spasm. *Clin. Exp. Ophthalmol.* **2014**, *42*, 254–261. [CrossRef] [PubMed]
23. Defazio, G.; Abbruzzese, G.; Girlanda, P.; Vacca, L.; Curra, A.; De Salvia, R.; Marchese, R.; Raineri, R.; Roselli, F.; Livrea, P.; et al. Botulinum toxin A treatment for primary hemifacial spasm: A 10-year multicenter study. *Arch. Neurol.* **2002**, *59*, 418–420. [CrossRef] [PubMed]

24. Kong, D.-S.; Park, K.; Shin, B.-G.; Lee, J.A.; Eum, D.-O. Prognostic value of the lateral spread response for intraoperative electromyography monitoring of the facial musculature during microvascular decompression for hemifacial spasm. *J. Neurosurg.* **2007**, *106*, 384–387. [CrossRef]
25. Czyz, C.N.; Burns, J.A.; Petrie, T.P.; Watkins, J.R.; Cahill, K.V.; Foster, J.A. Long-term Botulinum Toxin Treatment of Benign Essential Blepharospasm, Hemifacial Spasm, and Meige Syndrome. *Am. J. Ophthalmol.* **2013**, *156*, 173–177.e172. [CrossRef] [PubMed]
26. Miller, L.E.; Miller, V.M. Safety and effectiveness of microvascular decompression for treatment of hemifacial spasm: A systematic review. *J. Neurosurg.* **2012**, *26*, 438–444. [CrossRef] [PubMed]
27. Kurokawa, Y.; Maeda, Y.; Toyooka, T.; Inaba, K.-I. Microvascular decompression for hemifacial spasm caused by the vertebral artery: A simple and effective transposition method using surgical glue. *Surg. Neurol.* **2004**, *61*, 398–403. [CrossRef]
28. Masuoka, J.; Matsushima, T.; Kawashima, M.; Nakahara, Y.; Funaki, T.; Mineta, T. Stitched sling retraction technique for microvascular decompression: Procedures and techniques based on an anatomical viewpoint. *Neurosurg. Rev.* **2011**, *34*, 373–380. [CrossRef]
29. Lee, S.H.; Park, J.S.; Ahn, Y.H. Bioglue-Coated Teflon Sling Technique in Microvascular Decompression for Hemifacial Spasm Involving the Vertebral Artery. *J. Korean Neurosurg. Soc.* **2016**, *59*, 505–511. [CrossRef]
30. Møller, A.R.; Jannetta, P.J. Physiological abnormalities in hemifacial spasm studied during microvascular decompression operations. *Exp. Neurol.* **1986**, *93*, 584–600. [CrossRef]
31. Von Eckardstein, K.; Harper, C.; Castner, M.; Link, M. The significance of intraoperative electromyographic "lateral spread" in predicting outcome of microvascular decompression for hemifacial spasm. *J. Neurol. Surg. Part B Skull Base* **2014**, *75*, 198–203. [CrossRef]
32. Lee, J.-A.; Park, K. Short-term versus long-term outcomes of microvascular decompression for hemifacial spasm. *Acta Neurochir.* **2019**, *161*, 2027–2033. [CrossRef] [PubMed]
33. Fukuda, M.; Oishi, M.; Hiraishi, T.; Fujii, Y. Facial nerve motor-evoked potential monitoring during microvascular decompression for hemifacial spasm. *J. Neurol. Neurosurg. Psychiatry* **2010**, *81*, 519–523. [CrossRef] [PubMed]
34. Xiao, L.; Pan, L.; Li, B.; Zhou, Y.; Pan, Y.; Zhang, X.; Hu, Y.; Dressler, D.; Jin, L. Botulinum toxin therapy of hemifacial spasm: Bilateral injections can reduce facial asymmetry. *J. Neurol.* **2018**, *265*, 2097–2105. [CrossRef] [PubMed]
35. Cavus, H.; İşeri, P.; Öztürk, O.; Anık, Y. Evaluation of MR-Tractography Findings in Hemifacial Spasm Patients Injected with Botulinum Neurotoxin. *Neurol. India* **2022**, *70*, 543. [CrossRef]
36. Lolekha, P.; Choolam, A.; Kulkantrakorn, K. A comparative crossover study on the treatment of hemifacial spasm and blepharospasm: Preseptal and pretarsal botulinum toxin injection techniques. *Neurol. Sci.* **2017**, *38*, 2031–2036. [CrossRef]
37. Park, J.S.; Ahn, Y.H. Glossopharyngeal Neuralgia. *J. Korean Neurosurg. Soc.* **2022**, *66*, 12–23. [CrossRef]
38. Zhao, C.; Chai, S.; Xiao, D.; Zhou, Y.; Gan, J.; Jiang, X.; Zhao, H. Microscopic versus endoscopic microvascular decompression for the treatment of hemifacial spasm in China: A meta-analysis and systematic review. *J. Clin. Neurosci.* **2021**, *91*, 23–31. [CrossRef]
39. Flanders, T.M.; Blue, R.; Roberts, S.; McShane, B.J.; Wilent, B.; Tambi, V.; Petrov, D.; Lee, J.Y.K. Fully endoscopic microvascular decompression for hemifacial spasm. *J. Neurosurg.* **2018**, *131*, 813–819. [CrossRef]
40. Thirumala, P.D.; Altibi, A.M.; Chang, R.; Saca, E.E.; Iyengar, P.; Reddy, R.; Anetakis, K.; Crammond, D.J.; Balzer, J.R.; Sekula, R.F., Jr. The utility of intraoperative lateral spread recording in microvascular decompression for hemifacial spasm: A systematic review and meta-analysis. *Neurosurgery* **2020**, *87*, E473–E484. [CrossRef]

Disclaimer/Publisher's Note: The statements, opinions and data contained in all publications are solely those of the individual author(s) and contributor(s) and not of MDPI and/or the editor(s). MDPI and/or the editor(s) disclaim responsibility for any injury to people or property resulting from any ideas, methods, instructions or products referred to in the content.

Review

Lateral Spread Response: Unveiling the Smoking Gun for Cured Hemifacial Spasm

Kyung Rae Cho [1], Sang Ku Park [1] and Kwan Park [1,2,*]

1 Department of Neurosurgery, Konkuk University Medical Center, Seoul 05030, Republic of Korea; medicasterz@gmail.com (K.R.C.); heydaum@daum.net (S.K.P.)
2 Department of Neurosurgery, School of Medicine Sungkyunkwan University, Seoul 16419, Republic of Korea
* Correspondence: kwanpark@skku.edu

Abstract: Hemifacial spasm (HFS) is a rare disorder characterized by involuntary facial muscle contractions. The primary cause is mechanical compression of the facial nerve by nearby structures. Lateral spread response (LSR) is an abnormal muscle response observed during electromyogram (EMG) testing and is associated with HFS. Intraoperative monitoring of LSR is crucial during surgery to confirm successful decompression. Proper anesthesia and electrode positioning are important for accurate LSR monitoring. Stimulation parameters should be carefully adjusted to avoid artifacts. The disappearance of LSR during surgery is associated with short-term outcomes, but its persistence does not necessarily indicate poor long-term outcomes. LSR monitoring has both positive and negative prognostic value, and its predictive ability varies across studies. Early disappearance of LSR can occur before decompression and may indicate better clinical outcomes. Further research is needed to fully understand the implications of LSR monitoring in HFS surgery.

Keywords: lateral spread response; abnormal muscle response; hemifacial spasm

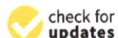

Citation: Cho, K.R.; Park, S.K.; Park, K. Lateral Spread Response: Unveiling the Smoking Gun for Cured Hemifacial Spasm. *Life* **2023**, *13*, 1825. https://doi.org/10.3390/life13091825

Academic Editors: Zuzanna Nowak and Aleksandra Nitecka-Buchta

Received: 29 June 2023
Revised: 11 August 2023
Accepted: 26 August 2023
Published: 29 August 2023

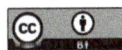

Copyright: © 2023 by the authors. Licensee MDPI, Basel, Switzerland. This article is an open access article distributed under the terms and conditions of the Creative Commons Attribution (CC BY) license (https://creativecommons.org/licenses/by/4.0/).

1. Introduction

Hemifacial spasm (HFS) is a rare neuromuscular disorder characterized by involuntary contractions of the facial muscles, predominantly affecting one side of the face. The underlying pathophysiology of HFS involves mechanical compression of the facial nerve at the root exit zone (REZ) by adjacent structures, including arteries, veins, and tumors. Identification of the offending vessel can be achieved through magnetic resonance imaging and confirmed during surgical intervention. However, in some cases, there may be multiple compressing structures, or they may elude detection during the surgical procedure. Therefore, it is crucial for surgeons to accurately identify the primary cause when manipulating the surface of the brainstem. Intraoperative monitoring can be valuable in confirming successful decompression while minimizing the risk of unnecessary manipulation near delicate structures.

Lateral spread response (LSR), an abnormal muscle response (AMR), represents a distinctive neurophysiological characteristic of HFS that remains undetectable under normal conditions. When one branch of the facial nerve is stimulated, an atypical response is observed on the electromyogram (EMG) in other branches of the facial nerve. This anomalous response was initially reported by Janetta and Moller [1,2], and subsequent studies have been conducted to elucidate its significance and its connection to the pathophysiology of HFS. Although LSR holds substantial importance during microvascular decompression surgery (MVD) for HFS, its precise implications are not yet fully understood. The presence of LSR indicates the existence of aberrant cross-connections between facial nerve branches or fibers, although the exact nature of these abnormal connections remains to be identified [3].

The objectives of this article are to provide a comprehensive review of the pathophysiology of LSR, the appropriate techniques for its accurate monitoring, and its clinical implications, and to address the controversies that have been previously discussed in the literature.

2. Methods for Monitoring Lateral Spread Response (LSR)

LSR monitoring is typically conducted throughout the entire surgical procedure, from the initiation of general anesthesia until its conclusion. The monitoring of LSR does not interfere with the surgical process, allowing for continuous observation while manipulating the facial nerve and adjacent vessels. Generally, monitoring of LSR begins after the insertion of electrodes, before dural opening, after dural opening, during REZ decompression, and after dural closure [4]. Even if LSR disappears immediately after dural opening or decompression, its recurrence may indicate unsuccessful decompression. Hence, continuous monitoring of LSR is recommended throughout the surgery, even if it disappears initially.

2.1. Anesthesia

Since LSR is an abnormal electromyogram (EMG), appropriate anesthetic agents must be used to avoid interfering with the accurate monitoring of this abnormal muscle response. During the induction of general anesthesia, anesthesiologists typically administer neuromuscular blockade (NMB) agents such as rocuronium or vecuronium to minimize patient stress during endotracheal intubation [5]. However, continuous administration of these agents can affect the precise detection of LSR. Therefore, careful titration of NMB is necessary, and many anesthesiologists prefer to delay its administration until the end of the surgery [6]. It is generally recommended that a train-of-four count of more than two be maintained, for accurate monitoring. However, maintaining partial NMB with a target T1/Tc ratio of 50% has proven to be clinically acceptable for LSR monitoring and surgical conditions during MVD [7]. Complete termination of NMB did not significantly enhance LSR monitoring when compared to maintaining a T1/Tc ratio of 50%; thus, it is not recommended in MVD surgery [8].

Inhalational anesthetics have the potential to inhibit or block LSR [9,10]. Studies have also demonstrated significant alterations in the chronaxie of human corticospinal axons when exposed to the inhalational anesthetic sevoflurane [10]. There are reports indicating that desflurane can suppress LSR amplitude by 43%, compared to total intravenous anesthesia alone [9].

2.2. Electrode Position

The accurate positioning of electrodes significantly affects the results of neuromonitoring. Misplaced electrodes may stimulate unintended structures, leading to monitoring artifacts instead of capturing meaningful waves. Therefore, ensuring correct electrode positioning is crucial for the precise monitoring of LSR. Typically, the stimulation electrode is placed between the ipsilateral tragus and the external canthus of the eye, where the zygomatic branches of the facial nerve are located. Since the zygomatic branch of the facial nerve innervates the orbicularis oculi muscle, the abnormal muscle response recorded in other facial muscles, such as the frontalis (temporal), orbicularis oris (buccal), and mentalis (marginal mandibular), is defined as LSR [11]. Some institutions have also explored stimulating the marginal mandibular branch, which is located at the border of the mandible and lateral to the mental tubercle, and recording from the orbicularis oculi muscle and the mentalis muscle [3,5].

The conventional stimulation method involves placing paired dermal electrodes in such a way that the cathode is positioned at the proximal branch and the anode is positioned at the distal branch, resulting in centripetal impulses toward the brainstem. However, Lee et al. [12] conducted a study in which they inverted this method by placing the cathode at the distal branch and the anode at the proximal facial nerve. They found that the innervated muscles responded more sensitively to this new stimulation method. In fact, the new method with the cathode at the distal branch demonstrated a higher detection rate for the disappearance of LSR than that of the conventional method. The conventional method achieved a detection rate of 61.8%, while the new method achieved a detection rate of 98.2%. Additionally, after surgical decompression, the conventional method still showed a remaining LSR rate of 29.1%, while the new method had a remaining LSR rate of only 1.8% (Figure 1).

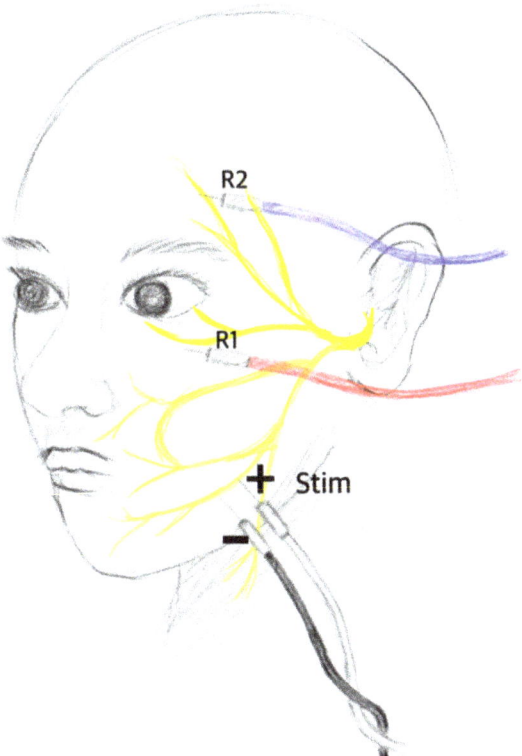

Figure 1. A paired dermal stimulation electrode was positioned either at the zygomatic branch or at the marginal mandibular branch to induce stimulation. Typically, in conventional practice, the cathode is placed proximally while the anode is placed distally to elicit a centripetal impulse. In contrast, Lee et al. conducted a study in which they reversed the placement of the cathode and the anode. Interestingly, this alternative configuration resulted in more sensitive recording of lateral spread response. Their findings suggested that the directionality of the electrode placement can significantly impact the quality and precision of LSR recordings.

2.3. Stimulation Parameters

Currently, there is no standardized guideline for the stimulation and recording methods used in LSR monitoring. Due to variations in nerve excitability thresholds among individuals and the potential influences of anesthesia and other conditions, establishing specific parameters for stimulation presents challenges. However, in most studies, a pulse wave with a duration of 0.2–0.3 ms and an intensity ranging from 5 to 25 mA have been commonly employed. Within this intensity range, LSR can be consistently detected [11].

Nevertheless, although the results have not yet been published, the authors of this review paper discovered the presence of superficially spreading artifacts that can be mistaken for LSR during high-intensity stimulation. In cases where LSR disappears early or goes undetected, examiners may be inclined to increase the stimulation intensity to reveal any hidden LSR. However, the authors' study revealed the presence of artifacts that mimic LSR, particularly when the abnormal muscle response appears with a very short latency—specifically, less than 10 ms. Therefore, it is advisable that the stimulation intensity not be increased in such cases, where the abnormal muscle response seems to appear too quickly, as it may be due to these artifact responses (Figure 2).

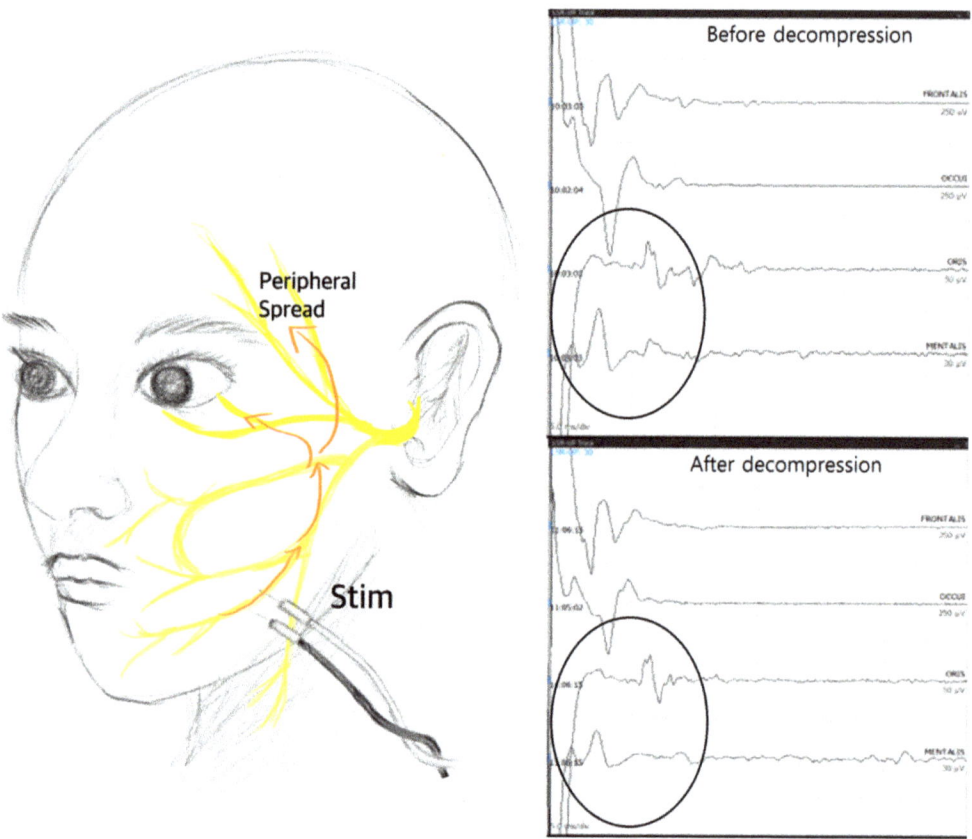

Figure 2. The study conducted by the authors revealed that when the intensity of stimulation surpassed its upper threshold, a direct spreading artifact resembling the low-threshold sensory afferent response (LSR) was observed that did not disappear, even after decompression. This exceeding intensity was quantified by a reduction in the latency of the abnormal muscle response, which was shorter than 10 milliseconds according to their findings. These results suggest that care must be taken to differentiate true LSR from artifacts caused by excessive stimulation intensity, as these artifacts can lead to misleading interpretations and, potentially, affect the accuracy of experimental outcomes.

3. Prognostic Value of LSR

Zhang et al. conducted a meta-analysis of 14 papers that investigated the prognostic value of lateral spread response (LSR) during microvascular decompression (MVD) [13]. Their findings indicated that the disappearance of LSR is highly associated with short-term outcomes. However, they did not find a significant predictive effect on long-term outcomes. Another systematic review, by Nugroho [4], also concluded that short-term outcomes are strongly correlated with the resolution of LSR. However, the resolution of LSR does not significantly impact long-term outcomes, as patient outcomes tend to improve over time with adequate decompression, even if LSR persists after surgery.

In contrast, a meta-analysis performed by Thirumala et al. [14] revealed that intraoperative LSR monitoring demonstrates high specificity but low sensitivity in predicting a postoperative hemifacial spasm (HFS)-free status at discharge, at 3 months after discharge, and at 1 year after discharge. According to their analysis, the sensitivity was calculated as 40%, 41%, and 40%, respectively, while the specificity was estimated as 89%, 90%, and 89%, respectively, at discharge, 3 months after discharge, and 1 year after discharge. They further calculated the negative predictive value, which indicates the probability of patients achieving LSR resolution, as 92.7%, 95.8%, and 96.0%, respectively, at discharge, 3 months after discharge, and 1 year after discharge. Additionally, the positive predictive value, representing cases where LSR persists, was determined as 47.8%, 40.8%, and 24.4%, respectively, at discharge, 3 months after discharge, and 1 year after discharge. These results suggest that both short-term and long-term outcomes can be predicted based on the resolution of LSR during surgery. However, it should be noted that even if LSR persists during surgery, long-term outcomes may still be positive.

3.1. Positive Prognostic Value

Lee et al. [12] reported that the AMR monitoring during MVD is beneficial for identifying the offending vessel and suggesting the most appropriate surgical endpoint. Kong et al. [15] reported that the monitoring of AMR is an effective tool when performing complete decompression, and it may help to predict the outcomes. Some patients still had residual spasm despite LSR disappearance. Various and complicated findings of the offending vessels, as stated in that report, may be the cause of spasm persistence. However, in follow-up visits at 1 year, the number of patients that were included in the category of HFS-free status increased remarkably, so that the correlation between LSR and outcome became significant. Nevertheless, divergent views on this issue have always existed.

Sekula et al. reported that the likelihood of achieving a cure is 4.2 times higher if LSR disappears during surgery than when it persists. However, it is important to note that that meta-analysis only evaluated the utility of LSR at the final follow-up visit and did not consider the postoperative measurements taken two days after surgery [16], Furthermore, there is a consensus among studies that there is a positive relationship between the resolution of LSR and the clinical outcome of HFS. Concerns regarding this relationship arise when there is no LSR observed or when there is early disappearance of LSR. Additionally, questions arise when LSR persists even after successful decompression. In cases where no LSR is observed, or where there is early disappearance, the predictive value becomes uncertain. It becomes challenging to determine the prognosis and the clinical outcome without the presence of LSR as a reliable indicator. Further research is needed to understand the implications and significance of these scenarios.

Similarly, when LSR persists despite successful decompression, the correlation between LSR and clinical outcomes becomes less straightforward. The persistence of LSR may indicate the presence of additional contributing factors or complexities that influence the overall outcome. These cases highlight the multifactorial nature of HFS and the need for a comprehensive assessment of various clinical factors to determine the prognosis and treatment outcomes accurately. However, the resolution of LSR followed by successful decompression of the vessel compressing the facial nerve REZ suggests a positive clinical outcome (Figure 3).

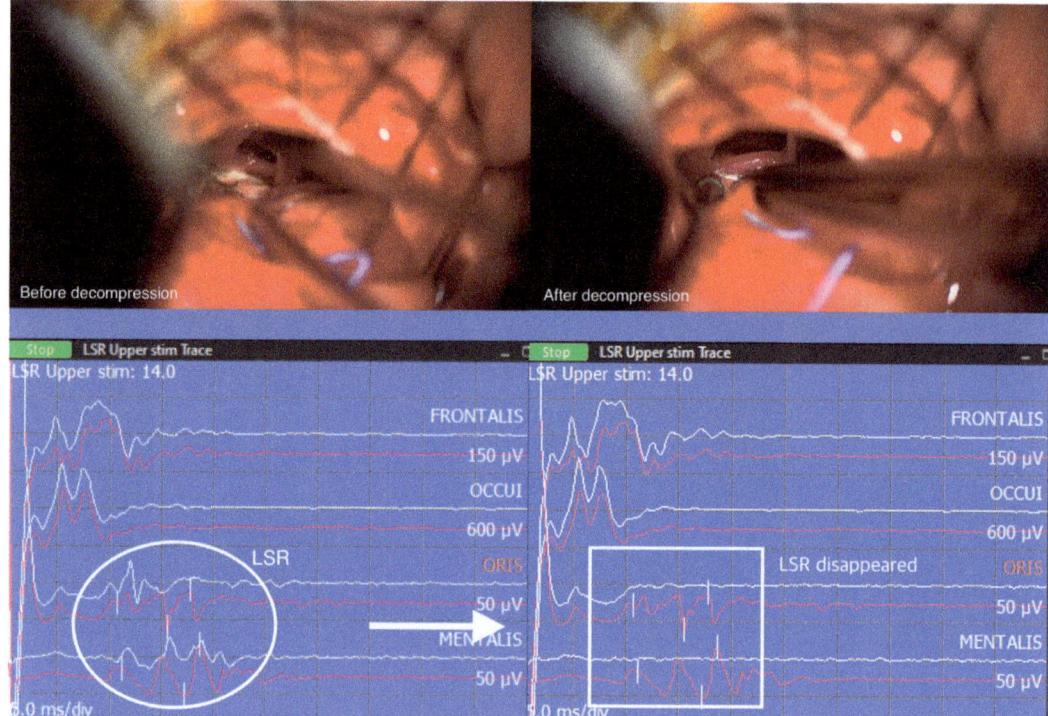

Figure 3. Captured image from intraoperative neuromonitoring program. The offending vessel was dissected from the facial nerve root exit zone, but teflon felt was not yet inserted. As a result, lateral spread response (LSR) is still seen (white oval). After placing teflon felt between the facial nerve and the dissected vessel, LSR disappeared (white rectangle).

3.2. Negative Prognostic Value

While most studies concur that the disappearance of lateral spread response (LSR) is associated with favorable outcomes in hemifacial spasm (HFS), there are some studies that demonstrate a lack of correlation between LSR resolution and clinical outcomes. This discrepancy may be attributed to intraoperative findings of multiple vessel compressions, as well as to the presence of vessels that are not easily visible behind the facial nerve or vessels coursing around the root exit zone without compressing the nerve. These factors can contribute to residual spasms following microvascular decompression (MVD) [15].

In a study by Wei et al. [17], the efficacy of intraoperative auditory brainstem response (AMR) monitoring in improving the outcomes of MVD for HFS was evaluated. However, the findings indicated that intraoperative AMR monitoring did not significantly enhance the efficacy of MVD for HFS, when performed by skilled surgeons.

Notably, studies by Kiya et al. [18] and Yamashita et al. [19] reported a high proportion of patients who exhibited LSR persistence but were free from HFS symptoms. This finding resulted in an insignificant correlation between LSR resolution and HFS relief. It should be acknowledged that these studies may have been limited by small sample sizes. Kiya et al.'s study lacked remaining spasms in both the LSR-disappearance and the persistence groups, rendering their 3 month follow-up analysis inconclusive. Similarly, Yamashita et al. found no significant correlation in the 1 year evaluation.

Indeed, there are studies that have reached different conclusions regarding the predictive value of intraoperative lateral spread response (LSR) monitoring in the outcomes of microvascular decompression (MVD) [20]. One such study, by El Damaty et al. [21], prospectively analyzed 100 patients with hemifacial spasm (HFS) and found that while LSR could guide the appropriate decompression of the facial nerve during MVD, it did not serve as a reliable predictor of postoperative efficacy. Similarly, Hatem et al. [22] observed that all 10 patients in their study achieved clinical cures despite the persistence of LSR during MVD. That finding raised doubts about the practical usefulness of LSR in the context of MVD.

These studies indicated that there is conflicting evidence regarding the predictive value of intraoperative LSR monitoring in MVD outcomes, highlighting the need for further research and consideration of multiple factors in surgical decision-making [3].

In a review conducted by Neves, the abolition of lateral spread response (LSR) and its correlation with clinical outcomes were examined in a group of 32 patients. The study reported a sensitivity of 100% and specificity of 94% in predicting long-term outcomes based on LSR abolition. However, there was no observed relationship between intraoperative LSR changes and relief from hemifacial spasm (HFS) on the first day after surgery.

These findings suggested that LSR abolition may serve as a reliable predictor of long-term outcomes in HFS patients. Additionally, the presence of increased temporal dispersion in the direct response at the stimulated nerve branch could provide valuable insights regarding LSR status, especially in patients with a history of botulinum toxin treatment [23].

Additionally, the clinical course of hemifacial spasm (HFS) after microvascular decompression (MVD) is characterized by high variability. Although many patients experience immediate relief from spasms following MVD, there are instances in which facial spasms continue to persist for several months or even years after surgery, despite the disappearance of LSR. This variability underscores the complex nature of HFS and indicates that factors other than LSR status contribute to the persistence or recurrence of symptoms [24].

3.3. Early Disappearance of LSR

Furthermore, it has been observed that the disappearance of lateral spread response (LSR) can occur early in the surgical procedure, even before any vascular decompression of the facial nerve takes place. This early LSR disappearance can be attributed to various factors, such as changes in the dynamics of cerebrospinal fluid (CSF) upon dural opening, CSF drainage, or minimal cerebellar retraction [25]. In some cases, there may be a transient disappearance of LSR followed by its reappearance at a later stage [5,26].

Jiang et al. [5] conducted a retrospective review of 372 patients. Among them, 33 patients exhibited early disappearance of LSR. The study found that the injection of muscle relaxants could diminish LSR and, importantly, that early disappearance of LSR was associated with better clinical outcomes. Several studies have explored the mechanism behind early loss of LSR before decompression in HFS surgery [5,26,27]. This early loss of LSR suggests that the compression force exerted by the offending blood vessels is relatively mild and can be easily influenced by subtle environmental changes, such as CSF egress. Kim et al. [28] suggested that the disappearance of LSR during dural opening or after CSF drainage, prior to decompression, was correlated with poorer outcomes. They emphasized the importance of surgeons carefully identifying the exact offending vessels in order to optimize surgical outcomes. These findings highlight the dynamic nature of LSR changes during HFS surgery and the potential significance of early LSR disappearance as a predictor of surgical outcomes. Surgeons should be attentive to the timing and patterns of LSR changes to improve identification of the responsible vessels and to optimize treatment strategies.

Figure 4 presents a flow chart that outlines the surgical decision-making process with LSR monitoring. This flow chart provides a visual representation of the sequential steps involved in making informed surgical interventions based on the observed LSR patterns.

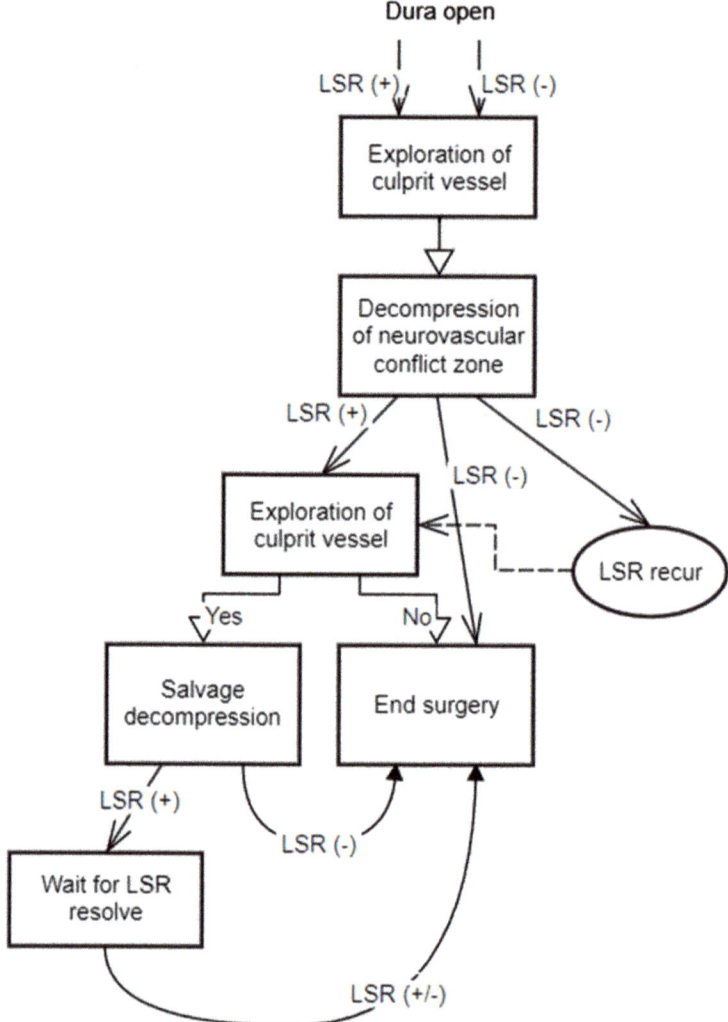

Figure 4. Flowchart for surgical decision-making based on lateral spread response (LSR) monitoring. If LSR disappears before decompression or persists after decompression, careful exploration is warranted. However, the delayed disappearance of LSR is common and, occasionally, early disappearance leads to better outcomes. Therefore, excessive exploration should be avoided to prevent unnecessary intervention.

3.4. LSR Monitoring in Secondary HFS

LSR constitutes an electrophysiological manifestation that arises not only from neurovascular conflicts, but also from influences encompassing the REZ and, potentially, other unidentified mechanisms. Consequently, LSR can manifest within secondary HFS, where lesions exert an impact along the trajectory of the facial nucleus and the facial nerve REZ.

However, within the context of tumors originating from the facial nerve, such as facial nerve schwannomas, reports of facial spasm presentation are conspicuously absent [29–31]. This discrepancy may be attributed to the propensity of facial nerve schwannomas to originate, predominantly, from the peripheral aspect of the facial nerve rather than from its intracranial segment. Consequently, the presence of abnormal electrophysiological signs such as LSR are not evident in such cases [32].

4. Pathophysiology of LSR

The exact pathophysiology of HFS remains unclear. While the most common cause is believed to be mechanical compression of the facial nerve at the REZ by an adjacent artery, there are cases where venous compression, or no specific vessel near the REZ, is identified. Thus, a more comprehensive explanation is needed beyond the direct compression of the REZ. Due to the vague nature of the disease's pathophysiology, the physiology of the AMR is also a subject of debate.

4.1. Peripheral Theory

The peripheral theory of HFS suggests an abnormal cross-transmission of facial nerve fibers at the site of vascular compression, known as the ephaptic transmission of neural impulses between different branches of the facial nerve [33]. Yamashita et al. [34] conducted a study using double stimulation of the AMR in 12 HFS patients to explain the pathophysiology of the condition. Their results showed a refractory period of 3.4 msec between stimulations, which remained constant within the same patients. This finding provided evidence of a peripheral mechanism underlying the pathophysiology of HFS, in contrast to the central nucleus theory. It indicated that the amplitude and latency intervals of the AMR stimulated at different time sequences remain consistent, suggesting no influence from the facial motor neuron. If the site of abnormal cross-transmission were in the facial nucleus, lateral spread responses would exhibit variable latency and amplitude, similar to the F wave [34]. Wilkinson used a strength–duration analysis to suggest that the AMR is likely mediated by antidromic afferent signaling along the facial nerve, as the chronaxies determined for the AMR and M wave were virtually identical [35].

4.2. Central Theory

The hyperexcitability of the facial nucleus has been proposed as a significant contributing factor in the pathogenesis of HFS, as suggested by Moller and Jannetta [36] and Poignonec et al. [37]. Yamakami et al. [38] suggested that the kindling-like hyperactivity of the facial nucleus induced by chronic electrical stimulation is the cause of the AMR. Several reports support the central theory, suggesting that the hyperexcitability of the facial nucleus is the origin of the lateral spread response. Ishikawa et al. [39–41] examined F waves pre- and postoperatively and during surgery, finding support for this central theory. By correlating F/M-wave amplitude ratios with lateral spread response F/M-wave amplitude ratios, they concluded that the origin of enhanced F waves is the same as that of the lateral spread response. The F wave exhibits variable latency and amplitude due to the hyperexcitability of the central nucleus [34,42].

5. Further Research

Thirumala and colleagues [14], in their meta-analysis, proposed that the definition of lateral spread response (LSR) resolution varies across different studies. They suggested that a prospective international multicenter study, with standardized and established definitions of LSR resolution, would yield more accurate and precise results regarding its prognostic value. This highlights the importance of having consistent criteria for determining LSR resolution in future research, to enhance the comparability and the reliability of findings.

Additionally, Kim's report [28] emphasized that the timing of LSR resolution may have prognostic significance. To further explore this aspect, more studies comparing the timing of LSR disappearance and its relationship to clinical outcomes should be conducted. Understanding the timing of LSR resolution in relation to patient outcomes can provide valuable insights into the prognostic implications of LSR changes during the course of hemifacial spasm (HFS) and subsequent microvascular decompression (MVD) surgeries.

6. Limitations

The primary aim of this paper was to provide a comprehensive overview of the monitoring methods, prognostic values, and pathophysiology of LSR. However, it is important to acknowledge certain limitations that were inherent in the scope and nature of this review. Unlike a traditional systematic review or meta-analysis, this study did not adhere to the conventional structure that includes detailed information about the methodology employed, such as the specific time frame of the literature search, the search terms used, and the inclusion and exclusion criteria. As this review focused on presenting a subjective overview of the topic rather than conducting an exhaustive analysis of the available literature, the absence of these methodological components is recognized. Therefore, it is acknowledged that the level of the evidence in the considered literature was limited, given that it did not fall within the domain of a systematic review or a meta-analysis. Nevertheless, significant efforts were made to maintain a neutral standpoint and to encompass a wide range of concerns related to LSR.

7. Conclusions

LSR monitoring has been used to identify the cause of HFS and to guide surgical interventions. This review article discussed the pathophysiology of LSR, the techniques for accurate monitoring, and the clinical implications. The presence and resolution of LSR were found to be associated with short-term outcomes, but their predictive value for long-term outcomes is less clear. Studies have shown conflicting results regarding the correlation between LSR resolution and HFS relief, highlighting the need for further research. Factors such as multiple vessel compressions and vessels that are not easily visible can contribute to residual spasms, even after successful decompression. The early disappearance of LSR before decompression can occur due to various factors. Overall, LSR monitoring is a valuable tool, but further research is needed to fully understand its implications and to optimize its use in HFS treatment.

Author Contributions: K.R.C. collected data, drafted the manuscript, and created the illustrations and figures. S.K.P. collected the electrophysiology data, interpreted the monitoring results, provided images from the monitoring device, and contributed to the conceptualization of the figures and the manuscript. K.P. collected data, revised the manuscript, and provided supervisory guidance on the literature. All authors have read and agreed to the published version of the manuscript.

Funding: This research received no external funding.

Institutional Review Board Statement: Not applicable.

Informed Consent Statement: Not applicable.

Data Availability Statement: Not applicable.

Conflicts of Interest: The authors declare no conflict of interest.

References

1. Moller, A.R.; Jannetta, P.J. Hemifacial spasm: Results of electrophysiologic recording during microvascular decompression operations. *Neurology* **1985**, *35*, 969–974. [CrossRef]
2. Moller, A.R.; Jannetta, P.J. On the origin of synkinesis in hemifacial spasm: Results of intracranial recordings. *J. Neurosurg.* **1984**, *61*, 569–576. [CrossRef]
3. Song, H.; Xu, S.; Fan, X.; Yu, M.; Feng, J.; Sun, L. Prognostic value of lateral spread response during microvascular decompression for hemifacial spasm. *J. Int. Med. Res.* **2019**, *47*, 6120–6128. [CrossRef] [PubMed]
4. Nugroho, S.W.; Perkasa, S.A.H.; Gunawan, K.; Manuhutu, Y.N.; Rahman, M.A.; Rizky, A. Predicting outcome of hemifacial spasm after microvascular decompression with intraoperative monitoring: A systematic review. *Heliyon* **2021**, *7*, e06115. [CrossRef]
5. Jiang, C.; Xu, W.; Dai, Y.; Lu, T.; Jin, W.; Liang, W. Early permanent disappearance of abnormal muscle response during microvascular decompression for hemifacial spasm: A retrospective clinical study. *Neurosurg. Rev.* **2017**, *40*, 479–484. [CrossRef] [PubMed]
6. Cho, M.; Ji, S.Y.; Go, K.O.; Park, K.S.; Kim, J.M.; Jeon, Y.T.; Ryu, J.H.; Park, S.; Han, J.H. The novel prognostic value of postoperative follow-up lateral spread response after microvascular decompression for hemifacial spasm. *J. Neurosurg.* **2021**, *136*, 1114–1118. [CrossRef]

7. Chung, Y.H.; Kim, W.H.; Lee, J.J.; Yang, S.I.; Lim, S.H.; Seo, D.W.; Park, K.; Chung, I.S. Lateral spread response monitoring during microvascular decompression for hemifacial spasm. Comparison of two targets of partial neuromuscular blockade. *Anaesthesist* 2014, *63*, 122–128. [CrossRef]
8. Chung, Y.H.; Kim, W.H.; Chung, I.S.; Park, K.; Lim, S.H.; Seo, D.W.; Lee, J.J.; Yang, S.I. Effects of partial neuromuscular blockade on lateral spread response monitoring during microvascular decompression surgery. *Clin. Neurophysiol.* 2015, *126*, 2233–2240. [CrossRef] [PubMed]
9. Wilkinson, M.F.; Chowdhury, T.; Mutch, W.A.; Kaufmann, A.M. Is hemifacial spasm a phenomenon of the central nervous system?—The role of desflurane on the lateral spread response. *Clin. Neurophysiol.* 2015, *126*, 1354–1359. [CrossRef]
10. Burke, D.; Bartley, K.; Woodforth, I.J.; Yakoubi, A.; Stephen, J.P. The effects of a volatile anaesthetic on the excitability of human corticospinal axons. *Brain* 2000, *123 Pt 5*, 992–1000. [CrossRef]
11. Thirumala, P.D.; Shah, A.C.; Nikonow, T.N.; Habeych, M.E.; Balzer, J.R.; Crammond, D.J.; Burkhart, L.; Chang, Y.F.; Gardner, P.; Kassam, A.B.; et al. Microvascular decompression for hemifacial spasm: Evaluating outcome prognosticators including the value of intraoperative lateral spread response monitoring and clinical characteristics in 293 patients. *J. Clin. Neurophysiol.* 2011, *28*, 56–66. [CrossRef] [PubMed]
12. Lee, S.H.; Park, B.J.; Shin, H.S.; Park, C.K.; Rhee, B.A.; Lim, Y.J. Prognostic ability of intraoperative electromyographic monitoring during microvascular decompression for hemifacial spasm to predict lateral spread response outcome. *J. Neurosurg.* 2017, *126*, 391–396. [CrossRef]
13. Zhang, J.; Li, Z.H.; Wang, J.F.; Chen, Y.H.; Wang, N.; Wang, Y. Prognostic Value of Abnormal Muscle Response During Microvascular Decompression for Hemifacial Spasm: A Meta-Analysis. *World Neurosurg.* 2020, *137*, 8–17. [CrossRef] [PubMed]
14. Thirumala, P.D.; Altibi, A.M.; Chang, R.; Saca, E.E.; Iyengar, P.; Reddy, R.; Anetakis, K.; Crammond, D.J.; Balzer, J.R.; Sekula, R.F. The Utility of Intraoperative Lateral Spread Recording in Microvascular Decompression for Hemifacial Spasm: A Systematic Review and Meta-Analysis. *Neurosurgery* 2020, *87*, E473–E484. [CrossRef] [PubMed]
15. Kong, D.S.; Park, K.; Shin, B.G.; Lee, J.A.; Eum, D.O. Prognostic value of the lateral spread response for intraoperative electromyography monitoring of the facial musculature during microvascular decompression for hemifacial spasm. *J. Neurosurg.* 2007, *106*, 384–387. [CrossRef]
16. Sekula, R.F., Jr.; Bhatia, S.; Frederickson, A.M.; Jannetta, P.J.; Quigley, M.R.; Small, G.A.; Breisinger, R. Utility of intraoperative electromyography in microvascular decompression for hemifacial spasm: A meta-analysis. *Neurosurg. Focus* 2009, *27*, E10. [CrossRef]
17. Wei, Y.; Yang, W.; Zhao, W.; Pu, C.; Li, N.; Cai, Y.; Shang, H. Microvascular decompression for hemifacial spasm: Can intraoperative lateral spread response monitoring improve surgical efficacy? *J. Neurosurg.* 2018, *128*, 885–890. [CrossRef]
18. Kiya, N.; Bannur, U.; Yamauchi, A.; Yoshida, K.; Kato, Y.; Kanno, T. Monitoring of facial evoked EMG for hemifacial spasm: A critical analysis of its prognostic value. *Acta Neurochir.* 2001, *143*, 365–368. [CrossRef]
19. Yamashita, S.; Kawaguchi, T.; Fukuda, M.; Watanabe, M.; Tanaka, R.; Kameyama, S. Abnormal muscle response monitoring during microvascular decompression for hemifacial spasm. *Acta Neurochir.* 2005, *147*, 933–937; discussion 937–938. [CrossRef]
20. Tobishima, H.; Hatayama, T.; Ohkuma, H. Relation between the persistence of an abnormal muscle response and the long-term clinical course after microvascular decompression for hemifacial spasm. *Neurol. Med. Chir.* 2014, *54*, 474–482. [CrossRef]
21. El Damaty, A.; Rosenstengel, C.; Matthes, M.; Baldauf, J.; Schroeder, H.W. The value of lateral spread response monitoring in predicting the clinical outcome after microvascular decompression in hemifacial spasm: A prospective study on 100 patients. *Neurosurg. Rev.* 2016, *39*, 455–466. [CrossRef] [PubMed]
22. Hatem, J.; Sindou, M.; Vial, C. Intraoperative monitoring of facial EMG responses during microvascular decompression for hemifacial spasm. Prognostic value for long-term outcome: A study in a 33-patient series. *Br. J. Neurosurg.* 2001, *15*, 496–499. [CrossRef]
23. Neves, D.O.; Lefaucheur, J.P.; de Andrade, D.C.; Hattou, M.; Ahdab, R.; Ayache, S.S.; Le Guerinel, C.; Keravel, Y. A reappraisal of the value of lateral spread response monitoring in the treatment of hemifacial spasm by microvascular decompression. *J. Neurol. Neurosurg. Psychiatry* 2009, *80*, 1375–1380. [CrossRef]
24. Jo, K.W.; Kong, D.S.; Park, K. Microvascular decompression for hemifacial spasm: Long-term outcome and prognostic factors, with emphasis on delayed cure. *Neurosurg. Rev.* 2013, *36*, 297–301; discussion 301–292. [CrossRef]
25. Moller, A.R.; Jannetta, P.J. Monitoring facial EMG responses during microvascular decompression operations for hemifacial spasm. *J. Neurosurg.* 1987, *66*, 681–685. [CrossRef] [PubMed]
26. Hirono, S.; Yamakami, I.; Sato, M.; Kado, K.; Fukuda, K.; Nakamura, T.; Higuchi, Y.; Saeki, N. Continuous intraoperative monitoring of abnormal muscle response in microvascular decompression for hemifacial spasm; a real-time navigator for complete relief. *Neurosurg. Rev.* 2014, *37*, 311–319; discussion 319–320. [CrossRef]
27. Haines, S.J.; Torres, F. Intraoperative monitoring of the facial nerve during decompressive surgery for hemifacial spasm. *J. Neurosurg.* 1991, *74*, 254–257. [CrossRef] [PubMed]
28. Kim, C.H.; Kong, D.S.; Lee, J.A.; Kwan, P. The potential value of the disappearance of the lateral spread response during microvascular decompression for predicting the clinical outcome of hemifacial spasms: A prospective study. *Neurosurgery* 2010, *67*, 1581–1587; discussion 1587–1588. [CrossRef]

29. Navarro-Olvera, J.L.; Covaleda-Rodriguez, J.C.; Diaz-Martinez, J.A.; Aguado-Carrillo, G.; Carrillo-Ruiz, J.D.; Velasco-Campos, F. Hemifacial Spasm Associated with Compression of the Facial Colliculus by a Choroid Plexus Papilloma of the Fourth Ventricle. *Ster. Funct. Neurosurg.* **2020**, *98*, 145–149. [CrossRef]
30. Ozaki, K.; Higuchi, Y.; Nakano, S.; Horiguchi, K.; Yamakami, I.; Iwadate, Y. Arachnoid cyst alone causes hemifacial spasm: Illustrative case. *J. Neurosurg. Case Lessons* **2022**, *3*, CASE2275. [CrossRef]
31. Cai, X.; Tang, Y.; Zhao, H.; Chen, Z.; Wang, H.; Zhu, W.; Li, S. A Case Report of Hemifacial Spasm Caused by Vestibular Schwannoma and Literature Review. *Brain Sci.* **2022**, *12*, 1347. [CrossRef] [PubMed]
32. Vrinceanu, D.; Dumitru, M.; Popa-Cherecheanu, M.; Marinescu, A.N.; Patrascu, O.-M.; Bobirca, F. Extracranial Facial Nerve Schwannoma—Histological Surprise or Therapeutic Planning? *Medicina* **2023**, *59*, 1167. [CrossRef]
33. Kameyama, S.; Masuda, H.; Shirozu, H.; Ito, Y.; Sonoda, M.; Kimura, J. Ephaptic transmission is the origin of the abnormal muscle response seen in hemifacial spasm. *Clin. Neurophysiol.* **2016**, *127*, 2240–2245. [CrossRef]
34. Yamashita, S.; Kawaguchi, T.; Fukuda, M.; Suzuki, K.; Watanabe, M.; Tanaka, R.; Kameyama, S. Lateral spread response elicited by double stimulation in patients with hemifacial spasm. *Muscle Nerve* **2002**, *25*, 845–849. [CrossRef]
35. Wilkinson, M.F.; Chowdhury, T.; Kaufmann, A.M. Using strength-duration analysis to identify the afferent limb of the lateral spread response in hemifacial spasm patients during microvascular decompression surgery. *J. Clin. Neurosci.* **2020**, *74*, 6–10. [CrossRef]
36. Moller, A.R.; Jannetta, P.J. Microvascular decompression in hemifacial spasm: Intraoperative electrophysiological observations. *Neurosurgery* **1985**, *16*, 612–618. [CrossRef] [PubMed]
37. Poignonec, S.; Vidailhet, M.; Lamas, G.; Fligny, I.; Soudant, J.; Jedynak, P.; Willer, J.C. Electrophysiological evidence for central hyperexcitability of facial motoneurons in hemifacial spasm. In *The Facial Nerve: An Update on Clinical and Basic Neuroscience Research*; Springer: Berlin/Heidelberg, Germany, 1994; pp. 216–217. [CrossRef]
38. Yamakami, I.; Oka, N.; Higuchi, Y. Hyperactivity of the facial nucleus produced by chronic electrical stimulation in rats. *J. Clin. Neurosci.* **2007**, *14*, 459–463. [CrossRef]
39. Ishikawa, M.; Namiki, J.; Takase, M.; Ohira, T.; Nakamura, A.; Toya, S. Effect of repetitive stimulation on lateral spreads and F-waves in hemifacial spasm. *J. Neurol. Sci.* **1996**, *142*, 99–106. [CrossRef]
40. Ishikawa, M.; Ohira, T.; Namiki, J.; Gotoh, K.; Takase, M.; Toya, S. Electrophysiological investigation of hemifacial spasm: F-waves of the facial muscles. *Acta Neurochir.* **1996**, *138*, 24–32. [CrossRef]
41. Ishikawa, M.; Ohira, T.; Namiki, J.; Ishihara, M.; Takase, M.; Toya, S. F-wave in patients with hemifacial spasm: Observations during microvascular decompression operations. *Neurol. Res.* **1996**, *18*, 2–8. [CrossRef]
42. Trontelj, J.V.; Trontelj, M. F-responses of human facial muscles. A single motoneurone study. *J. Neurol. Sci.* **1973**, *20*, 211–222. [CrossRef]

Disclaimer/Publisher's Note: The statements, opinions and data contained in all publications are solely those of the individual author(s) and contributor(s) and not of MDPI and/or the editor(s). MDPI and/or the editor(s) disclaim responsibility for any injury to people or property resulting from any ideas, methods, instructions or products referred to in the content.

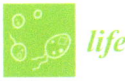

Article

Penetrating Offenders in Hemifacial Spasm: Surgical Tactics and Prognosis

Hyun-Seok Lee [1] and Kwan Park [1,2,*]

[1] Department of Neurosurgery, Konkuk University Medical Center, Seoul 05030, Republic of Korea; 20220205@kuh.ac.kr
[2] Department of Neurosurgery, Sungkyunkwan University School of Medicine, Seoul 06351, Republic of Korea
* Correspondence: kwanpark@skku.edu; Tel.: +82-2-2030-7357

Abstract: (1) Background: In cases of hemifacial spasm (HFS), there are various patterns related to the vascular compression of the facial nerve, including a very rare form that is seen when the offending vessel penetrates the facial nerve. However, there have been few reports in the literature regarding the associated surgical techniques and postoperative prognosis. (2) Methods: A retrospective review was conducted of 4755 patients who underwent microvascular decompression (MVD) surgery from April 1997 to June 2023. In total, 8 out of the 4755 patients (0.2%) exhibited a penetrating offending vessel; the medical and surgical records of these 8 patients were then analyzed. Surgery was then attempted to maximally decompress the penetrating offender. (3) Results: Seven out of the eight patients (87.5%) were spasm-free immediately after surgery, and one had only 10% residual spasm compared to their preoperative condition. That patient was also spasm-free one year later. Postoperative facial palsy occurred in one patient (12.5%) who was assessed as grade II in the House–Brackmann grading system. In another patient, the resection of a small facial nerve bundle did not result in facial palsy. There were no cases of hearing loss or other complications. (4) Conclusions: Decompressing the penetrating offender did not increase the incidence of facial palsy, and the prognosis for hemifacial spasms was good. Therefore, when a penetrating pattern was encountered during MVD surgery, decompression between the penetrating offender and the facial nerve may offer good results.

Keywords: hemifacial spasm; microvascular decompression; penetrating offender

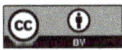

Citation: Lee, H.-S.; Park, K. Penetrating Offenders in Hemifacial Spasm: Surgical Tactics and Prognosis. *Life* 2023, 13, 2021. https://doi.org/10.3390/life13102021

Academic Editor: Alfredo Conti

Received: 3 August 2023
Revised: 22 September 2023
Accepted: 5 October 2023
Published: 7 October 2023

Copyright: © 2023 by the authors. Licensee MDPI, Basel, Switzerland. This article is an open access article distributed under the terms and conditions of the Creative Commons Attribution (CC BY) license (https://creativecommons.org/licenses/by/4.0/).

1. Introduction

Hemifacial spasm (HFS) is a form of neurovascular syndrome that is usually due to neurovascular compression in the root exit zone (REZ) of the facial nerve. The disease presents as an intermittent, involuntary facial twitching movement that usually begins in the eyelids and progresses to involve the entire system of ipsilateral facial muscles. The result is an asymmetrical appearance of the face, due to the strengthening of the facial muscles on the side of the spasm. The pathogenesis of HFS is thought to be derived from the vascular compression of the facial nerve that emerges close to the brain stem, leading to demyelination and ephaptic transmissions [1,2].

There are various treatments for HFS, such as medications and *Botulinum toxin* injections, but, compared to these treatments, MVD surgery is the most effective treatment and one that completely resolves the symptoms [3–9]. The overall rate of being spasm-free after MVD surgery in patients with HFS is approximately 90%, with the other 10% of patients experiencing a recurrence of facial spasm or surgical failure [3,10,11]. In the 10% of cases where this facial spasm did not resolve itself, in rare instances, the surgeons may have encountered unusual patterns of compression that would make for a very difficult surgical challenge. In 2007, we categorized six different patterns of facial nerve compression, describing their clinical implications and prognosis [12]. As the number of cases increased, we began to see other rare and difficult cases [11], one of which was the perforating pattern, where the offending vessel penetrated the facial nerve.

There are currently no reports as to how this pattern should be decompressed, whether complications such as postoperative facial palsy and hearing loss after decompression are likely, and with what factors they are associated; this is the focus of the current study.

2. Materials and Methods

2.1. Patient Cohort

We retrospectively analyzed the medical records of 4755 patients who underwent MVD with HFS from April 1997 to June 2023. All MVD surgeries were performed by a single surgeon (Kwan Park), with facial nerve motor-evoked potential (facial MEP), lateral spread response (LSR), and brain stem auditory evoked potential (BAEP) being monitored by an experienced neurophysiologist. The clinical information and details of the offending vessels of all 4755 patients are summarized in Table 1. Cases with 2 or 3 offending vessels present a sandwich pattern or a tandem pattern, in which the vessels are compressed together.

Table 1. Clinical characteristics of 4755 patients treated with MVD surgery for hemifacial spasm.

Clinical Characteristics	
Median age at MVD (range (years))	53 (17–75)
Sex (male:female)	1395: 3360
Operation side (left:right)	2441: 2314
Median duration of symptom (in months)	48
Average length of hospital stays, in days (range)	7.4 (3–185)
Penetrating offender type (%)	8 (0.2%)
Offending vessel, *n* (%)	
AICA	2635 (55.4%)
PICA	1011 (21.3%)
AICA-PICA common trunk	14 (0.3%)
VA	50 (1.1%)
AICA + PICA	275 (5.8%)
AICA + VA	469 (9.9%)
PICA + VA	162 (3.4%)
AICA + vein	21 (0.4%)
PICA + vein	5 (0.1%)
AICA + PICA + VA	61 (1.3%)
Vein only	44 (0.9%)
Other vessels	5 (0.1%)
Cannot be confirmed	3 (0.0%)

MVD: microvascular decompression, AICA: anterior inferior cerebellar artery, PICA: posterior inferior cerebellar artery, VA: vertebral artery.

Of these 4755 patients, 8 exhibited the penetrating type of pattern (0.2%). All penetrating offenders were confirmed via surgical microscopic findings. Of these 8 patients, 4 were male, 4 were female, 5 had right-sided lesions, and 3 had left-sided lesions. The median age of the patients was 41.5 years (an age range of 23–67). Of the 8 patients, the two oldest patients (67 and 55 years old) had underlying hypertension and were on anti-hypertensive medication, and the next-oldest patient (49 years old) was taking medication for diabetes mellitus. The other 5 patients had no underlying medical conditions.

The degree of preoperative facial spasm was analyzed using our previously published SMC grading system [13,14]. Grade I refers to situations when the spasm is localized to the periocular area, whereas grade II refers to situations when the involuntary movement spreads to other areas of the ipsilateral face and affects other muscles, such as the orbicularis oculi, frontalis, zygomaticus, mentalis, and platysma. Grade III represents the disruption of vision due to frequent spasms, whereas grade IV refers to a persistent spasm resulting in significant facial asymmetry. Among the 8 patients under study, the degree of preoperative spasm was classified as grade II in 3 patients (37.5%), as grade III in 3 patients (37.5%), and as grade IV in 1 patient (12.5%), whereas the grade of the final patient could not be determined.

The mean duration of postoperative spasm symptoms was 60.4 months (in a range of 18–120 months), with 4 patients being prescribed medication for preoperative treatment, 4 patients receiving botulinum toxin (Botox) injections, and 2 patients receiving both Botox injections and medication. One patient was prescribed medication and acupuncture at an oriental medicine clinic, whereas another received botulinum toxin treatment and acupuncture at an oriental medicine clinic. The final 2 patients received no other treatment prior to MVD surgery (see Table 2).

Table 2. Clinical characteristics of 8 patients with penetrating offenders.

No.	Sex	Age	Laterality	Preoperative Spasm Grade	Preoperative Treatment	Symptom Duration (Month)	Medical History
1	M	55	R	N/A	None	120	HTN
2	M	67	R	IV	Medication, Oriental Medicine	84	HTN
3	F	49	L	II	BTX injection, Oriental Medicine	48	DM
4	F	44	L	III	BTX injection	18	None
5	F	39	L	III	Medication	78	None
6	M	23	R	II	None	46	None
7	F	36	R	III	Medication, BTX injection	61	None
8	M	34	R	II	Medication, BTX injection	28	None

No: number, M: male; F: female, R: right, L: left, BTX: botulinum toxin, HTN: hypertension, DM: diabetes mellitus, N/A: not available or not mentioned.

2.2. Operative Technique and Intraoperative Monitoring

The patients underwent MVD surgery via a retromastoid suboccipital craniotomy (RMSOC) while in the park bench lateral position. All patients underwent MVD surgery with intraoperative neuromonitoring, which consists of a real-time BAEP monitoring method [14] and the facial motor evoke potential (fMEP) and lateral spread response (LSR), i.e., abnormal muscle response (AMR). The evaluations of intraoperative LSR disappearance were categorized as follows: disappearance after durotomy and cerebrospinal fluid drain from the lateral medullary cistern; disappearance after immediate decompression, where the amplitude of LSR decreases but does not disappear completely; and no disappearance. In all patients, decompression of the neurovascular conflict zone was performed using Teflon felt.

2.3. Assessment of Postoperative Outcomes

All patients underwent preoperative intra-auditory canal (IAC) magnetic resonance imaging (MRI) to identify the most likely offender, the results of which were reviewed by an experienced neuroradiologist. Preoperative audiometry, including pure tone audiometry (PTA) and speech audiometry (SA), was performed, and the patients also underwent preoperative lateral spread response (LSR) testing conducted by an experienced neurophysiologist. Computed tomography (CT) of the brain was performed immediately after the operation in all patients, and a temporal bone CT scan was also taken postoperatively on day three in all patients. Postoperative pure tone audiometry (PTA) and SA (speech audiometry) was performed postoperatively on days 4–5, and the results were then compared with the preoperative results. The patient's spasms were assessed preoperatively, immediately after surgery (until 5 days after surgery), 1 month after surgery, 1 year after surgery, and up to 2 years after surgery. The lateral spread response (LSR) was examined just before the patient's outpatient department visit after their discharge.

3. Results

In the eight patients identified, the offending vessels were as follows: the anterior inferior cerebellar artery (AICA) in six patients (75%), the branch of the AICA in one patient

(12.5%), and the posterior inferior cerebellar artery (PICA) in one patient (12.5%). The intraoperative LSR disappearance pattern was IIa (i.e., the vessel disappeared immediately after decompression) in seven patients (87.5%) and IIc (i.e., a 50% reduction with a residual presence) in one patient (12.5%).

An intraoperative change in BAEP was seen in three patients. Two had a 50% decrease in amplitude, prolonged by 1.6 ms and 2.0 ms, respectively, with full recovery by the end of surgery, and one exhibited the loss of all but wave I, with 80% recovery by the end of surgery. There was no long-term hearing loss after surgery. It is worth noting that three of the eight patients underwent surgery before our real-time BAEP monitoring method was established. All three exhibited no postoperative hearing loss.

Postoperative facial palsy was seen in one patient (12.5%). Immediately after surgery, the palsy was classified as House–Brackmann grade III–IV, and the patient showed gradual improvement to grade II but still demonstrated residual issues. The other seven patients (87.5%) exhibited no facial palsy.

The prognosis of postoperative spasm was evaluated immediately after surgery (around 5 days), 1 month after surgery, 1 year after surgery, and 2 years after surgery. In seven of the eight patients (87.5%), there was no spasm immediately after surgery. One patient had 10% residual spasms compared to their preoperative state. At 1 month after surgery, one of the seven patients who had no spasm immediately after surgery had 10% residual spasm compared to their preoperative state, and the one patient with 10% residual spasm had worsened slightly to 20%. At 1 year after surgery, one patient with a new 10% spasm at 1 month had similar symptoms, and one patient with symptoms shortly after surgery was then spasm-free. Of the other six patients who were asymptomatic immediately after surgery, three remained spasm-free, one patient was lost to follow-up, one patient with no spasm developed a spasm of approximately 10% compared to preoperative levels, and one had not yet reached the one-year postoperative mark. Upon follow-up in year 2, two patients with a residual 10% of spasms at 1 year after surgery were completely spasm-free after 2 years, and one patient who had spasms immediately after surgery and after 1 month remained spasm-free at 1 and 2 years after surgery. Of the three patients who were followed up, one was lost to follow-up, and two continued to be spasm-free (one of these two is a patient who developed facial palsy after MVD surgery) (see Table 3).

Table 3. Intraoperative findings and prognosis of 8 patients with penetrating offenders.

No.	Offender	LSR Disappearance	Intraoperative BAEP Change	Postoperative Spasm (%)				Postoperative Facial Palsy	Surgical Findings
				~5D	~1M	~1Y	~2Y		
1	AICA	Disappeared after decompression	No change	0	0	0	0	H-B II	N/A
2	AICA	Disappeared after decompression	No change	0	0	N/A	N/A	None	N/A
3	AICA	Disappeared after decompression	No change	0	0	0	0	None	N/A
4	AICA	Disappeared after decompression	50% decreased, delay to 2.0 ms, full recovery	0	10	10	0	None	Only the medial side was decompressed because the lateral side was difficult to decompress; LSR disappearance after decompression
5	PICA	Disappeared after decompression	All but wave I disappeared, recover to 80%	10	20	0	0	None	90% nerve fascicle on the medial side of the PICA, and 10% on the lateral side, with adhesion; therefore, a minor portion was resected after detachment. Weak response from the orbicularis oris when stimulated before resection.

Table 3. Cont.

No.	Offender	LSR Disappearance	Intraoperative BAEP Change	Postoperative Spasm (%)				Postoperative Facial Palsy	Surgical Findings
				~5D	~1M	~1Y	~2Y		
6	AICA	Decline amplitude, but not disappeared	50% decreased, delay to 1.6 ms, full recovery	0	0	0	N/A	None	On the lateral side, the AICA circled between CNs 7 and 8, penetrated the facial nerve medially, and exited laterally.
7	AICA	Disappeared after decompression	No change	0	0	10	0	None	The facial nerve was split, and the AICA passed through the center; a small piece of Teflon felt was placed inside the split to decompress the nerve.
8	Branch of AICA	Disappeared after decompression	No change	0	0	N/A	N/A	None	LSR disappeared when decompressing the penetrating vessel.

No: number, LSR: lateral spread response, BAEP: brain stem auditory evoked potential, D: day, M: month, Y: year, AICA: anterior inferior cerebellar artery, PICA: posterior inferior cerebellar artery, N/A: not available or not mentioned, H-B: House–Brackmann grade, CN: cranial nerve.

Illustrative Case

A 34-year-old man developed twitching of the right eye and mouth two and a half years prior to admission and was subsequently diagnosed with HFS. After medication and botulinum toxin treatments, he was referred for MVD surgery and visited our institution. His pre-operative spasm grade was SMC grade II; magnetic resonance imaging showed a complex REZ, which the radiologist interpreted as demonstrating that both the AICA and PICA were in contact in the REZ (Figure 1). LSR was observed in the right facial nerve during an examination with electrical stimulation (Figure 2a).

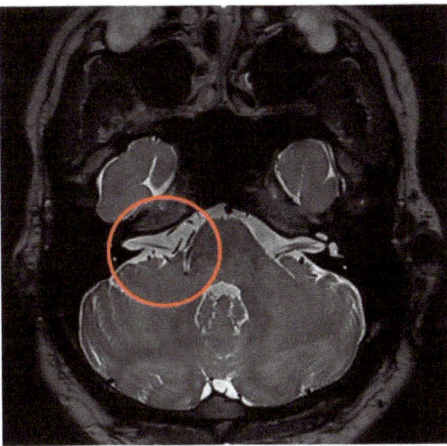

Figure 1. A 34-year-old man with right HFS, shown in a preoperative proton density-weighted (PD-weighted) magnetic resonance image (MRI). At the exit region of the right facial nerve root, the right anterior inferior cerebellar artery (AICA) and posterior inferior cerebellar artery (PICA) have a complex appearance (red circle).

Intraoperatively, the offending vessel was a branch of the AICA, which was penetrating the facial nerve (Figure 3a–c).

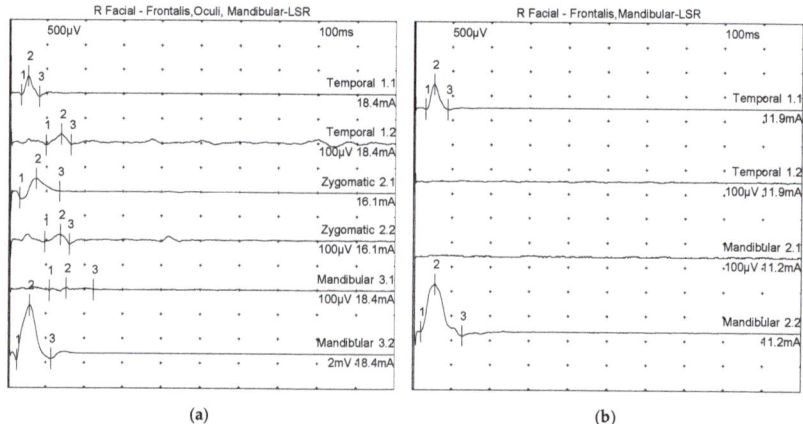

Figure 2. Right-side facial nerve conduction studies of a patient acting as an illustrative case. In both picture, each number is a reference point for measurement. '1' is onset latency, from '1' to '2' is onset to peak amplitude, and from '2' to '3' is peak to peak amplitude: (**a**) the preoperative examination showed lateral spread response (LSR); (**b**) in the postoperative examination, the LSR seen before surgery has disappeared.

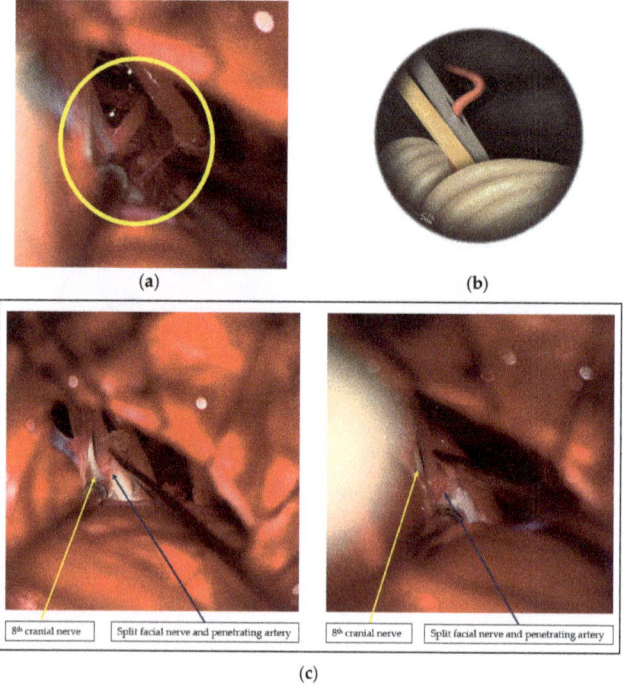

Figure 3. Intraoperative microscopic findings for the illustrative case: (**a**) a branch of the anterior inferior cerebellar artery (AICA) passing through the facial nerve, with no other indentations visible in the root exit zone (yellow circle); (**b**) illustration of the surgical visualization before decompression. The illustration shows the offending artery passing through the facial nerve; (**c**) Microscopic findings with decompression in progress on both the left and right sides. The yellow arrow is the 8th cranial nerve, and the navy arrow shows a branch of the AICA penetrating the facial nerve, both images.

First, we checked whether there was a space between the facial nerve and the penetrating artery and carefully dissected the facial nerve and the penetrating branch of the AICA to decompress in all directions (Figure 4a–c).

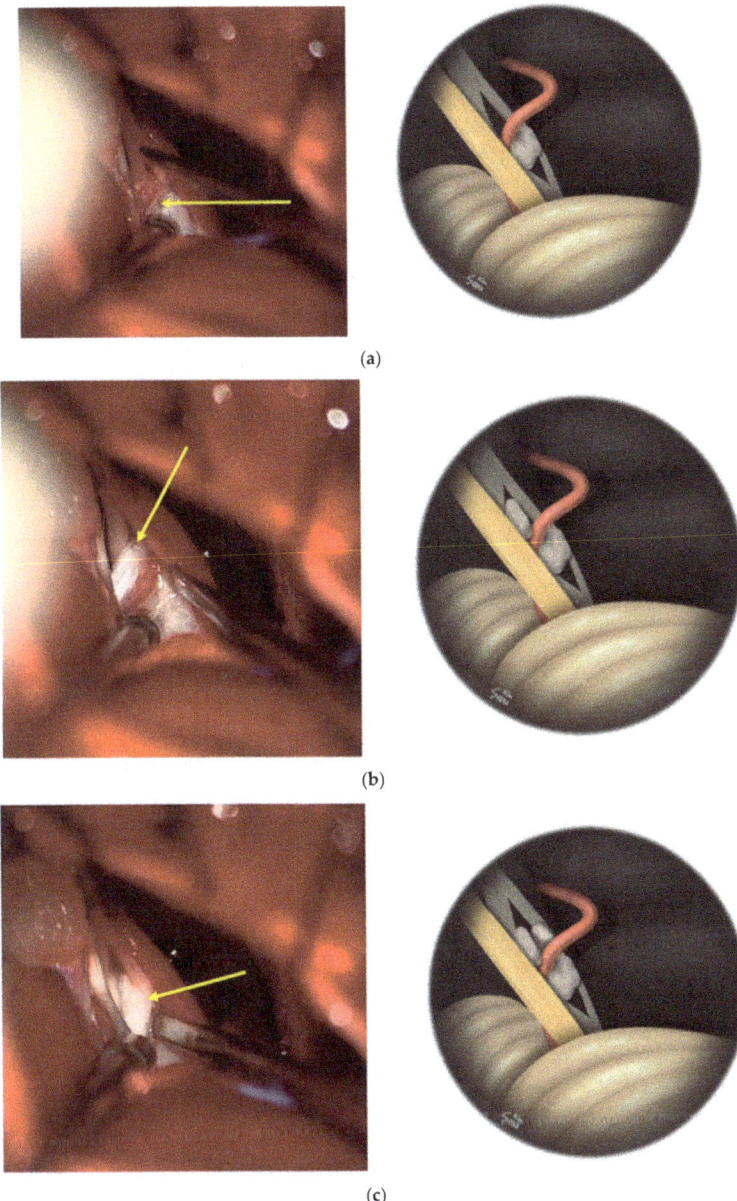

Figure 4. (**a**) First, decompression was started with small Teflon felt, from inferior side of the perforation site (yellow arrow); (**b**) Next, decompression was performed in supero-medial (supero-anterior) side (yellow arrow); (**c**) Lastly, the supero-lateral (supero-posterior) side decompression was performed (yellow arrow) to decompress in all directions of the perforation site, and the lateral spread response (LSR) subsequently disappeared.

Immediately after decompression, the LSR disappeared, and the surgery was completed. The patient in question had no spasms and no facial palsy immediately after surgery and was discharged on day 5 with no further complications. Postoperative audiometry showed no hearing difficulty. One month after surgery, the patient still had no spasms, and the disappearance of LSR was confirmed via a postoperative neurophysiological study (Figure 2b).

4. Discussion

In 2008, we analyzed 236 cases of HFS, reporting several patterns of neurovascular compression of the facial nerve [12]. At the time, we categorized the patterns into six types: arachnoid (28.0%), loop (4.7%), and perforator (24.6%), which are generally compressed by a single causative vessel, and branch (7.6%), sandwich (11.9%), and tandem (22.0%), which are compressed by two or more vessels [12]. There were also three cases (1.3%) in which the pattern category was not clear at the time. As the number of surgeries grew, we added new neurovascular compression patterns. One is the encircling pattern, in which the vessel encircles the facial nerve in a 270-degree or even 360-degree loop. Another is the penetrating type, in which the culprit vessel passes completely through the facial nerve [11]. These patterns of neurovascular compression are particularly challenging to operate on, especially the penetrating type, as they are often not clearly identifiable from a magnetic resonance image, and cases are so rare that there are no established decompression methods.

There is a very limited corpus of literature on HFS caused by a penetrating offender; however, a report was published for a single case in 2015. Oh et al. reported a left HFS presenting in a 20-year-old male patient. The penetrating offender in this patient was the AICA; after decompression, the spasm disappeared, but definite facial palsy occurred [15]. From this case report and from our study, it is apparent that HFS caused by the penetrating type occurs at a relatively young age compared to the general population. Typically, HFS is reported to be more prevalent in those in their 40s and 50s [16,17]. Similarly, when analyzing all 4755 of our cases, the median patient age was 53 years old (range: 17–75), and the median age of the eight patients with the penetrating type was 41.5 years (range: 23–67). This has the clinical implication that symptoms occur at a younger age in the case of penetrating offenders (Table 4). It is conceivable that the symptoms occur at a younger age because the causative vessels (mostly the AICA) directly irritate the facial nerve. It is also possible that if the facial nerve is separated, myelination is less well developed than if it is not separated. Reports of duplication of the facial nerve in the mastoid segment or its distal part are rare in the ENT department [18–20], but there are few reports of duplication in the intracranial portion from the root exit zone of the facial nerve to the entry point of the IAC; therefore, further anatomic and pathologic studies are required.

Table 4. Factors correlating with penetrating offenders and hemifacial spasm.

Factor	Univariate (p-Values)	Multivariate (p-Values)
Sex (female)	0.213	0.258
Age	0.038	0.052
Lesion side (Right)	0.439	0.435
Symptom duration	1.000	0.621
Hospital days	0.808	0.694

In general, the same trend is seen in our 4755 cases; the AICA is the most common offending vessel for HFS, whereas the second most common is the PICA, followed by the AICA and other vessel compressions in conjunction (see Table 1) [12,21]. The PICA originates in the VA and emerges from the ventral to the dorsal side of the brain stem, usually at the level of the lower cranial nerves (at the 9th, 10th, and 11th cranial nerves), forming a hairpin structure (caudal loop) downward [21,22]. Therefore, while it is possible for a vessel to loop and compress the root exit zone of the facial nerve or encircle the facial nerve, it is structurally difficult for the vessel to pass through the facial nerve. In the cases examined in this study, only one out of the eight (12.5%) showed penetration by the PICA, and almost all of them showed penetration by the AICA (87.5%) (see Table 3). The facioauditory primordium, the origin of the facial nerve, appears in the third week of gestation. It then splits into two sections at the end of the fourth week and is complete by the fifth or sixth week of gestation [15,23]. The AICA begins to develop later, in the gestational fourth or fifth month, when the facial nerve is already fairly well-developed [15,24]. Therefore, facial nerve penetration by the artery is thought to occur as the facial nerve attempts to pass through the divergence that appears after 5–6 weeks of gestation.

In all patients, we attempted complete decompression in all directions and a 360-degree inspection in all patients, as in the illustrative case. First, check for space in the perforating artery and facial nerves with a micro-dissector or micro-bayonet forceps. Then, carefully dissect, and, when space is made, put small Teflon felt in there to first decompress. Next, we decompressed in all possible directions (Figure 4a–c). Decompressing the location between the facial nerve and penetrating vessels was associated with a very low probability of postoperative facial palsy. In one case, we decompressed only the medial side in a patient presenting a difficult dissection. As the LSR improved when the medial side was decompressed in this patient, the lateral side, which was difficult to meticulous dissection and presented a high risk of facial nerve injury upon dissection, was left untreated, and the operation was terminated. Postoperatively, the facial spasm had been resolved. In another case, the fascicle of the facial nerves was divided into 90% and 10% divisions by a penetrating PICA. In this patient, decompression of the thin side of the divided nerve fascicle was not possible. We first stimulated the thin nerve fascicle with a direct nerve stimulator to check the facial muscle response, which showed a small response by the orbicularis oris muscle. The thin fascicle that could not be decompressed and dissected was then excised, and the neurovascular compression between the large fascicle and the offending vessel was decompressed with Teflon felt. Immediately after decompression, the LSR disappeared. After the surgery, facial spasms remained at 10–20% compared with preoperative conditions; notably, there was no postoperative facial palsy. The absence of facial palsy despite the resection of a portion of the facial nerve in this patient was thought to be related to the innervation of the distal branch of the facial nerve. The facial nerve has five branches, namely, the temporal, zygomatic, buccal, marginal, and cervical branches, each of which is known to have interconnections, and these connections vary considerably [25–28]. In addition, several studies have shown that facial nerve is anatomically connected to the trigeminal nerve [25,27–31], vestibulocochlear nerve [25,32], glossopharyngeal nerve [25,33], and vagus nerve [25], as well as the cervical plexus [25,34]. In particular, there are numerous interconnections and variations between the zygomatic and buccal branches of the facial nerve, which can confound LSR measurements; we have previously published a paper on how to measure LSR in this context [26]. As the orbicularis oris muscle is often innervated by both the zygomatic and buccal branches, we consider that facial palsy did not occur despite the partial resection of the nerve fascicle during the operation. Maximal decompression using Teflon felt placed between the penetrating vessel and the facial nerve was performed in all eight patients, as mentioned, and attempted decompression in all compression sites. One patient developed postoperative facial palsy that was classified as House–Brackmann grade II, but the other seven patients exhibited no facial palsy and had good prognoses regarding postoperative facial spasm (see Table 3). Therefore, even if the artery were going through the facial nerve, it is considered necessary to actively dissect and decompress it. Yet, the most important thing we and other very experienced surgeons of more than 4000 cases emphasize is to check the neurovascular conflict completely, it is important to check the full inspection of facial nerve and entire 360 degrees of REZ if possible [35]. Also, even if you encounter a perforating artery, you should look for offenders in the REZ. This is because MVD of HFS is not an emergency surgery, but a functional neurosurgery, and it is recommended to decompress all offenders safely.

There is also a nervus intermedius that can be confused with a split in the facial nerve. The nervus intermedius was first identified in 1563; it was first named "portio media intercommunicantem faciei et nervum auditorium" in 1777 by Heinrich August Wrisberg [36,37]. The nervus intermedius is thus named because it is located between the facial nerve and the superior portion of the vestibular cochlear nerve [37,38]. The nervus intermedius carries parasympathetic nerve fibers to the nasopalatine and lacrimal glands, conducting sensory information from facial areas such as the concha of the ear and the nose [37–41]. Irritation of the nervus intermedius can cause geniculate neuralgia, which is expressed as intermittent but severe sharp pains deep in the ear, accompanied by the disruption of salivation, the sense of taste, and lacrimation [42]. Geniculate neuralgia can also be caused by neurovascular compression, which is an indicator of the need for MVD surgery. Lovely and Jannetta reported on 14 cases of MVD surgery in patients with geniculate neuralgia [43]. In their paper, they reported that vascular compression of the nervus intermedius was present in the surgical findings and correlated with symptoms such as deep ear pain [43]. In surgical findings that appear to show a perforating offender, it is possible to differentiate between the perforating offender and the nervus intermedius by tracing the entire course of the facial nerve. It may be helpful to perform direct nerve stimulation to check the response of the facial muscles. As mentioned above, the nervus intermedius is mainly a sensory nerve; when stimulated, it manifests as ear pain [38], rather than as a facial muscle response. It is also thought to be helpful in the differentiation of preoperative symptoms.

A limitation of this study is the small cohort of eight cases. This refers to 8 out of 4755 cases, so a very small probability of 0.2%. This means that the chances of actually encountering a perforating offender during MVD surgery are very low. In addition, this study was based on data regarding the experiences of a single surgeon, and it was not possible to compare the findings with results from other institutions. This is because there are few reports regarding HFS with a perforating offender that are available from other institutions. However, this limitation also means that our surgical method can act as a reference for the operation. As more data are accumulated from continuing MVD surgeries, in the future, we expect to analyze the prognoses and casual factors in a large series.

5. Conclusions

In as little as 0.2% of the 4755 cases examined in this study, offenders of the penetrating type are very rare, but they do exist. Cases of penetrating offenders in the context of HFS have been reported very rarely, and there is no established policy for decompression. In our experience, when the penetrating offender and the facial nerve fascicle are delicately dissected and decompressed using a small piece of Teflon felt, the facial spasm is resolved, and the likelihood of postoperative facial palsy is very low. In the case where it was necessary to cut a minor portion of a facial nerve that was difficult to decompress, it was found that the patient recovered without exhibiting facial palsy.

The statistical analysis of the factors involved showed that such patients were treated at a relatively young age compared to the general age of HFS patients. For this reason, in HFS cases at a relatively young age, when the offending vessels in the root exit zone are unclear on an MRI scan, it is advisable to consider the possibility that the offending vessel is of the penetrating type. In addition, if encountering a penetrating offender during MVD surgery, it is recommended that the surgeon should not hesitate but instead conduct careful dissection and complete decompression.

Author Contributions: Conceptualization, K.P.; Writing—original draft, H.-S.L.; Writing—review & editing, H.-S.L.; Supervision, K.P. All authors have read and agreed to the published version of the manuscript.

Funding: This research received no external funding.

Institutional Review Board Statement: This study was conducted in accordance with the Declaration of Helsinki and was approved by the Institutional Review Board of Konkuk University Medical Center (2023-07-008).

Informed Consent Statement: Informed consent was obtained from all subjects involved in the study.

Data Availability Statement: All data included in this study can be provided by contacting hs5937@hanmail.net.

Conflicts of Interest: The authors declare no conflict of interest.

References

1. Gardner, W.J. Cross talk—The paradoxical transmission of a nerve impulse. *Arch. Neurol.* **1966**, *14*, 149–156. [CrossRef] [PubMed]
2. Nielsen, V.K. Pathophysiology of hemifacial spasm: I. Ephaptic transmission and ectopic excitation. *Neurology* **1984**, *34*, 418–426. [CrossRef] [PubMed]
3. Miller, L.E.; Miller, V.M. Safety and effectiveness of microvascular decompression for treatment of hemifacial spasm: A systematic review. *Br. J. Neurosurg.* **2012**, *26*, 438–444. [CrossRef] [PubMed]
4. Bigder, M.G.; Kaufmann, A.M. Failed microvascular decompression surgery for hemifacial spasm due to persistent neurovascular compression: An analysis of reoperations. *J. Neurosurg.* **2016**, *124*, 90–95. [CrossRef] [PubMed]
5. Sindou, M.; Mercier, P. Microvascular decompression for hemifacial spasm: Outcome on spasm and complications. A review. *Neurochirurgie* **2018**, *64*, 106–116. [CrossRef]
6. McLaughlin, M.R.; Jannetta, P.J.; Clyde, B.L.; Subach, B.R.; Comey, C.H.; Resnick, D.K. Microvascular decompression of cranial nerves: Lessons learned after 4400 operations. *J. Neurosurg.* **1999**, *90*, 1–8. [CrossRef]
7. Sindou, M.P. Microvascular decompression for primary hemifacial spasm. Importance of intraoperative neurophysiological monitoring. *Acta Neurochir.* **2005**, *147*, 1019–1026, discussion 1026. [CrossRef]
8. Kalkanis, S.N.; Eskandar, E.N.; Carter, B.S.; Barker, F.G., 2nd. Microvascular decompression surgery in the United States, 1996 to 2000: Mortality rates, morbidity rates, and the effects of hospital and surgeon volumes. *Neurosurgery* **2003**, *52*, 1251–1261, discussion 1261–1252. [CrossRef]
9. Barker, F.G., 2nd; Jannetta, P.J.; Bissonette, D.J.; Shields, P.T.; Larkins, M.V.; Jho, H.D. Microvascular decompression for hemifacial spasm. *J. Neurosurg.* **1995**, *82*, 201–210. [CrossRef]
10. Lee, S.; Park, S.K.; Joo, B.E.; Lee, J.A.; Park, K. Vascular Complications in Microvascular Decompression: A Survey of 4000 Operations. *World Neurosurg.* **2019**, *130*, e577–e582. [CrossRef]
11. Lee, S.; Joo, K.M.; Park, K. Challenging Microvascular Decompression Surgery for Hemifacial Spasm. *World Neurosurg.* **2021**, *151*, e94–e99. [CrossRef] [PubMed]
12. Park, J.S.; Kong, D.S.; Lee, J.A.; Park, K. Hemifacial spasm: Neurovascular compressive patterns and surgical significance. *Acta Neurochir.* **2008**, *150*, 235–241, discussion 241. [CrossRef] [PubMed]
13. Park, J.S.; Kong, D.S.; Lee, J.A.; Park, K. Chronologic analysis of symptomatic change following microvascular decompression for hemifacial spasm: Value for predicting midterm outcome. *Neurosurg. Rev.* **2008**, *31*, 413–418, discussion 418–419. [CrossRef]
14. Lee, J.A.; Jo, K.W.; Kong, D.S.; Park, K. Using the new clinical grading scale for quantification of the severity of hemifacial spasm: Correlations with a quality of life scale. *Stereotact. Funct. Neurosurg.* **2012**, *90*, 16–19. [CrossRef] [PubMed]
15. Oh, C.H.; Shim, Y.S.; Park, H.; Kim, E.Y. A case of hemifacial spasm caused by an artery passing through the facial nerve. *J Korean Neurosurg. Soc.* **2015**, *57*, 221–224. [CrossRef]
16. Tan, E.K.; Jankovic, J. Psychogenic hemifacial spasm. *J. Neuropsychiatry Clin. Neurosci.* **2001**, *13*, 380–384. [CrossRef]
17. Wang, A.; Jankovic, J. Hemifacial spasm: Clinical findings and treatment. *Muscle Nerve* **1998**, *21*, 1740–1747. [CrossRef]
18. Eide, J.; Isaac, A.; Maddalozzo, J. Facial Nerve Duplication and First Branchial Cleft Cysts: An Association in an Uncommon Pathology. *Otolaryngol. Head Neck Surg.* **2019**, *161*, 904–905. [CrossRef]
19. Hinson, D.; Poteet, P.; Bower, C. Duplicated facial nerve trunk with a first branchial cleft cyst. *Laryngoscope* **2014**, *124*, 662–664. [CrossRef]
20. Jakkani, R.K.; Ki, R.; Karnawat, A.; Vittal, R.; Kumar, A.D. Congenital duplication of mastoid segment of facial nerve: A rare case report. *Indian J. Radiol. Imaging* **2013**, *23*, 35–37. [CrossRef]
21. Mercier, P.; Bernard, F. Surgical anatomy for hemifacial spasm. *Neurochirurgie* **2018**, *64*, 124–132. [CrossRef] [PubMed]
22. Giotta Lucifero, A.; Baldoncini, M.; Bruno, N.; Tartaglia, N.; Ambrosi, G.; Marseglia, G.L.; Galzio, R.; Campero, A.; Hernesniemi, J.; Luzzi, S. Microsurgical Neurovascular Anatomy of the Brain: The Posterior Circulation (Part II). *Acta Biomed.* **2021**, *92*, e2021413. [CrossRef]
23. Sataloff, R.T. Embryology of the facial nerve and its clinical applications. *Laryngoscope* **1990**, *100*, 969–984. [CrossRef] [PubMed]
24. Osbor, A.G. *Diagnostic Cerebral Angiography*, 2nd ed.; LWW: Philadelphia, PA, USA, 1999.
25. Diamond, M.; Wartmann, C.T.; Tubbs, R.S.; Shoja, M.M.; Cohen-Gadol, A.A.; Loukas, M. Peripheral facial nerve communications and their clinical implications. *Clin. Anat.* **2011**, *24*, 10–18. [CrossRef]

26. Kim, M.; Park, S.K.; Lee, S.; Lee, J.A.; Park, K. Lateral spread response of different facial muscles during microvascular decompression in hemifacial spasm. *Clin. Neurophysiol.* **2021**, *132*, 2503–2509. [CrossRef] [PubMed]
27. Ouattara, D.; Vacher, C.; de Vasconcellos, J.J.; Kassanyou, S.; Gnanazan, G.; N'Guessan, B. Anatomical study of the variations in innervation of the orbicularis oculi by the facial nerve. *Surg. Radiol. Anat.* **2004**, *26*, 51–53. [CrossRef]
28. Raslan, A.; Volk, G.F.; Moller, M.; Stark, V.; Eckhardt, N.; Guntinas-Lichius, O. High variability of facial muscle innervation by facial nerve branches: A prospective electrostimulation study. *Laryngoscope* **2017**, *127*, 1288–1295. [CrossRef]
29. Kwak, H.H.; Park, H.D.; Youn, K.H.; Hu, K.S.; Koh, K.S.; Han, S.H.; Kim, H.J. Branching patterns of the facial nerve and its communication with the auriculotemporal nerve. *Surg. Radiol. Anat.* **2004**, *26*, 494–500. [CrossRef]
30. Odobescu, A.; Williams, H.B.; Gilardino, M.S. Description of a communication between the facial and zygomaticotemporal nerves. *J. Plast. Reconstr. Aesthet. Surg.* **2012**, *65*, 1188–1192. [CrossRef]
31. Tohma, A.; Mine, K.; Tamatsu, Y.; Shimada, K. Communication between the buccal nerve (V) and facial nerve (VII) in the human face. *Ann. Anat.* **2004**, *186*, 173–178. [CrossRef]
32. Ozdogmus, O.; Sezen, O.; Kubilay, U.; Saka, E.; Duman, U.; San, T.; Cavdar, S. Connections between the facial, vestibular and cochlear nerve bundles within the internal auditory canal. *J. Anat.* **2004**, *205*, 65–75. [CrossRef] [PubMed]
33. Salame, K.; Ouaknine, G.E.; Arensburg, B.; Rochkind, S. Microsurgical anatomy of the facial nerve trunk. *Clin. Anat.* **2002**, *15*, 93–99. [CrossRef] [PubMed]
34. Yang, H.M.; Kim, H.J.; Hu, K.S. Anatomic and histological study of great auricular nerve and its clinical implication. *J. Plast. Reconstr. Aesthet. Surg.* **2015**, *68*, 230–236. [CrossRef] [PubMed]
35. Zhong, J.; Zhu, J.; Sun, H.; Dou, N.N.; Wang, Y.N.; Ying, T.T.; Xia, L.; Liu, M.X.; Tao, B.B.; Li, S.T. Microvascular decompression surgery: Surgical principles and technical nuances based on 4000 cases. *Neurol. Res.* **2014**, *36*, 882–893. [CrossRef] [PubMed]
36. Clifton, W.E.; Grewal, S.; Lundy, L.; Cheshire, W.P.; Tubbs, R.S.; Wharen, R.E. Clinical implications of nervus intermedius variants in patients with geniculate neuralgia: Let anatomy be the guide. *Clin. Anat.* **2020**, *33*, 1056–1061. [CrossRef]
37. Tubbs, R.S.; Steck, D.T.; Mortazavi, M.M.; Cohen-Gadol, A.A. The nervus intermedius: A review of its anatomy, function, pathology, and role in neurosurgery. *World Neurosurg.* **2013**, *79*, 763–767. [CrossRef]
38. Rhoton, A.L., Jr.; Kobayashi, S.; Hollinshead, W.H. Nervus intermedius. *J. Neurosurg.* **1968**, *29*, 609–618. [CrossRef]
39. Rowed, D.W. Chronic cluster headache managed by nervus intermedius section. *Headache* **1990**, *30*, 401–406. [CrossRef]
40. Smith, J.J.; Breathnach, C.S. Functions of the seventh cranial nerve. *Ear Nose Throat J.* **1990**, *69*, 688–691.
41. Burmeister, H.P.; Baltzer, P.A.; Dietzel, M.; Krumbein, I.; Bitter, T.; Schrott-Fischer, A.; Guntinas-Lichius, O.; Kaiser, W.A. Identification of the nervus intermedius using 3T MR imaging. *Am. J. Neuroradiol.* **2011**, *32*, 460–464. [CrossRef]
42. Headache Classification Committee of the International Headache Society. Classification and diagnostic criteria for headache disorders, cranial neuralgias and facial pain. Headache Classification Committee of the International Headache Society. *Cephalalgia* **1988**, *8* (Suppl. S7), 1–96.
43. Lovely, T.J.; Jannetta, P.J. Surgical management of geniculate neuralgia. *Am. J. Otol.* **1997**, *18*, 512–517. [PubMed]

Disclaimer/Publisher's Note: The statements, opinions and data contained in all publications are solely those of the individual author(s) and contributor(s) and not of MDPI and/or the editor(s). MDPI and/or the editor(s) disclaim responsibility for any injury to people or property resulting from any ideas, methods, instructions or products referred to in the content.

MDPI
St. Alban-Anlage 66
4052 Basel
Switzerland
www.mdpi.com

Life Editorial Office
E-mail: life@mdpi.com
www.mdpi.com/journal/life

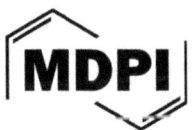

Disclaimer/Publisher's Note: The statements, opinions and data contained in all publications are solely those of the individual author(s) and contributor(s) and not of MDPI and/or the editor(s). MDPI and/or the editor(s) disclaim responsibility for any injury to people or property resulting from any ideas, methods, instructions or products referred to in the content.

www.ingramcontent.com/pod-product-compliance
Lightning Source LLC
LaVergne TN
LVHW070715100526
838202LV00013B/1097